SECOND EDITION

The New Prescriber

An Integrated Approach to Medical and Non-medical Prescribing

Edited by

T0329679

Joanne Lymn BSc PhD NTF
Professor of Healthcare Education, University of Nottingham

Alison Mostyn BSc Biomedical Sciences (Pharmacology) PhD PGCHE SFHEA
Professor in Pharmacology Education for Health, University of Nottingham

Roger Knaggs BSc BMedSci PhD EDPM FHEA FFRPS FRPharmS FFPMRCA
Professor of Pain Management, University of Nottingham;
Specialist Pharmacist in Pain Management;
Primary Integrated Community Solutions

Michael Randall MA PhD FBPhS SFHEA
Professor of Pharmacology, University of Nottingham

Dianne Bowskill RN DPSN(DN) BSc DHSci
Associate Professor of Prescribing Education, University of Nottingham;
Professor of Healthcare Education, University of Nottingham

WILEY Blackwell

Registered Offices
John Wiley & Sons, Inc., 111 River Street, Hoboken, NJ 07030, USA
John Wiley & Sons Ltd, The Atrium, Southern Gate, Chichester, West Sussex, PO19 8SQ, UK

For details of our global editorial offices, customer services, and more information about Wiley products visit us at www.wiley.com.

Wiley also publishes its books in a variety of electronic formats and by print-on-demand. Some content that appears in standard print versions of this book may not be available in other formats.

Library of Congress Cataloging-in-Publication Data applied for:

Paperback ISBN:9781119833154

Cover Design: Wiley
Cover Image: © calvindexter/Getty Images

Set in 9.5/12pt STIXTwoText by Straive, Pondicherry, India

The New Prescriber

Contents

2 Accountability and Prescribing   14

Matthew Boyd, Stephanie Bridges, and Helen Boardman

3 Prescribing and the Law   23

Richard Griffith

4	The Ethics of Prescribing	36

Matthew Boyd, Stephanie Bridges, and Helen Boardman

SECTION 2 Pharmacology 63

7 General Principles of Pharmacology 67

Joanne Lymn and Alison Mostyn

8 Pharmacokinetics 1: Absorption and Distribution 79

Joanne Lymn and Alison Mostyn

11 | Variations in Drug Handling 114

Michael Randall

12 | Polypharmacy and Medicines Optimisation 124

Daniel Shipley

13 | Adverse Drug Reactions and Interactions 134

Alison Mostyn and Daniel Shipley

14 | Introduction to the Autonomic Nervous System 144

Joanne Lymn

15 Clinical Application of the Principles of the Autonomic Nervous Systems 157

Joanne Lymn

16 The Gastrointestinal System 167

Michael Randall

17 | Cardiovascular Drugs and Diseases 177

Richard Roberts

18 Haemostasis and Thrombosis 196

Michael Randall

19 The Renal System 208

Michael Randall

20 The Respiratory System 221

Richard Roberts

21   Introduction to the Central Nervous System   235

Yvonne Mbaki

22 Neurodegenerative Disorders 245

David Kendall

23 Depression and Anxiety 256

Yvonne Mbaki

24 Schizophrenia 267

David Kendall

25 Epilepsy and Antiseizure Drugs 277

Michael F O'Donoghue and Christina Giavasi

26 | Pain and Analgesia   293

Roger Knaggs

27 | Drugs of Misuse   308

Michael Randall

28   Antibacterial Chemotherapy   **315**

Tim Hills

33 | Cancer Pharmacotherapy 381

Michael Randall

List of Contributors

Alison Mostyn, Professor of Pharmacology Education for Health, School of Health Sciences, University of Nottingham

Anna Soames, Sexual Health Nurse Training Lead Nottingham University Hospitals Nurse Representative FSRH Practice Learning and Development Board

Christina Giavasi, Consultant Neurologist, Nottingham University Hospital Trust

Daniel Shipley, Senior Clinical Pharmacist

David Kendall, Professor Emeritus of Pharmacology, University of Nottingham

David Andrew Walsh, Professor of Rheumatology, School of Medicine, University of Nottingham

Dianne Bowskill, Associate Professor of Prescribing Education, School of Health Sciences, University of Nottingham

Frank Coffey, Consultant in Emergency Medicine, Nottingham University Hospitals NHS Trust; Clinical Consultant to the Postgraduate Clinical Skills Programme, School of Health Sciences, University of Nottingham

Helen Boardman, Associate Professor in Pharmacy Practice, School of Pharmacy, University of Nottingham

Joanne Lymn, Professor of Healthcare Education, School of Health Sciences, University of Nottingham

Katharine Whittingham, Associate Professor, School of Health Sciences, University of Nottingham

Matthew Boyd, Professor of Medicines Safety, School of Pharmacy, University of Nottingham

Michael F O'Donoghue, Neurology Consultant, Nottingham University Hospital Trust and Honorary Assistant Professor in Neurology, University of Nottingham

Michael Randall, Professor of Pharmacology, School of Life Sciences, University of Nottingham

Michael Watson, Trustee, Institute of Health Promotion and Education

Richard Griffith, Senior Lecturer in Law, School of Health & Social Care, University of Swansea

Richard Roberts, Associate Professor and Lecturer in Pharmacology, School of Life Sciences, University of Nottingham

Roger Knaggs, Professor of Pain Management, University of Nottingham; Specialist Pharmacist in Pain Management; Primary Integrated Community Solutions

Sana Awan, Assistant Chief Pharmacist & Head of Operations, Sherwood Forest Hospitals NHS Foundation Trust

Stephanie Bridges, Associate Professor, Clinical Pharmacy Practice, School of Pharmacy, University of Nottingham

Tim Hills, Senior Pharmacist - Microbiology & Infection Control, Nottingham University Hospitals NHS Trust

Yvonne Mbaki, Associate Professor in Medical Physiology, School of Life Sciences, University of Nottingham

Foreword

Since the publication of the first edition of *The New Prescriber* in 2010, more allied health professionals, including paramedics and dieticians, have gained independent or supplementary prescribing rights, expanding the variety of practitioners who can prescribe and ensuring patients have timely access to medicines.

This second edition of *The New Prescriber* has been fully updated and restructured to meet the needs of all clinicians who are new to prescribing. New chapters on polypharmacy and medicines optimisation, cancer pharmacotherapy, drugs of misuse and musculoskeletal prescribing have been included to address these common challenges. The book remains focussed on the new prescriber, with a friendly and clear tone to develop confident and safe prescribers.

ALISON MOSTYN

As a Paramedic Advanced Clinical Practitioner, I felt a lot of pressure to do well, and using *The New Prescriber* textbook as a key text made the journey even better. *The New Prescriber* contains all the information you will need to successfully compete the course and to succeed in practice. Since completing the non-medical prescribing course, my role has become more exciting and more autonomous, giving me all the skills and knowledge to practice at a high level.

CRAIG PRENTICE

Preface

While there are a number of current textbooks that deal with individual aspects of prescribing, this book uses an integrated approach providing important information across the broader aspects of prescribing.

The book is divided into two sections dealing with the patient, and pharmacology and therapeutics. The initial section, on the patient, explores the consultation and outlines the legal, professional and ethical frameworks that guide medical and non-medical prescribing. The second section is concerned with pharmacology. Here, the reader is introduced to the basic concepts of pharmacodynamics and pharmacokinetics, adverse drug reactions and variability of response. These concepts are important as the reader progresses through the rest of the section exploring the therapeutic use of drugs for the treatment of disease.

Throughout the text, the reader will find 'Stop and think' and 'Practice application' boxes. These are intended to help the reader link theory to practice but in different ways. The 'Stop and think' boxes are designed to do exactly what they say and encourage the reader to stop and reflect on the knowledge gained and how this might be applied in practice, thus developing greater understanding. Ideal answers to the questions in these boxes are not presented in the book but should be drawn from an integration of all the relevant information presented within the chapter itself, previous chapters of the book and clinical practice. 'Practice application' boxes take a more factual approach by providing a direct link from theory to clinical practice.

Definitions of key terms used in the book can be found in the relevant section glossary.

Acknowledgements

We would like to thank everyone who has contributed to both the first and this second edition of *The New Prescriber*. The breadth of clinical and academic expertise that we have been able to call on across both editions has been tremendous and means we have been able to ensure a contemporary output.

In addition to these contributors, we would like to thank Lianne Nachmias for her support with the initial development of this edition.

Perhaps most importantly we would like to thank Sue Evans, who has been our key administrative support, managing the production of this edition for us. She has kept us all on track, helped with editing, formatting and proof-reading, and liaising with the publishers. This edition has been possible only because of Sue's ongoing support. Thank you, Sue.

JO, ALISON, ROGER, MICHAEL, AND DIANNE

The Patient

SECTION INTRODUCTION

In this first section we focus on the practical aspects of prescribing for patients. As a new prescriber you will find there are many factors specific to your patient, your profession and your employer that influence both your decision to prescribe and the prescribing decisions you make. Throughout this section you will be encouraged to think about prescribing in practice and we begin with the consultation, the starting point for prescribing. All prescribers must practice within the law and in a manner consistent with the professional and public expectations of a prescriber. The legal framework of medical and non-medical prescribing is defined in this section and new prescribers are encouraged to think about their prescribing role in relation to these aspects. Your actions as a prescriber will reach far beyond the patients you prescribe for, and this section encourages you to explore the ethical and public health issues associated with prescribing authority. As your prescribing experience grows, you will find it useful to revisit the definitions and questions raised in this section.

The term non-medical prescriber is used throughout the book and refers to nurses, pharmacists and allied health professionals who, following successful completion of a programme of formal prescribing education, are on the professional record as a prescriber.

The New Prescriber: An Integrated Approach to Medical and Non-medical Prescribing, Second Edition.
Edited by Joanne Lymn, Alison Mostyn, Roger Knaggs, Michael Randall, and Dianne Bowskill.
© 2024 John Wiley & Sons Ltd. Published 2024 by John Wiley & Sons Ltd.

The Consultation

Frank Coffey and Dianne Bowskill

CHAPTER 1

LEARNING OUTCOMES

By the end of this chapter the reader should be able to:

- recognise and analyse the important elements of a consultation

- identify the components of the traditional medical history

- appreciate the diagnostic process and distinguish between the treatment of symptoms and the treatment of a disease or condition

- identify the elements of the consultation essential for safe prescribing (bottom liners)

- refine their professional assessment/consultation for the prescribing role

- have insight into the impact of technological advances on assessment, diagnosis and treatment.

As you begin your prescribing education you already have a wealth of professional experience in your own area of practice. The assessment and consultation skills learnt as part of professional registration are well practised but may need to be refined as you take on prescribing. We are not suggesting that you need to adopt a new or medical model of consultation, although this might be desirable in certain advanced practice roles. For the majority of new prescribers, the focus will be on analysing their current framework of assessment or consultation and identifying adaptations required to support prescribing decisions. In this chapter we will ask you to think about the elements of the consultation that you may need to adapt or work on. We will give practice tips and point out common errors that can affect the quality of a consultation.

Prescribing inherently brings with it a greater requirement to make a diagnosis. This responsibility may be new and quite daunting. Prescribers need to understand the diagnostic process. In most circumstances, the key factor for accurate diagnosis is eliciting a good history. For this reason, we will look in detail at the elements of a history. Examination and investigations are directed by and supplement the history. The depth and focus of the history and examination will vary depending on the setting and your role. Wherever you work, however, it is essential to be thorough and systematic, and above all to know the bounds of your competence. History taking, examination and clinical decision making are skills that need to be continuously practiced under expert supervision.

Ideally your prescribing will be effective, but above all it should be safe. The primary dictum of all healthcare practice is 'primum non nocere' (above all do no harm). We will outline the elements of the consultation that are essential for safe prescribing, the 'bottom liners' of a prescribing consultation.

In the final part of the chapter, we will explore the potential impact of technological and scientific advances on assessment and clinical decision making and outline the increasing emphasis on health improvement and prevention in consultations.

The New Prescriber: An Integrated Approach to Medical and Non-medical Prescribing, Second Edition.
Edited by Joanne Lymn, Alison Mostyn, Roger Knaggs, Michael Randall, and Dianne Bowskill.
© 2024 John Wiley & Sons Ltd. Published 2024 by John Wiley & Sons Ltd.

THE CONSULTATION

The consultation is a two-way interaction between a healthcare practitioner and a patient. Your role will influence the types of patients you treat, the environment in which you see them and your approach to the consultation. As a non-medical prescriber your focus is on diagnosis. Assessment for diagnosis in a typical consultation comprises the history, examination and investigations. Factors to consider include the urgency and seriousness of the presentation, time constraints and the personalities, culture, language and medical knowledge of both the patient and the clinician. Previous contact with the patient, autonomy, and confidence are further influences on the consultation. Communication and consultation skills are inextricably interlinked. There are many excellent textbooks available for prescribers who wish to enhance their communication skills (Brown et al. 2016; Silverman et al. 1998; Berry 2004).

ELEMENTS OF A CONSULTATION

Although consultations differ in specifics, there are common elements and generic skills that are applicable in varying degrees to any given situation. Numerous consultation models have been developed over the years, for example Neighbour (2005), Pendleton et al. (2003) and Calgary Cambridge in Silverman et al. (1998). Rather than dwelling on the theory underpinning consultations, we will describe a practical framework for the consultation (see Box 1.1). This includes an assessment component (see I to (j) in Box 1.1) and other elements which can be applied in varying degrees to all consultations.

It is important for consultations to have a degree of structure. The skill in consulting is to maintain a structure and system that includes all the vital elements and yet does not feel like a

---

BOX 1.1   **ELEMENTS OF A CONSULTATION**

a. Preparing for the consultation and setting goals for it.

b. Establishing an initial rapport with the patient.

c. Identifying the reason(s) for the consultation.

d. Exploring the patient's problem(s) and ascertaining their ideas, concerns and expectations about it.

e. Focusing questions to obtain essential information.

f. Gathering sufficient information relating to the patient's social and psychological circumstances to ascertain their impact.

g. Coming up with a diagnosis or a number of differential diagnoses in order of likelihood.

h. Performing a focused physical examination and near-patient tests to support or refute the differential diagnoses.

i. Reaching a shared understanding of the problem with the patient.

j. Interpreting the information gathered and re-evaluating the problem.

k. Considering further investigations if necessary.

l. Deciding what treatment options, pharmacological and non-pharmacological, are available.

m. Advising the patient about actions needed to tackle the problem.

n. Explaining these actions and the time of follow-up if required.

o. Inviting and answering any questions.

p. Summarising for the patient and terminating the consultation.

q. Making a written record of the consultation.

r. Presenting your findings to another health professional.

straitjacket for the patient or clinician. In the following section we will analyse the different elements of the consultation in more detail and highlight those that are likely to change or need more emphasis for you as you take on prescribing.

STOP AND THINK

Using Box 1.1 as a framework, reflect on your current consultations and identify elements you are less confident with. Make a note of these to inform learning and development needs.

(A) PREPARING FOR THE CONSULTATION AND SETTING GOALS

Take time to study all the information available to you about the patient prior to the consultation. Study referral letters and available medical records for vital information, including the patient's past history, medications and allergies. Set goals for the consultation and ensure that the environment is set up appropriately with adequate lighting and privacy.

(B) ESTABLISHING THE INITIAL RAPPORT

First impressions are especially important and will influence your subsequent relationship with the patient. If you have not encountered the patient before, introduce yourself by name and explain your role. Check the patient's details (name, date of birth, address). Observe the patient's demeanour and physical appearance. The patient will invariably be feeling nervous. Put them at ease by projecting confidence and warmth, and they are more likely to open up to you during the consultation.

(C) TO (G) HISTORY TAKING/DIAGNOSIS HYPOTHESIS

Elements (c) to (g) in Box 1.1 are primarily concerned with the taking of a history and the consideration of differential diagnoses. The importance of the history cannot be overstated. In the vast majority of cases (>70%) the history will provide an accurate diagnosis or differential diagnosis even before the examination and investigations are performed. A good history will therefore facilitate effective prescribing. Certain minimum information *must* be elicited to ensure safe prescribing,

The history is a two-way process. In reality, we do not 'take' a history. Rather, we 'make' a history with the patient. The result is influenced by both the practitioner's and the patient's prior knowledge, experiences and understanding of language. Where understanding of language is a barrier, clinical risk is significantly increased and an interpreter should be considered. There are psychodynamic processes at play during any consultation which the practitioner needs to be aware of. These are explored in detail in other publications (Berry 2004).

The scope and depth of the history will depend on the role of the practitioner and the circumstances surrounding the consultation. Whatever the nature of the history, it is essential to be systematic and as far as possible follow the same sequence of questioning each time. In this way vital information will not be overlooked. This becomes particularly important when the patient has multiple symptoms and/or a complicated medical history.

Most patient histories will contain some or all the elements of a traditional medical history. This structure has limitations and has been criticised for being practitioner rather than patient centred. A full history is too time-consuming in most situations. However, we believe that it is important for prescribers to understand the elements of the traditional history before considering some of the modified and/or abbreviated versions that are used in practice.

THE TRADITIONAL MEDICAL HISTORY

PRESENTING COMPLAINT (PC)

Consider the symptom(s) or problem(s) that has brought the patient to seek medical attention and its duration. The presenting complaint should ideally be written or presented orally in the patient's own words, for example 'tummy ache for 3 hours' 'dizzy spells for 2 years'.

Remember that the complaint that the patient seeks medical advice about might not be their main concern, for example a man concerned about impotence might attend on the pretext of back pain. The true presenting problem will be elucidated by an empathetic and skilled interviewer.

HISTORY OF THE PRESENTING COMPLAINT (HxPC)

This is where you clarify the presenting complaint. It is the most important part of the history and is essential for the formulation of a differential diagnosis. Explore the patient's symptoms and try to build a clear picture of the patient's experience. Avoid leading questions as far as possible. At some point, however, you will need to move to focused questioning to elicit essential information and fill in gaps in the patient's story. When there are a number of symptoms, it is important to complete the questioning around each symptom in a systematic fashion before moving on to the next one. Pain is one of the most common presenting symptoms. The following information should be elicited about pain: its onset (gradual or sudden), location, radiation, character, periodicity (does it come and go?), duration, aggravating and relieving factors, and associated features (secondary symptoms). Similar questioning with modifications can be applied to most symptoms, for example for diarrhoea the character (amount, colour, etc.), timing, aggravating and relieving factors, and associated symptoms (e.g., abdominal pain) are all relevant. Several mnemonics have been created as an *aide mémoire* for symptom analysis (see Boxes 1.2 and 1.3 for examples).

BOX 1.2	SYMPTOM ANALYSIS MNEMONIC

PQRST
P – provocation or palliation
Q – quality and quantity: what does the symptom look, feel, sound like?
R – region/radiation
S – severity scale, may be rated on a scale of 1–10, which is useful for subsequent evaluation and comparison
T – timing

BOX 1.3	SYMPTOM ANALYSIS MNEMONICS

SQITARS
S – site and radiation
Q – quality
I – intensity
T – timing
A – aggravating factors
R – relieving factors
S – secondary symptoms

SOCRATES
S – site
O – onset
C – character
R – radiation
A – associated symptoms
T – time intensity relationship
E – exacerbating/relieving
S – severity

PRACTICE APPLICATION

As a new prescriber using a mnemonic/acronym is an effective approach to remembering key questions to ask in a consultation

Always ask about the cardinal symptoms in any system potentially involved, for example for chest pain, ask about the cardinal symptoms relating to the cardiovascular and respiratory systems. The cardinal respiratory symptoms are cough, dyspnoea, wheeze, chest pain, sputum production and haemoptysis. Include within the history of the presenting complaint the presence of risk factors for conditions that may be the cause of the presenting symptom(s), for example if ischaemic chest pain is in the differential, hypertension, smoking and a positive family history examples of such risk factors. Similarly, oral contraceptive pill (OCP) therapy or prolonged immobilisation would be risk factors for pulmonary embolism.

PAST MEDICAL AND SURGICAL HISTORY (PMHx)

The past medical history, along with medications, drug history and allergies, provides the background to the patient's current health or disease. Record previous illnesses, operations and injuries in chronological order. Include the duration of chronic conditions, for example diabetes mellitus or asthma, in your record and, where appropriate, the location of treatment and the names of the treating clinicians. Remember that many medical conditions may impact on your choice and/or dose of drug treatment.

FAMILY HISTORY (FamHx)

Information regarding the age and health or the cause of death of the patient's relatives can be invaluable and provide vital clues in the diagnostic process. Many conditions have a well-defined mode of inheritance. Enquire specifically about the following common conditions: hypertension, coronary artery disease, high cholesterol, diabetes mellitus, kidney or thyroid disease, cancer (specify type), gout, arthritis, asthma, other lung disease, headache, epilepsy, mental illness, alcohol or drug addiction, and infectious diseases such as tuberculosis. Depending on the clinical area, you may need to explore the family history of sensitive areas such as mental health, drug misuse or sexual health in more detail. The family history may also throw light on the patient's ideas, fears and expectations, for example a patient whose sibling has died from a brain tumour is likely to be genuinely concerned about a headache that is persisting.

MEDICATIONS, DRUG HISTORY AND ALLERGIES

The drug and allergy history are an extremely important part of the medical history. The presenting symptoms may result from the side effects or complications of drug therapy. Current medications and previous allergies will influence prescribing. Ask the patient to list the medications that they are taking on medical advice or otherwise. Ask to see a recent medication list or prescription. Ideally, you should see the medications. Note the name, dose, route, frequency of use and indications for all medications. It is also important to establish if the patient is taking the medicines prescribed. List over-the-counter drugs, and complementary and herbal medicines. The oral contraceptive pill is often not perceived as a medication. Ask specifically about it in women of the appropriate age. Patients may omit to mention medications that are not tablets (e.g., inhalers, home oxygen, creams, eye or ear drops, pessaries, suppositories). Ask specifically about such agents.

Enquire about allergies or adverse reactions to medications, foods, animals, pollen or other environmental factors. If the patient gives a history of allergy, record the exact nature and circumstances of the reaction and the treatment given.

PERSONAL AND SOCIAL HISTORY

The personal and social history is a critical aspect of the history. All illnesses, treatments and rehabilitation must be seen in the context of the patient's personality, spirituality, and personal and social circumstances. Occupation, habitation, hobbies and lifestyle habits can have a profound impact on health and disease. Where appropriate, do not neglect to ask about recent travel abroad and sexual history. Ascertain whether the patient smokes or has smoked in the past and quantify their smoking. Enquire about alcohol intake and, where appropriate, the use of illicit drugs. Some patients may be reluctant to reveal the full extent of their smoking, alcohol consumption or recreational drug use. Maintain a non-judgmental attitude to encourage such patients to share information.

SYSTEMS REVIEW

The systems review (SR), which is undertaken at the end of the history, involves a series of screening questions that systematically cover all the body systems. It is usually done in a head-to-toe sequence. Its purpose is to elicit any further information that might be relevant to the current illness or to uncover present or past problems that the patient has overlooked. The SR may provide information that leads you to suspect a multisystem disease process such as systemic lupus erythematosus or may demonstrate associated symptoms in another system, for example arthritis associated with inflammatory bowel disease. A comprehensive list of SR questions can be found in Coffey, Wells and Stone (2024).

(H) PHYSICAL EXAMINATION/NEAR-PATIENT TESTS

The purpose of the physical examination and near-patient tests is to supplement your findings from the history and to support or refute your diagnostic hypotheses. The extent of your examination will depend on your training and experience. It is not essential to be able to perform a physical examination to be a competent prescriber in a specialised area. Increasingly, however, healthcare practitioners are taking on advanced examination skills. It is important that these are taught and assessed appropriately.

Perform vital signs, including temperature. Consider vital signs in the context of the patient's age, physical fitness and medication, and always seek a reason for abnormal vital signs. Perform a thorough examination and avoid taking shortcuts. In most cases, your examination will be a focused one, concentrating on a specific area of the body. It is important to expose adequately the area to be examined and always compare limbs with the contralateral one.

Near-patient tests are tests that produce immediate results, for example electrocardiograms, urinalyses, arterial blood gases and blood glucose. Increasingly other investigations such as the full blood count and urea and electrolytes are becoming available as near-patient tests. These tests can be invaluable for diagnosis and can also direct or influence the prescription of medications. Remember always to check glucose level in a patient with confusion or altered consciousness.

(I) TO (K) DIAGNOSIS

Diagnosis is the process of ascertaining the nature and cause of a disease. This enables the practitioner to target treatments effectively. The diagnosis is made by evaluating the symptoms, signs and investigation results, which together constitute the diagnostic criteria. The information is considered in the context of the patient's physical, social and psychological status. A treatment plan is then formulated, ideally in partnership with the patient, who should be kept informed throughout the diagnostic procedure.

Increasingly healthcare practitioners other than doctors are involved in the diagnostic process. The advent of non-medical prescribing has accelerated this trend. Practitioners moving into the diagnostic arena need to understand the process and be aware of potential pitfalls. The way clinicians diagnose alters as they become more experienced. The word *diagnosis* comes from the Greek words for 'through' *(dia)* and 'knowledge' *(gnosis)* and fundamental to the process for any practitioner is a thorough knowledge of the presenting features, examination and investigation findings of conditions likely to present to their area of practice. Some of this knowledge is gained through experience with patients (pattern recognition) and much of it is book learned. The practitioner must apply their knowledge to extract information from the patient that will make conditions in the potential differential diagnosis more or less likely, for example eliciting the presence of haemoptysis, oral contraceptive pill therapy and a previous deep vein thrombosis in a 39-year-old woman presenting with pleuritic chest pain would make the diagnosis of pulmonary embolism extremely likely. If these features were absent and the same patient with pleuritic chest pain had fever and cough with purulent sputum, chest infection or pneumonia would be a more likely diagnosis. The presence of breathlessness, while an important symptom, would not help to differentiate between these two diagnoses. The speed of onset of breathlessness might help, however, as an acute onset would be more typical of a pulmonary embolism.

STOP AND THINK

What are the red flags you look out for during consultations in your area of practice?

Practitioners should know the 'red flag' features, suggesting serious pathology or high risk, in conditions likely to present to them. Examples of these would be new onset of back pain with urinary incontinence, anticoagulant therapy in a patient with a head injury or a suicide note written by a patient who has overdosed. Examples of generic red flag symptoms are unexplained weight loss, night sweats, unexplained chronic pain or pain that keeps the patient awake at night. You should also be aware of classic atypical presentations in your area of practice, for example myocardial infarction presenting with jaw, arm or abdominal pain or ectopic pregnancy masquerading as shoulder tip pain and collapse.

One of the common errors made by practitioners new to diagnosis is premature closure, that is, establishing a diagnosis early in the consultation and being blinkered to evidence that might refute that diagnosis or suggest an alternative, for example attributing colicky abdominal pain with frequent loose stools to gastroenteritis and ignoring the radiation of unilateral loin to groin pain which would increase the probability of a urological cause. It is important to weigh up *all* the evidence from the history, examination and any investigations carried out. The consideration of risk factors is also an important part of this process. Even though the chest pain of a 40-year-old man may not sound typical for cardiac pain, the fact that his brother died of a heart attack aged 38 will significantly alter your index of suspicion and consequently your management.

STOP AND THINK

What is the difference between treating a symptom and a disease?
Identify examples from your practice.

SYMPTOM VERSUS DISEASE/CONDITION

In the context of diagnosis, prescribing practitioners should have a clear understanding of the difference between a symptom and a disease or condition. A *symptom* is a manifestation of a disease described by the patient, for example chest pain, breathlessness and haemoptysis are symptoms associated with pneumonia. A symptom may give a clue as to the nature of the disease, but it Is not in itself a diagnosis. A *diagnosis* is the recognition of a disease or condition by its outward symptoms and signs. These are supplemented by the findings from near-patient testing, imaging and other investigations. Pneumonia, for example, might be diagnosed based on symptoms (cough, dyspnoea, pleuritic chest pain, rusty coloured sputum), signs (tachypnoea, pyrexia, decreased breath sounds, crackles, bronchial breathing) and imaging (chest X ray).

Medications can be prescribed to treat symptoms or conditions/diseases, for example morphine can be used to treat the symptoms of severe chest pain without knowledge of the underlying diagnosis. An ECG and troponin might reveal the diagnosis of myocardial infarction subsequently, necessitating a range of pharmacological and non-pharmacological interventions.

In many situations the diagnosis also includes the underlying physiological, biochemical or microbiological cause(s) of a disease or condition, for example pneumococcal pneumonia suggests not only the diagnostic criteria for pneumonia but also the causative microorganism. Where causality is known, it is usually possible to target prescribing more effectively to treat or cure the condition. There are conditions, however, where the underlying cause has yet to be discovered. In such situations, palliative treatment targeted at reducing the symptoms may be the best that the clinician can achieve. It is vital, however, that symptoms are not treated without looking for an underlying diagnosis. Pain, the most common symptom for which patients seek healthcare advice, is frequently treated before the underlying diagnosis is identified. Constipation is another example of a symptom that may be treated without an effort being made to find a cause for it. You need to understand as a prescriber that it is not sufficient to treat a symptom. If, for example, the underlying diagnosis is bowel cancer for a patient who presents with constipation, failing to seek a cause may have disastrous consequences. You must seek to make a diagnosis and if the diagnostic reasoning lies outside your area of expertise, you must refer on to another appropriate health professional.

(L) TREATMENT

When you have made a diagnosis consider the various treatment options. Non-pharmacological options, for example weight loss and salt reduction for hypertension, should be considered before prescribing drugs with potentially debilitating side effects. Take into account the patient's age, lifestyle, mobility, dexterity and potential compliance when prescribing. Ensure that the patient is not allergic to the treatment that you are considering and that it does not interact with other medications or worsen any existing medical conditions.

(M) TO (P) SUMMARISING AND CLOSING THE CONSULTATION

When you have all the information required, share your conclusions with the patient in language appropriate to their intellectual and educational level, avoiding medical jargon. Ensure that the patient has understood the information that you have given and agreed to the treatment plan. This will improve concordance. Give the patient verbal and, ideally, written information about the administration and common side effects of any prescribed medications.

Illnesses evolve. Initial mild viral-like symptoms may develop rapidly into a full-blown meningococcal septicaemia. A patient may progress from having abdominal pain with minimal abdominal tenderness to obvious appendicitis with peritonism a few hours later. Give the patient a realistic timeframe for the resolution of symptoms and ask them to return or contact you if things deteriorate or do not improve as anticipated. Record this advice clearly in your notes.

Always offer the patient the opportunity to ask questions. If you are unable to answer, be honest. Tell the patient that you will need to look up the answer or consult with another colleague. Finally, summarise the findings and treatment for the patient and finish the consultation.

(Q) AND (R) RECORDING AND PRESENTATION OF CONSULTATION FINDINGS

The written record is a medico-legal document that may be required to justify your diagnosis and choice of treatment. A satisfactory record of a consultation should include the presenting problem and the main features, including important negatives (e.g., haemoptysis or the absence of risk factors for thromboembolic disease for a patient with pleuritic chest pain). The examination findings should also contain relevant negatives. It is good practice to write an impression after the history and examination with a list of differential diagnoses in order of likelihood. The investigations (and results if available) should then be recorded followed by a final diagnosis and management plan. When prescribing medication(s), document the name(s) of the drug(s), the dosage and the length of prescription. Also record the names of healthcare practitioners with whom you have communicated in relation to the case. It is a useful exercise to critique your documentation, imagining that you are standing in a courtroom defending the contents 2 or 3 years after you have written them.

The ability to present the findings from a consultation in a systematic and concise fashion is vital in a busy practice area and when making referrals or requesting advice over the telephone. It is a difficult skill, which requires a great deal of practice. As you take on the role of prescribing, encourage your medical mentors and colleagues to critique your oral presentation skills.

STOP AND THINK

What do you consider to be essential components of a consultation to ensure safe prescribing?

'BOTTOM LINERS' WHEN PRESCRIBING

Much of this chapter has related to factors that contribute to effective prescribing, for example the formulation of an accurate diagnosis. In this section we will highlight the elements of the consultation that are essential for *safe* prescribing.

a. Ascertain that you have the right patient by checking name, date of birth, address, hospital or National Health Service (NHS) number.

b. Check weight where appropriate, particularly when prescribing for children.

c. Ascertain that the patient is not allergic to the medication and that there are no interactions with other medications that the patient is taking.

d. Ensure that the patient is not suffering from any medical condition that might be exacerbated by the medication (e.g., peptic ulcer disease by non-steroidal anti-inflammatory drugs) or require a different dosage (e.g., antibiotics in patients with renal failure).

e. Inform the patient of both nuisance and serious side effects of the medication and advise them to return if serious side effects occur or if the medication is not working as anticipated.

STOP AND THINK

What will consultations look like in 10 years' time?

FUTURE ADVANCES IN CONSULTATION

Future consultations will evolve as the delivery of healthcare adapts to technological and other scientific advances, as well the changing demographics of the patient population and the move to a more blended, multiprofessional workforce. As more evidence emerges on the contribution of inequality and lifestyle risk factors to injury and illness, prevention and health improvement will become more integrated into all consultations, with a philosophy of making every contact count (MECC). As initiatives such as social prescribing become more prevalent, integrating questions around the wider determinants of health such as housing or financial worries will become a standard in consultations.

Increasing numbers of older, frailer patients presenting with multiple comorbidities and polypharmacy will undoubtedly lead to more challenging consultations. Prescribers will need to be skilled in the assessment and treatment of this population and appreciate the impact the medications prescribed may have on cognition and function. The exponential growth in healthcare knowledge is likely to lead to a more integrated use of guidelines and clinical decision tools in consultations. Developments in genomics will refine both diagnosis and treatment, with targeted, personalised medicine becoming the dominant paradigm.

Advances in artificial intelligence (AI) have the potential to move much of the diagnostic decision making away from the clinician. There will still be a requirement for skilled history taking, but there is likely to be more direct interpretation of patient histories by AI clinical decision support systems.

SUMMARY

- The consultation is made up of a number of elements. As a prescriber, you need to analyse your professional assessment, refine current skills and, where appropriate, develop new ones.

- The history is central to making a diagnosis. Incorporate the elements of traditional medical history into your consultation. A systematic approach is required for gathering essential information. Combine this with a collaborative patient-centred approach.

- Diagnosis is important in prescribing. To diagnose, you should have an in-depth knowledge of conditions presenting to your practice. You need to integrate this knowledge with information systematically obtained from the history, examination and investigations. Be aware of red flags and early diagnostic closure.

- Both symptoms and conditions or diseases can be treated. It is important to understand the difference and to seek the underlying cause of any symptom you treat.

- 'Bottom liners' for safe prescribing are the reason for the prescription, date of birth, weight, past medical history, medications, allergies and the provision of appropriate information to the patient.

- Changing demographics with an ageing, more frail population presenting with conditions of increased complexity, aligned with the challenges of polypharmacy will require healthcare workers to upskill their consultation skills with older patients.

- A focus on lifestyle risk factors and other wider determinants of health in consultations in the future will allow a greater emphasis on health improvement and injury and illness prevention.

- Advances in science and technology, particularly in genomics and in AI and clinical decision support, will alter the landscape of consultations in the future.

ACTIVITY

What sort of preparation should you make in advance of a patient consultation?

1. List the seven elements of a traditional medical history.

2. The purpose of the physical examination and near-patient tests is diagnosis. Is this statement true or false?

3. Identify two generic 'red flag' features.

4. There are a number of 'bottom liners' that are considered essential elements for safe prescribing. List as many bottom liners as you can.

REFERENCES

Berry, D. (2004) *Risk, Communication and Health Psychology*. Open University Press, Berkshire.

Brown, J., Noble, L., Papageorgiou, A. and Kidd, J. (2016) *Clinical Communication in Medicine*. Wiley, Chichester.

Coffey, F., Wells, A., and Stone, S. (2024) *Oxford Handbook of Clinical Skills in Adult Nursing*, 2nd edn. Oxford University Press, Oxford.

Neighbour, R. (2005) *The Inner Consultation. How to Develop Effective and Intuitive Consulting Styles*. Radcliffe Medical Press, Abingdon.

Pendleton, D., Schofield, T., Tate, P. and Havelock, P. (2003) *The New Consultation. Developing Doctor–Patient Communication*. Oxford University Press, Oxford.

Silverman, J., Kurtz, S. and Draper, J. (1998) *Skills for Communicating with Patients*. Radcliffe Medical Press, Abingdon.

FURTHER READING

Bailey, P. (2014) *The New Doctor, Patient, Illness Model: Restoring the Authority of the GP Consultation*. CRC Press, Taylor & Francis Group, New York.

Bickley, L.S. (2020) *Bates' Guide to Physical Examination and History Taking*, 13th edn. Wolters Kluwer, Alphen aan Rijnthe.

Donovan, C. Sucking, H. and Walker, Z. (2004) *Difficult Consultations with Adolescents*. Radcliffe Medical Press, Abingdon.

Hastings, A. and Redsell, S. (2006) *The Good Consultation Guide for Nurses*, Radcliffe Medical Press, Abingdon.

Meskó, B. and Görög, M. (2020) A short guide for medical professionals in the era of artificial intelligence. *NPJ Digital Medicine* 3:126.

Pollock, K. (2016) *Concordance in Medical Consultations. A Critical Review*. Radcliffe Medical Press, Abingdon.

Public Health England (2016) *Making Every Contact Count (MECC): Consensus statement*. Public Health England, London.

WEBSITES

Health Education England (2022) *Making Every Contact Count (MECC)*. https://www.hee.nhs.uk/our-work/population-health/our-resources-hub/making-every-contact-count-mecc.

NHS England (2020) *Using online consultations in primary care: implementation toolkit*. https://www.england.nhs.uk/publication/using-online-consultations-in-primary-care-implementation-toolkit/

CHAPTER 2

Accountability and Prescribing

Matthew Boyd, Stephanie Bridges, and Helen Boardman

LEARNING OUTCOMES

By the end of the chapter the reader should be able to:

- define professional accountability and responsibility

- identify the spheres of accountability which underpin clinical practice

- discuss how clinical governance and frameworks of accountability underpin clinical practice

- discuss how clinical governance and frameworks of accountability may be used to ensure good prescribing practice

- apply the principles of accountable practice to the prescribing role.

STOP AND THINK

Prescribing takes many forms, not only prescribing of medicines. Take a moment to think about your current and potential future roles and note down the variety of prescribing activities you are likely to do.

As a registered healthcare practitioner, you will know that you are accountable for the care provided to your patients. In developing your role to include prescribing, you must also consider your accountability in the context of prescribing. This chapter explores definitions of responsibility and accountability, and considers the relationship between accountability, quality and clinical governance. Having determined what accountability is, the chapter analyses the spheres of accountability and the process by which the practitioner is held to account. We present a model of this process which we use to stimulate your professional thinking about accountability and prescribing.

With responsibility comes accountability. There are those who will argue that they are one and the same; even so, you could be responsible for an action but may not be held accountable.

PRACTICE APPLICATION

For example, a learner may be responsible for the care they provide the patient, but the registered practitioner supervising the learner is likely to be professionally accountable for the care provided.

At this point it is appropriate to consider what we mean by accountability.

The New Prescriber: An Integrated Approach to Medical and Non-medical Prescribing, Second Edition.
Edited by Joanne Lymn, Alison Mostyn, Roger Knaggs, Michael Randall, and Dianne Bowskill.
© 2024 John Wiley & Sons Ltd. Published 2024 by John Wiley & Sons Ltd.

DEFINING ACCOUNTABILITY

Accountability is a difficult concept to define. Many will state that it is an ethical concept associated with other concepts such as liability, responsibility, answerability or in terms of an expectation to give account of one's actions or omissions. Hence practitioners may associate accountability with a culture of blame. However, accountability is not necessarily a negative concept (Savage and Moore 2004) and should promote good practice. It is about considering what the outcomes may be according to your actions or decisions.

STOP AND THINK

Spend a few moments developing your definition of accountability. You may find it helpful to identify what you consider to be the key attributes of accountable practice.

As a prescriber you will be required to assess, diagnose, plan and act (which may or may not include prescribing a medicine) within your scope of practice and area of competence. You therefore need to be able to foresee probable or possible consequences of your actions, non-actions or omissions and have the freedom to act based on your clinical decision making (Batey and Lewis 1982). Accountability is the cornerstone of professional practice; it is in being accountable that health professionals are able to respond to patient needs, ensuring that their practice is evidence based, efficient and effective (McSherry and Pearce 2011).

STOP AND THINK

Identify factors which will assist you in becoming an accountable prescriber. What potential challenges might you face as a prescriber?

ASSURING QUALITY

Health professionals, through their regulatory bodies, are held accountable to deliver safe and effective care based on current evidence, best practice and, where appropriate, validated research. The structures and standards of accountability are created and implemented through a variety of different authorities and organisations, for example in England, the National Institute for Health and Care Excellence, National Service Frameworks, NHS Litigation Authority, NHS England and the Care Quality Commission. These organisations evolved and continue to evolve as a response to the public's perception of systemic failings in the National Health Service (NHS) and a consequent lack of confidence in professional self-regulation. Numerous inquiries have highlighted these failings of leadership that led to organisational cultures which allowed poor practices and behaviours to be seen as acceptable. When this poor-quality care was challenged by patients or health professionals, the organisations were not willing to listen or take responsibility for these systemic failings. The inquiries have investigated a wide range of services, including children's services, such as Victoria Climbié (Laming 2003); hospital care standards, such as Alder Hey (Redfern 2000), the Bristol Royal Infirmary Enquiry (Kennedy 2001) and Mid-Staffordshire (Francis 2013); and maternity services, such as Morecambe Bay (Kirkup 2015), East Kent (Kirkup 2022), and Telford and Shrewsbury (Ockenden 2022). Several have made key recommendations related to the accountability for prescribing and administration of medicines, including the Shipman Reports (Smith 2002, 2003a,b), Wayne Jowett (Toft 2001) and Gosport (Gosport Independent Panel 2018). The healthcare organisations act to ensure that both practitioners and their employers are held accountable for the care they provide.

CLINICAL GOVERNANCE

Clinical governance is the means by which care providers ensure that patients receive good-quality care. It was first defined in the consultation document A First-Class Service: Quality in the New NHS (Department of Health 1998) as a framework through which NHS organisations are accountable for continuously improving the quality of their services and safeguarding high standards of care. This is achieved by creating a culture and environment in which excellence in clinical care will flourish. Scally and Donaldson (1999) recognise clinical governance as a framework through which NHS organisations are accountable for quality assurance activities that ensure that predetermined clinical standards are maintained by practitioners and are evident within the health and social care settings. Clinical governance should be a practice-based, value-driven approach, with the goal of delivering the highest possible quality care and ensuring the safety of patients. In particular, clinical governance should be led and owned by frontline practitioners, supported by effective operational structures (Veenstra et al. 2017).

STOP AND THINK

Not all patients wish to be involved in making decisions about their care. Identify the strategies you may use to manage these situations when prescribing.

This highlights the importance of ensuring that prescribing practice is in keeping with governance principles. These include ensuring patients are involved in decisions about their care, that clear procedures are in place for risk reporting and that as a prescriber you maintain your knowledge and competence, and, importantly, practise only within the limits of your competence and responsibility (Royal Pharmaceutical Society 2021; Health and Care Professions Council 2019).

All professional regulatory bodies clearly identify that patient safety and protecting society are fundamental principles that are achieved through working in line with legislative and regulatory body guidance. For further discussion on policy and the legal framework for prescribing see Chapters 3 and 5.

THE FIVE SPHERES OF ACCOUNTABILITY

In undertaking your professional clinical practice, you are accountable to:

- your patient
- yourself
- the wider public and society
- your employer
- your profession.

These five spheres of accountability provide a framework by which we may analyse accountable prescribing practice.

PROFESSIONAL ACCOUNTABILITY

All prescribers are accountable to their professional regulator, which will be the Nursing and Midwifery Council for nurses and midwives, the General Pharmaceutical Council for pharmacists, the General Optical Council for optometrists, and the Health and Care Professions Council for other non-medical professionals. These regulators work to protect the well-being of people who use the services of health professionals, including, for example, nurses, midwives, physiotherapists, pharmacists, optometrists, chiropodists/podiatrists, paramedics and therapeutic radiographers. The regulatory bodies set standards of education for entry to the professions and standards of conduct for their members. It is against these standards that 'fitness for practise' is judged. These standards are applicable to all aspects of practice, including prescribing.

Issues of professional competency are appropriate to all practitioners (see Chapter 3 for the legal framework for prescribing). Practitioners should only prescribe within the sphere of their own competence; for many prescribers this will mean prescribing from a limited formulary of drugs that will be familiar to them from their clinical experience. All practitioners should base their prescribing guidance on the Royal Pharmaceutical Society prescribing framework (Royal Pharmaceutical Society 2021), whose principles determine that prescribers must have sufficient knowledge and competence to:

- assess a patient's/client's clinical condition
- undertake a thorough history, including medical history and medication history, and diagnose where necessary, including over-the-counter medicines and complementary therapies
- decide on the management of the presenting condition and whether or not to prescribe
- identify appropriate products if medication is required
- advise the patient/client about effects and risks
- prescribe if the patient/client agrees
- monitor the response to medication and lifestyle advice.

What is evident is that your accountability extends to the whole of the prescribing process from assessment to diagnosis, as well as the decision whether or not to prescribe. The decision not to prescribe can in practice be a difficult one for the practitioner when faced with a patient who expects a prescription. We will consider this issue again later in this chapter, but the example serves to highlight the fact that as a practitioner you are accountable for not only your actions but also your omissions to act, your decision making and your clinical skills. This brings us to your responsibilities in law and your responsibilities to your patient.

ACCOUNTABILITY TO YOUR PATIENT

All practitioners would accept that the patient or client is central to healthcare provision and that they are therefore accountable to them. Accountability to patients for one's actions or failure to act is outlined in two specific frameworks. These are:

1. The Health Service Ombudsman or, for privately funded patients, the Independent Sector Complaints Adjudication Service (ISCAS). This facilitates the patient or family in making a complaint to the NHS trust or private healthcare provider about the care provided. While the process is formal, the emphasis is placed on the local resolution of complaints.

2. The patient taking a civil legal action under the tort of negligence. It is worth noting that patients who purchase their health services privately would pursue a similar action under contract law. The basis of the civil action in negligence is that there has been a breach of the duty of care owed to the patient which has caused foreseeable damage.

In the second case, the relationship between the practitioner and patient is significant in determining whether a duty of care exists. Indeed, it is this duty of care which is the basis of healthcare law. A duty of care exists immediately from the point a practitioner agrees to consult with a patient and continues until that episode of treatment concludes. What is more appropriate is to identify the standard of care that is to be associated with prescribing practice. The case of *Bolam v. Friern Barnet Hospital Management Committee* (1957) set the test for the standard of care owed to the patient. This case concerned a patient who received fractures to his hips through the electroconvulsive therapy procedure used for treatment of his depressive illness. In determining whether the doctor had breached the duty of care, it was determined that there is no breach of the standard of care if a responsible body of professional opinion would accept the practice as being proper, even if they would have adopted a different practice.

The test has been criticised as favouring the professional, who may only need to find others who would be supportive of their practice. The more recent case of *Bolitho v. City & Hackney Health Authority* (1996) identified that it is no longer sufficient for healthcare professionals to rely solely on the Bolam test. Rather, evidence needs to be presented to the court. In rare cases where it can be demonstrated that professional opinion is not capable of withstanding logical analysis, the judge is entitled to conclude that the body of opinion is neither responsible nor reasonable. What we can therefore conclude is that prescribing practice must be responsible and reasonable, and to the standard normally associated with a prescriber. The prescriber should consequently be able to provide evidence for their prescribing practice to a court if required to do so.

A further consideration in preventing potential negligence claims is that of informed consent, particularly in the light of the Montgomery case (*Montgomery v. Lanarkshire Health Board* [2015] SC 11 [2015] 1 AC 1430), which concerned a woman with diabetes and of small stature, whose baby developed cerebral palsy through complications of a difficult vaginal delivery. Her obstetrician had not disclosed the increased risk, despite Montgomery asking if the baby's size was a potential problem and she had therefore made her decision about delivery based on the information provided to her at the time. The ruling established that, rather than being a matter of clinical judgment to be assessed by professional medical opinion, a patient should be told whatever they want to know, not what the doctor thinks they should be told.

The final aspect of the negligence action is that the breach of duty caused the damage. This is often considered using the 'but for' your actions (or omissions to act) test or the material contribution test, that is, the actions or omissions of the practitioner materially contributed to the damage sustained by the claimant.

ACCOUNTABILITY TO THE PUBLIC/SOCIETY

Society has expectations about the role of professional healthcare staff. While the standard of care provided by healthcare professionals is generally an issue for the civil courts, there are occasions where a health professional's conduct may attract criminal liability, for example a drug error that results in the death of a patient. In this situation the coroner would, in the first instance, undertake a postmortem and hold an inquest into the patient's death. Following this, the police may investigate the death and refer their findings to the Crown Prosecution Service, which would consider whether there were grounds for prosecution.

ACCOUNTABILITY TO THE EMPLOYER

Healthcare professionals are accountable in contract to their employers. The expectations of employers are stated in contracts of employment via organisational policies and procedures. A failure to follow policy could amount to a breach of the employment contract and result in disciplinary action. Prescribers must therefore follow the procedures of their employers, who are ultimately vicariously liable for the torts or wrongs of their employees, if the employee is acting in the course of their employment and doing the job they are employed to do.

ACCOUNTABILITY TO SELF

In many ways this aspect of accountability may be the most important to the practitioner providing care, in that it raises the issue of one's own moral and ethical viewpoints. Beauchamp and Childress (2019) advocate four principles of medical ethics: autonomy, beneficence, non-maleficence and justice, which are described in more detail in Chapter 4.

STOP AND THINK

Having explored the five spheres of accountability, how will you ensure that your prescribing practice meets the required professional standards?

USING THE FIVE SPHERES OF ACCOUNTABILITY

We need to recognise that the different spheres of accountability may at times conflict with one another. It is possible (although unlikely, perhaps), that what your employer wants you to do in a particular situation would not be in keeping with your professional standards, or that your patient requests treatment which is not in keeping with your professional judgement. We find it useful in these instances to recognise the different demands being placed on the practitioner. We have represented the process of accountability in Figure 2.1.

THE PROCESS OF ACCOUNTABLE PRACTICE

As an accountable prescriber you will need to use your knowledge and skills in determining the most appropriate professional practice that is both lawful and ethical to meet the needs of your patient and acceptable standards of practice. Figure 2.1 shows the elements of accountable practice.

What the practitioner considers to be ethical may, however, be unlawful and vice versa. Professional accountable practice is also influenced by national and local policy, clinical guidelines, codes of practice and clinical standards, all of which influence clinical decision making. Alongside that, the practitioner's clinical skills used in implementing the prescribing decision must also be considered. For example, in prescribing for your patient it is important to share and discuss information with them about your recommended course of action. The challenge for the

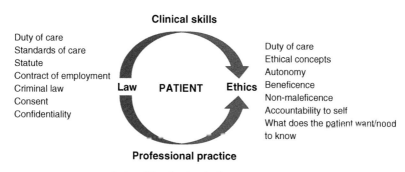

FIGURE 2.1   Model of accountable practice (Plant and Pitt 2010). DHSC, Department of Health and Social Care; NICE, National Institute for Health and Care Excellence.

prescriber is to provide meaningful information to the patient, who may be anxious and in pain. This process all takes place in the context of the relationship between the patient and the prescriber.

ACCOUNTABLE PRESCRIBING

The following scenario will be familiar to many practitioners who are not prescribers.

PRACTICE APPLICATION

We are sure many of us have asked a colleague to prescribe something for our patient based on our own patient assessment and s/he may or may not have done so. The question is, how will you respond when a colleague, recognising that you can now prescribe, requests that you prescribe a drug for their patient?

In considering your decision, your accountability comes to the fore. Perhaps a good starting point is to consider the law. Is the drug you are being asked to prescribe authorised? You will find further discussion of the prescribing framework in Chapter 5. It is clear that your colleague holds a duty of care to the patient, but it is debatable as to whether at this time you also share that duty. It is conceivable that in fact you do and you therefore have a legal responsibility to the patient for the decision you make.

In making your decision, you should also consider the relevant codes of practice, appropriate clinical guidelines and local policies that are in place to guide your decision making. Also consider the potential consequences of your actions. For example, what could be the effect on the patient, ensuring that their health needs are met and the wider impact on system resources. This falls under the domain of healthcare ethics as discussed in Chapter 4. Perhaps an appropriate approach, in recognising the clinical judgement of your colleague and your responsibilities for teamwork, would be to see the patient with them in making your clinical judgement. You are accountable for the decision you take. Also consider the skills you use, not only to make your prescribing decision, but also in exercising your accountability, in maintaining your professional relationship with your colleague, respecting the relationship between your colleague and their patient, and in involving the patient (who is now also your patient) in the decision-making process.

CONCLUSION

In exercising your accountability as a prescriber, it is necessary to view accountability as a process that requires each prescribing situation to be considered on its own merits. We have presented here the five spheres of accountability that provide a means for analysing your responsibility as an accountable prescriber. While it is evident that defining accountable practice is difficult, we have presented a process of accountable practice that may provide you with a framework to analyse your accountability in your day-to-day practice.

SUMMARY

- As a practitioner, you are accountable for both your actions and omissions to act.

- There are five spheres of accountability. You are accountable to your patient, yourself, the wider public and society, your employer and your profession.

- You are accountable professionally, ethically and legally for your prescribing practice.

- As a prescriber, you owe your patient a duty of care. You should be able to provide evidence to support your prescribing decisions.

ACTIVITY

Answer true or false to the following:

1. The Health and Care Professions Council, the Nursing and Midwifery Council and the General Pharmaceutical Council all act to protect the interests of the professions they represent. True/False

2. You cannot be held accountable for omissions in your prescribing. True/False

3. Maintaining your clinical knowledge and competence is only a professional requirement. True/False

4. The Bolam test means that as a prescriber, you have not breached your duty of care if other prescribers would have done the same thing. True/False

5. An error in prescribing resulting in a patient's death may result in criminal proceedings against the prescriber. True/False

6. Tort of negligence is covered by criminal law. True/False

7. In ethical practice I can always act with no harm to the patient. True/False

REFERENCES

Batey, M.V. and Lewis, F.M. (1982) Clarifying autonomy and accountability in nursing service. Part 1. *J Nursing Admin* 12:13–18.

Beauchamp, T.L. and Childress, J.K. (2019) *Principles of Biomedical Ethics*, 8th edn. Oxford University Press, Oxford.

Bolam v. *Friern Barnet Hospital Management Committee* (1957) 2All ER 118; 1 WLR 528.

Bolitho v. *City & Hackney Health Authority* (1996) 7 Med LR 1; (1997). 3WLR 1151; (1998) AC 232.

Department of Health (1998) *A first class service: Quality in the new NHS*. Department of Health, London.

Francis, R. (2013) *Report of the Mid Staffordshire NHS Foundation Trust Public Inquiry*. The Stationery Office, London.

Gosport Independent Panel (2018) *Gosport War Memorial Hospital: The Report of the Gosport Independent Panel*. The Stationery Office, London.

Health and Care Professions Council (2019) *Medicines and Prescribing*. https://www.hcpc-uk.org/standards/standards-relevant-to-education-and-training/standards-for-prescribing/

Kennedy, I. (2001) *The Report of the Public Inquiry into children's heart surgery at the Bristol Royal Infirmary 1984–1995*. The Stationery Office, London.

Kennedy, I. (2001) *Learning From Bristol: the Report of the Public Inquiry into Children's Heart Surgery at the Bristol Royal Infirmary 1984–1995, Cm5207*. Stationery Office, London.

Kirkup, B. (2015) *The Report of the Morecambe Bay Investigation*. The Stationery Office, London.

Kirkup, B. (2022) *Maternity and neonatal services in East Kent: 'Reading the signals' report*. The Stationery Office, 2022.

Laming, H. (2003) *The Victoria Climbié inquiry*. The Stationery Office, London.

McSherry, R. and Pearce, P. (2011) *Clinical Governance: A Guide to Implementation for Healthcare Professionals*, 3rd edn. Blackwell Science, Oxford.

Montgomery v. *Lanarkshire Health Board* (2015) SC 11 (2015) 1 AC 1430.

Ockenden, D. (2022) *Ockenden Report – Final. Findings, conclusions and essential actions from the independent review of maternity services at The Shrewsbury and Telford Hospital NHS Trust*. https://assets.publishing.service.gov.uk/media/624332fe8fa8f527744f0615/Final-Ockenden-Report-web-accessible.pdf.

Plant, N. and Pitt, R. (2010) Accountability and prescribing. Chapter 2 in Lymn, J, S. Bowskill, D. Hextall-Bath, F. Knaggs, R. The New prescriber, Wiley. Chichester.

Redfern, M. (2000) *Report of The Royal Liverpool Children's Inquiry*. Stationery Office, London.

Royal Pharmaceutical Society of Great Britain (2021) *Professional Standards and Guidance for Pharmacist Prescribers*. Royal Pharmaceutical Society of Great Britain, London.

Savage, J. and Moore, L. (2004) *Interpreting Accountability*. Royal College of Nursing, London.

Scally, G. and Donaldson, L. (1999) Clinical governance and the drive for quality improvement. *BMJ* 317:61–65.

Smith, J. (2002) *Shipman Inquiry First Report: Death Disguised*. The Shipman Inquiry, Manchester.

Smith, J, (2003a) *Shipman Inquiry Second Report: The Police Investigation of March 1998*. The Shipman Inquiry, Manchester.

Smith, J. (2003b) *Shipman Inquiry Third Report: Death and Cremation Certification*. The Shipman Inquiry, Manchester.

Toft, B. (2001) *External Inquiry into the adverse incident that occurred at Queen's Medical Centre, Nottingham, 4th January 2001*. Department of Health, London.

Veenstra, G.L., Ahaus, K., Welker, G.A., Heineman, E., van der Laan, M.J. and Muntinghe, F.L.H. (2017) Rethinking clinical governance: healthcare professionals' views: a Delphi study. *BMJ Open* 7:e012591.

FURTHER READING

Caulfield, H. (2005) *Accountability*. Blackwell, Oxford.

Ieraci, S. (2007) Responsibility versus accountability in a risk-averse culture. *Emerg Med Australasia* 18:63–64.

Royal Pharmaceutical Society (2021) *Professional Standards and Guidance for Pharmacist Prescribers*. Pharmaceutical Press, London.

USEFUL WEBSITES

The Medicines and Healthcare Products Regulatory Agency (MHRA) provides information about medicines regulation. www.gov.uk/government/organisations/medicines-and-healthcare-products-regulatory-agency.

The National Institute for Health and Care Excellence (NICE) provides some helpful information about prescribing. www.nice.org.uk

The Health and Care Professions Council is an independent, UK-wide health regulator. It sets standards of professional training, performance and conduct for 15 professions. It maintains a register of health professionals who meet its standards and takes action if registered health professionals do not meet those standards. www.hcpc-uk.org/

Prescribing and the Law

Richard Griffith

CHAPTER 3

LEARNING OUTCOMES

By the end of this chapter the reader should be able to:

- define the requirements for a lawful prescription and patient-specific direction

- identify when it would be lawful to prescribe unlicensed and off-label medicines to patients

- describe the risks and the measures taken to address them when prescribing and remote prescribing

- define a prescriber's duty of care

- outline the requirements of lawful consent.

INTRODUCTION

Non-medical prescribing has been a successful development for the National Health Service (NHS). There is no evidence of the grave dangers to patient safety predicted by the *Lancet* (Horton 2002) when non-medical prescribing was expanded in 2002, but there is no room for complacency.

Independent prescribing has increased the non-medical prescriber's exposure to litigation. Most claims for prescribing errors are settled out of court so the extent of that exposure to litigation can be difficult to measure, but when the Royal College of Nursing (RCN) changed its indemnity scheme in 2012 to exclude RCN members working in GP practices it did obliquely provide evidence of increased liability. The RCN argued the change was necessary because of the excessive drawdown from the scheme for this group of nurses, some £5 million a year, some 90% of the scheme's expenditure. The bulk of claims related to prescribing and medication errors (Jacques 2011).

Prescribing and medication errors are the second most common cause of claim for compensation in the NHS, behind slips, trips and falls (Urquart et al. 2021). Prescribing and medication errors are also the main clinical reason for a health professional facing a fitness to practice investigation.

The law seeks to protect patients and provide them with a means of redress by imposing standards on non-medical prescribers. Put simply, the law requires medicines to be prescribed, dispensed and administered to a person safely. That is, they are given to:

- the right person

- at the right time

- in the right form

- using the right dose

- via the right route.

Where these requirements are not met then harm can occur to the patient.

The New Prescriber: An Integrated Approach to Medical and Non-medical Prescribing, Second Edition.
Edited by Joanne Lymn, Alison Mostyn, Roger Knaggs, Michael Randall, and Dianne Bowskill.
© 2024 John Wiley & Sons Ltd. Published 2024 by John Wiley & Sons Ltd.

PRACTICE APPLICATION

In *Horton v. Evans & another* (2006) a prescriber issued a woman with a prescription for 4 mg of dexamethasone daily, eight times the daily dose she had usually taken to treat a minor ailment. The prescription was dispensed by a pharmacist without further inquiry despite the record showing the previous seven prescriptions were for 0.5 mg of the drug. A further prescription for 4 mg was issued while the woman was on holiday in the USA. The overdose eventually caused her health to deteriorate, and she sued the prescriber and pharmacy. The prescriber admitted they had been careless, and the pharmacy was also found liable by the court. The woman received some £1.4 million in damages.

PROFESSIONALISM

Professionalism is the term that encompasses the standards, values, skills and behaviour expected of a non-medical prescriber. It requires strict adherence to the prescriber's professional code and that prescribers act with honesty and integrity.

Professionalism is underpinned by accountability that protects patients and preserves public confidence in non-medical prescribing by making prescribers legally answerable for their personal acts or omissions to a range of higher authorities. Four areas of law are drawn together to provide maximum protection for patients:

- Accountable to society through the criminal law

  Practice application A non-medical prescriber was given a police caution for theft for stealing six boxes of painkillers and changing the records to cover it up.

- Accountable to the profession through their professional code of standards

  Practice application A non-medical prescriber was removed from their professional register for prescribing without proper authority, beyond the scope of practice and without seeing patients or keeping accurate records

- Accountable to their employer through the contract of employment

  Practice application A non-medical prescriber was dismissed by her employer for errors in the prescribing of medicine and acting outside the scope of their practice, together with further serious allegations that related to falsifying records and acting dishonestly when giving an account of her actions to her employer.

- Accountable to the patient through the civil law

  Practice application Some £400 million of the £2.3 billion paid in clinical negligence claims in 2021 for prescribing and medication errors that harmed patients (NHS Resolution 2021).

These spheres of accountability are not mutually exclusive: they can individually or collectively impose sanctions on a non-medical prescriber who fails to discharge their duties. Non-medical prescribers commonly face multiple jeopardy situations with investigations into complaints, compensation claims, disciplinary procedures and professional regulator concerns being launched into a single incident (Medical Defence Union 2022).

STOP AND THINK

Do you have the authority to prescribe the medicine and are you confident that you are prescribing within the scope of your practice to the standard required by the law and professional code to ensure that patients are protected from harm?

AUTHORITY TO PRESCRIBE

The Medicines Act 1968, sections 58 and 58A, requires that medicines that represent a danger to the patient are classified as prescription only and their administration be supervised by an appropriate practitioner.

Regulation 8 of the Human Medicines Regulations 2012 defines non-medical prescribers and regulation 214 sets out the prescribing authority of all prescribers.

Regulation 214 requires that a prescription-only medicine is sold or supplied in accordance with a prescription issued by an appropriate practitioner. Nurse and pharmacist independent prescribers are held to be appropriate practitioners for any prescription-only medicine; other non-medical prescribers have restrictions on their prescribing authority (see Table 3.1).

Table 3.1 Nonmedical prescriber summary of prescribing authority

Class of drug	Nurse and pharmacist independent prescriber	Community practitioner prescribers	Optometrist independent prescriber	Paramedic independent prescriber	Physiotherapist independent prescriber
Licensed drugs	Any prescription-only medicine	Only medicines listed in schedule 13 of the HMR 2012	Any prescription-only medicine	Any prescription-only medicine	Any prescription-only medicine for conditions within their competence
Off-label or off-licence	Drugs within the scope of practice and competence	Only nystatin for neonates	Drugs within the scope of practice and competence but discouraged by GOC	Drugs within the scope of practice and competence	Drugs within the scope of practice and competence
Unlicensed medicines	Can prescribe where this is accepted clinical practice	No	No	No	No
Controlled drugs	Can prescribe any schedule 2, 3, 4 or 5 controlled drug other than diamorphine, dipipanone or cocaine for the treatment of addition	No	No	**(a)** Morphine sulphate by oral administration or by injection; **(b)** Diazepam by oral administration or by injection; **(c)** Midazolam by oromucosal administration or by injection; **(d)** Lorazepam by injection; **(e)** Codeine phosphate by oral administration	Limited to diazepam, dihydrocodeine, lorazepam, morphine, oxycodone and temazepam by oral administration, morphine for injectable administration and fentanyl for transdermal administration
Borderline substances	Have authority to prescribe	No	Yes	Yes	Yes, but should not need to
For parenteral administration	Have authority to prescribe	Only if listed in schedule 13 of the HMR 2012	No	Yes	Yes

Source: Human Medicines Regulations 2012 (SI 2012/1916).

Table 3.2 Key areas of medicines law covered by the Human Medicines Regulations 2012

Definition and classification of medicinal products
Oversight and administration of medicines law
Manufacturing and wholesale dealing of medicinal products
Licensing of medicines
Homeopathic medicines
Herbal medicines
Borderline products
Unlicensed medicines
Medicines safety and pharmacovigilance
Dealings with medicinal products, including the sale, supply and administration of prescription-only medicines and authorised exemptions from the general law
Patient Group Directions
Patient Specific Directions
Packaging and information leaflets

Source: Human Medicines Regulations 2012 (SI 2012/1916).

The Human Medicines Regulations 2012 are the largest change to medicines legislation since the Medicines Act 1968. As well as consolidating medicines law under one set of regulations the Medicines and Healthcare products Regulatory Agency (MHRA) have also introduced some policy changes to ensure the 2012 regulations are fit for purpose and reflect current practice.

The regulations are now the main source of medicines law and contain provisions ranging from product development and clinical trials through to requirements for the use, supply and administration of homeopathic remedies, herbal compounds and prescription-only medicines (see Table 3.2).

The MHRA (2012) argue that the Human Medicines Regulations 2012 simplified medicines law by bringing the key provisions into one set of regulations. It remains the case, however, that several sections of the Medicines Act 1968 remain in force and controlled drugs continue to be regulated by the Misuse of Drugs Act 1971 and its regulations, particularly the Misuse of Drugs Regulations 2001, which set the requirements for the therapeutic use of controlled drugs, and the Misuse of Drugs (Amendment No.2) (England, Wales and Scotland) Regulations 2012, which extended wider controlled-drug prescribing authority to non-medical prescribers.

The Human Medicines Regulations 2012 do not radically alter medicines law. Their main objective is to consolidate the wide range of and often piecemeal orders, regulations and European directives that had built up over 40 years since the enactment of the Medicines Act 1968. These are now largely drawn together into a single legal framework set out in the 2012 regulations. Non-medical prescribers will use the Human Medicines Regulations 2012 as their main source of medicines law.

REQUIREMENTS FOR A LAWFUL PRESCRIPTION

The requirements for a valid prescription are set out in the Human Medicines Regulations 2012, regulation 217 (see Box 3.1).

SUPPLYING A PRESCRIPTION-ONLY MEDICINE WITHOUT A PRESCRIPTION

As a rule, prescription-only medicines will be supplied and administered in accordance with the directions of an appropriate practitioner set out in a valid prescription (Human Medicines Regulations 2012, regulation 214(1)(a)). This strict regime protects patients from the harmful effects of medicines but can delay treatment because of the need to visit an appropriate practitioner or a pharmacy before the medicine can be supplied or administered. To overcome this inflexible process

BOX 3.1	REQUIREMENTS OF A VALID PRESCRIPTION

- **Condition A** requires that the prescription is signed in ink by the appropriate practitioner giving it.
- Appropriate practitioners include independent prescribers, supplementary prescribers and community practitioner prescribers (Human Medicines Regulations 2012, regulation 214)
- **Condition B** requires that the prescription is written in ink or is otherwise indelible. For medicines other than controlled drugs this includes a prescription generated by the use of carbon paper etc.

  To reflect modern practice, the regulations allow conditions A and B to be replaced where the form and advanced signature are generated and sent electronically to the dispenser (Human Medicines Regulations 2012, regulation 219).
- **Condition C** requires that the prescription contains the address of the appropriate practitioner, the appropriate date, the kind of appropriate practitioner giving the prescription, the name and address of the patient and the patient's age if they are under 12.
- **Conditions D and E** require that a prescription or an initial repeat prescription are not dispensed where 6 months have passed from the appropriate date given by the prescriber on the prescription.

while still ensuring the safety of patients, the Human Medicines Regulations 2012 allow prescription-only medicines that would normally require a prescription to be supplied for administration through the use of Patient Specific Directions (PSDs).

PATIENT SPECIFIC DIRECTIONS

A PSD is a written instruction for prescription-only medicines to be supplied for administering to a named patient without a prescription. PSDs are routinely used in hospital settings where instructions for the supply and administration of a prescription-only medicine to a patient are issued by any appropriate practitioner on the patient's drug chart and administration record.

The Human Medicines Regulations 2012, regulation 229('), provides that a prescription is not required if the supply of a prescription-only medicine is provided by an NHS body under the written directions of a doctor, dentist, nurse independent prescriber, optometrist independent prescriber or pharmacist independent prescriber.

STOP AND THINK

Do you have authority to issue a Patient Specific Direction (PSD)? When might it be appropriate for you to use a PSD instead of a prescription? Are there local policies on the use of PSDs in your practice?

A PSD differs from a prescription. To be lawful a prescription must meet the requirements of the Human Medicines Regulations 2012, regulation 217.

To be valid the PSD must:

- be in writing
- relate to the particular person to whom the medicine is to be supplied for administration
- be issued by a person who is an appropriate practitioner with authority to issue a PSD in that setting.

Any appropriate practitioner can therefore issue a PSD in hospital or in a health centre to authorise the supply of a prescription-only medicine to be administered to a named patient (Human Medicines Regulations 2012, regulation 223). Only a nurse independent prescriber, optometrist independent prescriber or pharmacist independent prescriber can issue a PSD in a community setting such as a care home or the patient's own home.

Liability for harm rests with the independent prescriber, who will be accountable for the appropriateness of PSD and the appropriateness of any delegation of the administration of the medicine to another person.

PRESCRIBING CONTROLLED DRUGS FROM SCHEDULES 2–5 BY INDEPENDENT NURSE AND PHARMACIST PRESCRIBERS

The Misuse of Drugs Regulations 2001 (as amended by the Misuse of Drugs (Amendment No.2) (England, Wales and Scotland) Regulations 2012) extended the range of controlled drugs independent nurse and pharmacist prescribers can prescribe.

The 2012 regulations also:

- clarified the law on the compounding of medicines that include controlled drugs prior to administration

- authorised the supply of morphine and diamorphine by registered nurses and pharmacists under a Patient Group Direction in any setting

- authorised the possession of specific controlled drugs by healthcare professionals, including paramedics under a Patient Group Direction

The Misuse of Drugs Regulations 2001 regulations allow both nurse and pharmacist independent prescribers to prescribe any controlled drug from schedules 2–5 of the Misuse of Drugs Regulations 2001 for conditions that fall within the individual competence of the prescriber (regulation 6B). They are also able to requisition controlled drugs and are lawfully able to possess, supply, offer to supply and administer the drugs they are able to prescribe (regulation 14).

The authority of nurse and pharmacist independent prescribers to prescribe controlled drugs is not wholly unfettered as they cannot prescribe diamorphine, cocaine and dipipanone for the treatment of addiction.

AUTHORITY TO COMPOUND MEDICINES

The Medicines (Exemptions And Miscellaneous Amendments) Order 2009, paragraph 2, allows nurse and pharmacist independent prescribers to prescribe unlicensed medicines and to mix or authorise the mixing of medicines into a third unlicensed medicine.

STOP AND THINK

Do you have the authority to give instructions for the compounding of medicines? When might it be appropriate for you to require the compounding of medicines?

The authority to mix, or compound, two licensed products even though it produces a third unlicensed product allows nurse and pharmacist independent prescribers to meet the needs of patients who receive their medicines through such means as syringe drivers. This technique is well-established practice where patients have the need for several medicines to be administered over time. It is employed particularly in palliative care, where the medicines often contain controlled drugs.

The Misuse of Drugs Regulations 2001 (as amended), regulations 8 and 9, give independent nurse and pharmacist prescribers authority to compound two or more medicines prior to administration to a patient, including those listed in schedules 2–5 of the Misuse of Drugs Regulations 2001.

PRESCRIBING CONTROLLED DRUGS BY OTHER INDEPENDENT PRESCRIBERS

Currently, the prescribing of controlled drugs by other independent prescribers is limited to the following:

- physiotherapist independent prescribers, who are able to prescribe controlled drugs for the treatment of organic disease or injury provided but are limited to diazepam, dihydrocodeine, lorazepam, morphine, oxycodone and temazepam by oral administration, morphine for injectable administration and fentanyl for transdermal administration

- podiatrist independent prescribers, who have the authority to prescribe diazepam, dihydrocodeine, lorazepam and temazepam for oral administration only.

- since the 31st December 2023 a therapeutic radiographer independent prescriber and paramedic independent prescriber have been given the authority to prescribe and administer a limited range of controlled drugs set out in regulation 6D of the Misuse of Drugs Regulations 2001

STANDARD OF PRESCRIBING

While the authority to prescribe is regulated by statute law, the standard of prescribing is regulated by a combination of the prescriber's duty of care, professional code and local policies. The standards are drawn together by the Competency Framework for all Prescribers (Royal Pharmaceutical Society 2021), which emphasises a patient-centred approach to safe, evidence-based prescribing.

The Royal Pharmaceutical Society and the Nursing and Midwifery Council et al. (2019), along with the other health regulators and organisations, have also produced a set of high-level principles for remote prescribing and consultation that establish best practice to follow when prescribing remotely (see Table 3.3).

Table 3.3   High-level principles for remote prescribing

UK-registered healthcare professionals must follow 10 high-level key principles when providing remote consultations and prescribing remotely to patients
1.   Make patient safety the first priority
2.   Understand how to identify vulnerable patients
3.   Tell patients your name, role and (if online) professional registration details
4.   Explain that:
(a) You can only prescribe if it is safe to do so
(b) It is not safe if you do not have sufficient information about the patient's health or if remote care is unsuitable to meet their needs
(c) It may be unsafe if relevant information is not shared with other healthcare providers involved in their care
(d) If you cannot prescribe because it is unsafe you will signpost to other appropriate services
5.   Obtain informed consent and follow relevant medical capacity law and codes of practice
6.   Undertake an adequate clinical assessment
7.   Give patients information about all the options
8.   Make appropriate arrangements for aftercare
9.   Keep notes
10. Stay up to date

PRESCRIBER'S DUTY OF CARE

The competency framework sets out the standards that underpin the prescriber's duty of care. The relationship between a non-medical prescriber and their patient gives rise to a duty situation (*Kent v. Griffiths* (2001)), which gives rise to a legal obligation not to harm their patient through carelessness. The duty of care owed by a non-medical prescriber has been defines as:

> *A single comprehensive duty covering all the ways they are called on to exercise skill and judgement to improve the physical and mental condition of their patients.*
>
> (*Rogers v. Whitaker* (1992) at 483)

This comprehensive duty includes the standards set out in the competency framework but also encompasses the prescriber's handwriting, which must be clear enough for a careless or busy person to be able to read it.

PRACTICE APPLICATION

In *Prendergast v. Sam & Dee Ltd* (1988) a prescriber was liable for breaching their duty of care to a patient when a pharmacist dispensed the drug Daonil instead of the prescribed Amoxil because of the prescriber's poor handwriting.

RESPECTING PATIENT AUTONOMY

Non-medical prescribers regularly need to touch their patients to examine them or provide care and treatment. The right to touch an individual is limited in law and there is an initial presumption that it must not occur without permission in the form of a real consent (*F v. West Berkshire HA* (1990)).

The law recognises that adults have a right to determine what will be done to their bodies (*Schloendroff v. Society of New York Hospitals* (1914)). Touching a person without consent is generally unlawful and will amount to unprofessional behaviour, trespass to the person or, more rarely, a criminal assault. Bodily integrity is held in very high regard by the law. Unlike other civil wrongs, such as negligence, which requires harm, any unlawful touching is actionable even if done with the best of motives. The right to determine what shall be done with one's own body is a fundamental right and the bedrock of self-determination and individual autonomy (*Airedale NHS Trust v. Bland* (1993)).

In *Aintree University Hospitals Foundation Trust v. James* (2013), Lady Hale held that a patient's consent makes care and treatment lawful. It is not lawful to treat a patient who has capacity and refuses that treatment.

THE PROPRIETY OF TREATMENT

Permission to touch a patient by obtaining consent is an important defence to a claim of unlawful touching or trespass to the person. Consent, however, provides more than a defence to a claim of trespass to the person: it goes to the very heart of the propriety, the rightness, of care and treatment.

In *Airedale NHS Trust v. Bland* (1993), Lord Mustill held that bodily invasions in the course of proper treatment stand completely outside the criminal law. Consent is important because it not only provides healthcare professionals with a defence, but because it is usually essential to the propriety of treatment. If the consent is absent, the acts of the healthcare professional will lose their immunity.

ELEMENTS OF A REAL CONSENT

In *Chatterton v. Gerson* (1981) the Court held that once the patient is informed in broad terms of the nature of the care and treatment, and gives consent, that consent is real.

To be real, consent needs to satisfy three key elements. It must be:

- full
- freely given
- reasonably informed.

FULL CONSENT

When obtaining consent, non-medical prescribers must ensure that the patient agrees to all the treatment they intend to carry out. Proceeding with treatment that the patient is unaware of, or has refused to agree to, will be unprofessional behaviour, a trespass to the person and actionable in law (*Williamson v. East London and City HA* (1998)).

Non-medical prescribers must therefore take care to explain all the treatment or touching that will occur when obtaining consent from a patient and ensure that additional treatment or touching is subject to further consent.

FREELY GIVEN CONSENT

Consent is an expression of autonomy and must be the free choice of the individual. It cannot be obtained by undue influence. This does not mean that a non-medical prescriber cannot influence a patient's decision. Indeed, part of the role is to explain the benefits of treatment to patients to obtain consent. In law, to be undue the influence must erode the free will of the patient. It must be so forceful that the patient excludes all other considerations when making their choice, such as in situations where a threat of force or harm forces a patient to accept treatment.

REASONABLY INFORMED CONSENT

Non-medical prescribers have a duty to give advice and information to a patient so that the patient understands the nature of the proposed treatment and can make a choice (*Hills v. Potter* (1983)). The courts do not distinguish between advice given in therapeutic and non-therapeutic contexts (*Gold v. Haringey HA* (1987)).

The basis of the duty to give Information is derived from two areas of law: the law of trespass and the law of negligence.

TRESPASS TO THE PERSON

In trespass a real consent requires an explanation, in broad terms, of the nature of the treatment to the patient. If the broad nature of the care and treatment has been explained, no cause of action in trespass will arise.

PRACTICE APPLICATION

In *Potts v. NWRHA* (1983), a patient successfully sued for battery when she was led to believe that she was having a routine postnatal vaccination. In fact, she was given the long-acting contraceptive Depo-Provera. If a prescriber gives misinformation or false information to a patient, consent will be negated and liability in trespass will arise.

NEGLIGENCE

The second type of information concerns the risks inherent in any treatment. A failure to disclose risks does not vitiate a real consent and no action is possible in trespass (*Hills v. Potter* (1983)). The proper cause of action in disclosure of risks cases falls in negligence.

Non-medical prescribers owe a duty to their patients to take reasonable care not to cause harm. Advising patients about the risks associated with treatment and about less risky available options for treatment forms part of that duty (*Sidaway v. Bethlem Royal Hospital* (1985))

In *Montgomery v. Lanarkshire Health Board* (2015) the Supreme Court held that to discharge this duty prescribers must have a meaningful dialogue with their patients about the risks of the treatment and the availability of less risky treatment. The standard of disclosure is based on what a reasonable or prudent person in the patient's position would want to know about the risks of treatment. The decision of the Supreme Court in *Montgomery v. Lanarkshire Health Board* (2015) places much greater emphasis on the importance of involving the patient in decisions relating to treatment.

OBTAINING CONSENT

Non-medical prescribers lawfully obtain real consent in two ways. A patient may express their consent by making known their willingness to be touched. Express consent can be written or oral. Written consent is usually obtained where a procedure is invasive or perceived to carry a material risk. A consent form provides a degree of evidential certainty that the patient agreed to treatment but is only as good as the understanding of the person signing it (*Re T (Adult: Refusal of Treatment)* (1992))

The second form of consent is an implied consent. This is permission implied through the actions of the patient in response to a request to give treatment. It does not mean that agreeing to come to hospital or allowing a district nurse into their home implies that a patient agrees to treatment. Every episode of care or treatment must be subject to a real consent.

Consent is a continuous process and may be withdrawn at any time. A withdrawal of consent is as indistinguishable as an initial refusal to consent (*Ciarlariello v. Schacter* (1993)). If a patient changes their mind and refuses to continue with treatment, then it must cease or trespass to the person will occur.

SUMMARY

- A non-medical prescriber is accountable for their practice to four areas of law.

- The Human Medicines Regulations 2012 represent the most significant change in medicines legislation since the Medicines Act 1968.

- The Human Medicines Regulations 2012 are now the main source of medicines law and must be applied by non-medical prescribers when supplying or administering medicines to their patients.

- Controlled drugs continue to be regulated by the Misuse of Drugs Act 1971 and its regulations.

- Independent nurse, pharmacist and optometrist prescribers can issue Patient Specific Directions in community setting as well as in hospitals and health centres.

- The right to touch an individual is limited in law and requires consent.

- Real consent must be full, freely given and reasonably informed.

- Real consent makes treatment lawful.

- It is not lawful to treat a patient who has capacity and refuses that treatment.

- Non-medical prescribers owe their patients a duty of care that includes a duty to warn of risks.

ACTIVITY

1. Which one of the following is a non-medical prescriber not accountable to?

   - Society
   - Themselves
   - The patient
   - Their employer

2. What is now regarded as the main source of medicines law in the UK?

   - The Medicines Act 1968
   - The Consumer Protection Act 1987
   - The Prescription Only Medicines (Human Use) Order 1997
   - The Human Medicines Regulations 2012

3. The main source of law regulating a non-medical prescriber's authority to prescribe controlled drugs is:

   - The Misuse of Drugs Act 1971
   - The Misuse of Drugs Regulations 2001
   - The Misuse of Drugs (Amendment No 2) Regulations 2012
   - The Human Medicines Regulations 2012

4. Which of the following non-medical prescribers can issue a Patient Specific Direction in a community setting?

   - A community practitioner prescriber
   - A physiotherapist independent prescriber
   - A paramedic independent prescriber
   - A pharmacist independent prescriber

5. Consent is a defence against an allegation of trespass to the person.

   - True
   - False

6. The element(s) of a real consent are:

   - It is free, full and reasonably informed.
   - It is specific, the patient's choice and in writing.
   - The patient tells the prescriber what treatment they want.
   - Prescriber's professional judgement, patient's permission, consent form.

7. A patient with capacity who refuses treatment can be treated if it is in their best interests.

   - True
   - False

8. The duty to warn of risks is based on:

   - What a reasonable body of prescribers would mention to a patient with this condition.
   - What a reasonable person in the patient's situation would want to know about risks.
   - Whether the patient would be too afraid to have treatment if told about risks.
   - Whether the patient askes specific questions about specific risks.

9. Which of the following forms part of a non-medical prescriber's duty of care?

   - The standard of their handwriting.
   - Giving advice about medicines and adverse reactions.
   - Acting on allergy information.
   - All of the above.

10. The condition for a lawful prescription requires a prescriber to handwrite their signature

    - True
    - False

REFERENCES

Jacques, H. (2011) GPs could bear cost of changes to nurse indemnity. *BMJ* 343:d7151

Horton, R. (2002) Nurse prescribing in the UK: right but also wrong. *Lancet* 359:1875–1876.

Medical Defence Union (2022) Nurse practitioners face multiple investigations into single incident, according to MDU analysis. https://www.themdu.com/press-centre/press-releases/nurse-practitioners-face-multiple-investigations-into-single-incident-according-to-mdu-analysis.

MHRA (2012) *Simplified Medicines Regulations Come into Force*. London: Medicines and Healthcare Products Regulatory Agency.

NHS Resolution (2021) *NHS Resolution Annual Report 2020–2021*. London: NHS Resolution.

Nursing and Midwifery Council, Academy of Medical Royal Colleges, Care Quality Commission, Faculty of Pain Medicine, General Dental Council, General Medical Council, General Optical Council, General Pharmaceutical Council, Healthcare Improvement Scotland, Healthcare Inspectorate Wales, Pharmaceutical Society of Northern Ireland, Royal Pharmaceutical Society and Regulation and Quality Improvement Authority (2019) *High level principles for good practice in remote consultations and prescribing*. https://www.nmc.org.uk/globalassets/sitedocuments/other-publications/high-level-principles-for-remote-prescribing-.pdf.

Royal Pharmaceutical Society (2021) *A competency framework for all prescribers*. https://www.rpharms.com/Portals/0/RPS%20document%20library/Open%20access/Prescribing%20Competency%20Framework/RPS%20English%20Competency%20Framework%203.pdf?ver=mctnrKo4YaJDh2nA8N5G3A%3d%3d.

Urquart, A., Yardley, S., Thomas, E., Donaldson, L. and Carson-Stevens, A. (2021) Learning from patient safety incidents involving acutely sick adults in hospital assessment units in England and Wales: a mixed methods analysis for quality improvement. *J R Soc Med* 114(12):563–574.

CASE LAW

Aintree University Hospitals Foundation Trust v. James (2013) UKSC 67.

Airedale NHS Trust v. Bland (1993) AC 789.

Chatterton v. Gerson (1981) QB 432.

Ciarlariello v. Schacter (1993) 2 SCR 119.

Horton v. Evans & another (2006) EWHC 2808 (QB)

Kent v. Griffiths (2001) QB 36 (CA).

Montgomery v. Lanarkshire Health Board (2015) UKSC 11.

Prendergast v. Sam & Dee Ltd (1988) *Times Law Report*, 24 March (QBD).

Re T (Adult: Refusal of Treatment) (1992) 3 WLR

Rogers v. Whitaker (1992) 175 CLR 479.

Sidaway v. Bethlem Royal Hospital (1985) AC 871.

LEGISLATION

Misuse of Drugs Regulations 2001 (SI 2001/3998).

Medicines (Exemptions and Miscellaneous Amendments) Order 2009 (SI 2009/3062).

Human Medicines Regulations 2012 (SI 2012/1916).

Misuse of Drugs (Amendment No.2) (England, Wales and Scotland) Regulations 2012 (2012/973).

FURTHER READING

Human Medicines Regulations 2012. The Human Medicines Regulations 2012 (legislation.gov.uk).

The Medicines (Exemptions and Miscellaneous Amendments) Order 2009. The Medicines (Exemptions and Miscellaneous Amendments) Order 2009 (legislation.gov.uk).

The competency framework for all prescribers. A Competency Framework for all Prescribers | RPS (rpharms.com).

WEBSITES

Department of Health (2023) *Legislation covering medicines.* https://www.health-ni.gov.uk/articles/legislation-covering-medicines.

Association of the British Pharmaceutical Industry. *Policy position, the use of 'unlicensed specials'*

to treat NHS patients. https://www.abpi.org.uk/publications/policy-position-the-use-of-unlicensed-specials-to-treat-nhs-patients/.

CHAPTER 4

The Ethics of Prescribing

Matthew Boyd, Stephanie Bridges, and Helen Boardman

LEARNING OUTCOMES

By the end of this chapter the reader should be able to:

- describe three key ethical theories

- understand how ethical theory may be applied in prescribing practice

- consider ethics in relation to conscience, law and ethical codes

- reflect on unique ethical problems in prescribing.

You will be presented with situations in which you may feel conflicted about your responsibilities and decisions. The law and professional guidance do not always provide a clear way forward and this is where ethical decision making might be required.

Ethics, or moral philosophy as it is also known, is concerned with questioning and justifying what individuals do, and particularly what actions are thought right or wrong. Traditionally, this involved concerns about individuals' virtues but more recently the focus has shifted to justifying individual acts. The aim in this chapter is to focus on ethical theories that have been influential in the healthcare setting – deontology, utilitarianism and the four principles of bioethics – and to consider how ethical decision making occurs in practice.

DEONTOLOGY

Deontological ethical theories are concerned with duty and with what acts are right. They put forward several specific acts which individuals are expected to follow regardless of the consequences of these actions. The most influential deontological theory was that of Immanuel Kant (1998), who argued that acts are right only if they are in accordance with the 'categorical imperative'. There are two key statements of the categorical imperative: to act only in ways that can be accepted by everyone (universalised) and to treat individuals not as a means to an end but to respect them as individuals. Deontological theories do not allow the consequences of a proposed act to have any influence.

PRACTICE APPLICATION

The prescriber who prescribes a medicine, for example, to assist in suicide acts wrongly because to universalise such an act would threaten society. The prescriber who lies to a patient about a medicine's side effects to ensure they take it also acts wrongly according to the deontologist. Lying is not something that everyone would agree to if everyone were allowed to do it, and it does not respect the patient who is lied to.

Deontological, duty-based ethical theories have been criticised. First, these duties are very demanding and because every action must comply with the categorical imperative statements, they cannot be avoided. Second, it is not always obvious how to apply these rules in everyday situations.

The New Prescriber: An Integrated Approach to Medical and Non-medical Prescribing, Second Edition.
Edited by Joanne Lymn, Alison Mostyn, Roger Knaggs, Michael Randall, and Dianne Bowskill.
© 2024 John Wiley & Sons Ltd. Published 2024 by John Wiley & Sons Ltd.

UTILITARIANISM

In contrast to deontological theories based on duties, there are consequentialist theories that value the outcome or good of actions. The most influential of these, utilitarianism, involves a calculation of the overall measure of utility or good. The utilitarian must consider how a proposed act will affect everyone but, crucially, not allow anyone a greater weighting. Furthermore, the utilitarian can only be concerned with a single measure of utility and the best known, developed originally by Mill (1992), is happiness. The result is an ethical theory that is impartial in terms of individuals. One cannot give greater weighting to some (like family or friends) and one cannot exclude particular acts (like lying or suicide) if they result in the greatest overall welfare.

Utilitarianism has been influential for political and policy-based decisions but has been criticised since it can justify in certain circumstances acts usually considered wrong, such as torture and killing.

PRACTICE APPLICATION

Taking a utilitarian approach, a prescriber might limit the prescribing of expensive medicines that only benefit a minority of patients when greater happiness could be gained from prescribing a different drug for a larger number of patients. Utilitarian justification cannot give any extra weighting to the suffering that would result from the minority denied a medicine.

Whilst utilitarian and deontological ethical theories have been influential within healthcare, a principle-based theory has been highly influential too.

FOUR PRINCIPLES OF BIOETHICS

Principlism is a form of ethical justification that recognises that certain principles should guide individuals in deciding on what acts are right. Beauchamp and Childress (2019) proposed four principles: autonomy, beneficence (doing good), non-maleficence (avoiding harm) and justice. Whilst acknowledging that these were not the only principles that should guide individuals in life more generally, they were argued to be sufficient to allow ethical decisions within healthcare to be made.

AUTONOMY

Autonomy is the principle that patients should be self-directing or self-determining about what happens to them. This also applies to relatives, carers and healthcare professionals. The concept of autonomy encapsulates issues of consent, appropriate level of information giving and decision making. For prescribers, this principle would require consideration of patients' decisions and wishes, but also the prescriber's autonomy, including concerns about not being coerced into prescribing. The prescriber is therefore engaging the patient or client in the decision-making process, sharing information with the patient who themselves understands their symptoms to arrive at a decision. Ultimately, however, autonomy allows a patient to make their own decision, which may be in conflict or agreement with that of the health professional treating them.

BENEFICENCE

Beneficence implies that healthcare should be provided for the benefit of the patient or client. While this may not be controversial, in practice identifying the patient's best interest can be difficult, especially when patients may choose to exercise their autonomy in a way which the practitioner believes compromises their interest, for example by not taking prescribed medicines.

NON-MALEFICENCE

Non-maleficence is the duty not to harm the patient. Beneficence and non-maleficence seem similar and that to not harm is to do good. Non-maleficence is considered the more demanding principle and that not harming may take precedence over helping. For prescribers, this might involve consideration of not harming patients in prescribing and always prescribing to help them. This can be difficult for prescribers when, for example, the prescribed drug is known to have harmful side effects.

JUSTICE

The principle of justice suggests that health professionals should provide care that is equitable. It involves the notion of the fair and equitable distribution of treatment according to needs – prescribers considering this principle would need to appreciate conflicting demands on who would benefit most from medicines and how to allocate scarce resources in healthcare systems. While we are familiar with the notion of the 'postcode lottery', prescribers may have to consider what 'just' prescribing entails.

We find that these concepts are helpful in determining the nature of ethical dilemmas in practice and in recognising the complexities involved in meeting the needs of a diverse population with diverse needs.

It is obvious that these four principles may conflict at times. For example, a patient's autonomous wish for an unproven or expensive medicine cannot always be respected, since this may deprive other patients of treatment (a justice concern) or harm the patient (non-maleficence). Whereas Kantian deontological duties require all categorical imperatives to be observed and utilitarian theory involves only one consistent calculation, the four principles accept that all four cannot necessarily be applied in all situations and that a process of deciding which to use or what weighting to give each must be used.

The answer to how to decide which principles to apply involves what is termed a process of reflective equilibrium, following the liberal theory of Rawls (1979). This requires individuals to engage in a process of specifying and balancing the respective principles – choosing which might apply, together with their relative importance, in a given situation, all whilst considering these in relation to their own intuition. If the choice of one principle cannot be accommodated with one's own intuition, then one must return to the problem and reconsider the available principles again.

STOP AND THINK

If there are several conflicting theories, which one should the new prescriber use in practice?
Can you be a utilitarian when you want a patient to take a beneficial medicine that they do not want, but a deontologist when you want to give a patient medicine usually denied on cost grounds?

MAKING ETHICAL DECISIONS

To answer these questions, it is helpful to consider reasoning that is either 'top down' or 'bottom up'. The difference between these approaches is that 'top down' reasoning works from an ethical theory and seeks to apply it consistently to all cases. 'Bottom up' reasoning starts from a problem and applies theories to solve it. The bottom up approach is not the intended use of individual theories, but the approach is argued to be helpful in the practical aspect of resolving ethical problems. This approach also allows the practitioner to apply ethical theories alongside other factors, such as

BOX 4.1	BRITISH MEDICAL ASSOCIATION STAGES OF ETHICAL DECISION MAKING

1. Recognise that you are facing an ethical question.

2. Identify the ethically important components.

3. Where necessary, seek additional information.

4. Identify relevant legal and professional guidance.

5. Critically analyse the question.

6. Support the decision with sound arguments.

laws, codes and personal beliefs. Although this seems to be a convenient 'having your cake and eating it' approach, it is recognised that certain ethical problems can be considered in relation to different theories and so selecting them accordingly is relevant (Seedhouse 1998).

There is another approach to making ethical decisions that prescribers might find useful. It recognises that ethical theories are rather abstract and perhaps hard to apply in practice. This involves the development of several practical models of decision making (Cooper 2007; Wingfield and Badcott 2007). These may be contrasted with the three key ethical theories described so far in this chapter, in that they provide a series of steps or stages which individuals should work through to arrive at an ethical decision. Unfortunately, none of them does away with the fundamental need to apply some form of ethical reasoning to the problem at hand, but for the prescriber, such models may help in the gathering of relevant information and balancing other demands. Several models have been developed, but as an example, the British Medical Association (2023) stages of ethical decision making are shown in Box 4.1.

Whilst such models might seem unduly reductive and raise concerns as to whether all decision making can be reduced to such discrete and convenient stages, they are appealing in providing an *aide-mémoire* to allow the prescriber to gain confidence and perhaps conceptualise what is needed to resolve each ethical problem. However, individuals must be prepared to consider not only ethical arguments but also relevant law and this is now considered in terms of additional influences on decision making in prescribing.

CONSCIENCE, CODES AND LAW

An ethical decision in prescribing unfortunately does not involve considering ethical theory alone and it is usually accepted that the prescriber must also consider their own personal beliefs and conscience, as well as relevant laws and professional codes of ethics. In relation to personal beliefs, it is recognised that all individuals will have such thoughts, perhaps about issues that they have considered over time, or they may be one's first thoughts about a new situation, which may be referred to as one's intuition or even one's conscience.

STOP AND THINK

What sorts of beliefs or feelings might conflict with making an ethical decision?

Should such beliefs and convictions be given any weight? Or should the three key ethical theories considered so far always be used instead?

What are the implications of your own views on your practice?

ETHICS AND THE INDIVIDUAL

As noted, 'top down' approaches maintain that only one ethical theory applies and there can be no room for personal beliefs, but others have recognised the appeal of such personal beliefs. Beauchamp and Childress (2019), for example, believed that accommodating principles within one's own beliefs is a necessary process. Indeed, within healthcare, personal beliefs – be they religious or secular – are frequently (although not always) respected by the inclusion of conscience clauses in professional codes. However, there is a tension between accommodating personal beliefs and giving them primacy, since the latter introduces what is known as relativism. This is yet another ethical approach that, in various forms, maintains that different beliefs are possible amongst different individuals and, significantly, that these should all be valued. However, opponents have argued that this may mean that no agreement might be reached on anything if individuals hold many different views.

PRACTICE APPLICATION

Applied to prescribing and healthcare, relativism and appeals to personal beliefs are therefore problematic because they may lead to different outcomes for different prescribers and may be hard to justify to others.

Despite such problems, appeals to conscience are often accepted in healthcare in relation to issues such as abortion, for example, and these are supported in ethical codes and also law (General Pharmaceutical Council 2017a). However, although these are distinct from more extreme views that all healthcare professionals must undertake tasks that are part of their professional role (Savulescu 2006), caveats apply and conscientious objectors are usually required to provide details of where alternative services can be found. Hence, the prescriber who does not wish to prescribe contraception should indicate where such services are available, even if this is ethically problematic for them (Cooper et al. 2008).

ETHICS AND PROFESSIONAL CODES

As well as personal beliefs, prescribers must also consider relevant ethical codes. The role of professional codes of ethics is to offer guidance to practitioners, and they often include principles similar to those described above and may be identified in those issued by the Nursing and Midwifery Council (2018) and the General Pharmaceutical Council (2017b), for example. They have certain advantages over general ethical theories like utilitarianism and deontology in that they are usually specific to particular professions and hence offer potentially more specific advice related to practice. They also represent a formalisation of the standards of practice expected of a profession and may be used to measure standards of practice. They are therefore of importance in ethical justification in prescribing, but two problems should be mentioned: first, they appear not to be of relevance in ethical decision making in practice (Cooper 2007; Holm 1997) and, second, their contemporary and contextual nature means they are subject to revision and the criticism that they carry less ethical force than normative theories. Importantly, professional codes do not allow divestment of responsibility when there is personal conscientious objection. The patient must take priority, which may be against a prescriber's own personal beliefs.

ETHICS AND THE LAW

The relationship between ethics and the law is also potentially problematic for the prescriber. As considered in Chapter 3, prescribing is circumscribed by laws that permit only certain individuals to issue prescriptions. Furthermore, legal restrictions on which medicines may be prescribed and in what way are also in place and these carry potential penalties of prosecution if contravened. However, ethics can place conflicting demands on prescribers, for example should the prescriber who is asked for a prescription for a regular medicine for a patient, but the medicine is outside the scope of clinical competence for the prescriber make the patient wait for an urgently needed medicine? In such cases, ethical considerations about the welfare of the patient come into conflict with legal and professional requirements. Many factors, including clinical judgement and the details of each situation, are important but these may be considered analogous to the scenario of stopping at a red light whilst driving a car, then seeing an ambulance behind that can only proceed if you drive through the red light to let it pass. In such cases, ethical considerations are often thought to override legal ones and for the prescriber, this is something that should be considered on occasion. However, when considering more extreme examples such as assisted euthanasia, for example, whilst one can develop strong ethical arguments – often utilitarian – to support prescribing medicines that will hasten death and prevent suffering, the courts may not be prepared to accept such ethical arguments, mainly due to the gravity of the situation in such cases. Hence, the balance between following laws and making an ethically informed decision is both difficult and dependent on the exact nature of the problem.

STOP AND THINK

What ethical problems might you as a new prescriber encounter that are different from your previous clinical practice?

EXAMPLE OF AN ETHICAL PROBLEM IN PRESCRIBING

DISTRIBUTIVE JUSTICE: WHO SHOULD GET WHAT MEDICINE?

Although all services and treatments within the NHS in the UK are limited by costs and time, this is particularly evident in relation to medicines due to the economic impact they have on the NHS overall. Hence, as well as considering the necessary clinical and therapeutic aspects of prescribing, all prescribers must be aware of the impact that their prescribing has upon overall costs. The availability of primary care prescribing analyses and cost data about prescribing has led to an increased understanding of costs, but in relation to ethics there may be situations where budgetary restrictions and local formularies prevent some medicines being available. For example, the well-documented cases of 'postcode prescribing' arise due to different trusts taking different decisions about what medicines may be prescribed and these may lead to ethical concerns. Such decisions are often considered utilitarian, since they are intended to maximise the overall benefits for all patients, rather than provide help to specific individuals.

SUMMARY

- There are several important ethical theories for healthcare: utilitarian, deontological and the four principles approaches.

- Such theories often offer conflicting justification for ethical decisions in healthcare but the use of 'bottom-up' approaches together with practical decision-making models can be helpful in applying theory and reaching ethical decisions.

- The influence of conscience, ethical codes and the law may also be relevant and should be considered before making final ethical decisions.

- Ethical decision making remains variable and potentially difficult, and this chapter offers a starting point for prescribers to develop the skills and confidence to make ethical decisions in their work.

- New prescribers are encouraged to explore ethics texts and although some are difficult for beginners (Kant 1998), many are commendably approachable (Singer 1993).

ACTIVITY

Answer true or false to each of the following.

1. Prescribers must never act in an ethically justifiable way that is contrary to the law.   True/False

2. Duty-based deontological justification involves considering the overall consequences of a proposed action.   True/False

3. 'Top down' ethical reasoning involves applying a particular ethical theory consistently to different problems.   True/False

4. If a prescriber conscientiously objects to prescribing a certain medicine, they may still have to appropriately refer the patient to an alternative prescriber.   True/False

5. If using the four principles of bioethics, only one principle can be considered at a time when making an ethical decision.   True/False

USEFUL WEBSITES

British Medical Association. Children and Young People ethics toolkit. https://www.bma.org.uk/advice-and-support/ethics/children-and-young-people/children-and-young-people-ethics-toolkit

Association of the British Pharmaceutical Industry. https://www.abpi.org.uk/value-and-access/appropriate-prescribing/

REFERENCES

Beauchamp, T. and Childress, J. (2019) *Principles of Biomedical Ethics*, 8th edn. Oxford University Press, Oxford.

British Medical Association (2023) *How to approach an ethical question*. British Medical Association, London. https://www.bma.org.uk/media/7089/bma-how-to-approach-an-ethical-dilemma-final.pdf.

Cooper, R.J. (2007) *Ethical Problems and their Resolution by Community Pharmacists: a Qualitative Study*. PhD thesis, University of Nottingham.

Cooper, R.J., Bissell, P. and Wingfield, J. (2008) Ethical decision-making, passivity, and pharmacy. *J Med Ethics* 34:441–445.

General Pharmaceutical Council (2017a) *In practice: Guidance on religion, personal values and beliefs.* General Pharmaceutical Council, London.

General Pharmaceutical Council (2017b) *Standards for pharmacy professionals*. General Pharmaceutical Council, London

Holm, S. (1997) *Ethical Problems in Clinical Practice: The Ethical Reasoning of Health Care Professionals*. Manchester University Press, Manchester.

Kant, I. (1998) *Groundwork of the Metaphysics of Morals*. Cambridge University Press, Cambridge.

Mill, J.S. (1992) *On Liberty and Utilitarianism*. David Campbell, London.

Mill, J.S. (1863) *Utilitarianiam*. Parker, Son & Bourn, London.

Nursing and Midwifery Council (2018) *The Code: Professional standards of practice and behaviour for nurses, midwives and nursing associates*. Nursing and

Midwifery Council, London. https://www.nmc.org.uk/standards/code/.

Rawls, J.A. (1979) *Theory of Justice*. Harvard University Press, Cambridge, MA.

Savulescu, J. (2006) Conscientious objection in medicine. *BMJ* 332:294–297.

Seedhouse, D. (1998) *Ethics: The Heart of Healthcare*. Wiley, New York.

Singer, P. (1993) *Practical Ethics*. Cambridge University Press, Cambridge.

Wingfield, J. and Badcott, D. (2007) *Pharmacy Ethics and Decision Making*. Pharmaceutical Press, London.

FURTHER READING

Hawley, G. (ed.) (2007) *Ethics in Clinical Practice: An Interprofessional Approach*. Pearson Education, Harlow.

Norman, R. (1998) *The Moral Philosophers: An Introduction to Ethics*. Oxford University Press, Oxford.

CHAPTER 5

Prescribing in Practice

Dianne Bowskill and Daniel Shipley

LEARNING OUTCOMES

By the end of the chapter the reader should be able to:

- understand the difference between independent and supplementary prescribing and know when to use them in practice

- understand the importance and influence of both clinical guidelines and local drug commissioning when undertaking prescribing practice

- identify barriers and potential pitfalls concerned with prescribing practice and consider strategies to overcome them

- identify factors which promote, hinder or prevent prescribing in teams and consider strategies to manage and reduce barriers.

This chapter spans the process of prescribing from education to the integration of prescribing in clinical practice. As a new prescriber, you may need to revisit the definitions and questions raised here from time to time. The transition to prescriber takes time and achieving a license to prescribe is like passing a driving test, in that learning really begins after qualification.

INDEPENDENT AND SUPPLEMENTARY PRESCRIBING

These two types of prescribing form the legal framework for medical and non-medical prescribing. They originate from the second Crown Report (Department of Health 1999) in which Dr June Crown proposed two types of prescribers, independent and dependent. The term 'dependent' was quickly replaced by the term 'supplementary prescriber' and introduced as a type of prescribing in 2003 (Department of Health 2003). Understanding the difference between the types and knowing how and when to use them in practice is the foundation of safe and accountable prescribing.

- *Independent prescribing*: Prescribing by a practitioner responsible and accountable for the assessments of patients with undiagnosed or diagnosed conditions and for decisions about the clinical management required, including prescribing. (Department of Health 2006:7)

- *Supplementary prescribing*: A voluntary partnership between an independent prescriber (a doctor or dentist) and a supplementary prescriber to implement an agreed patient specific Clinical Management Plan with the patient's agreement. (Department of Health 2005:8)

STOP AND THINK

Look carefully at the descriptions of independent and supplementary prescribing. Can you identify the differences between them?

The New Prescriber: An Integrated Approach to Medical and Non-medical Prescribing, Second Edition.
Edited by Joanne Lymn, Alison Mostyn, Roger Knaggs, Michael Randall, and Dianne Bowskill.
© 2024 John Wiley & Sons Ltd. Published 2024 by John Wiley & Sons Ltd.

The key difference between the two types of prescribing lies in the accountability and responsibility for diagnosis. Under independent prescribing, it is the independent prescriber (doctor, dentist, nurse, pharmacist, physiotherapist, podiatrist, paramedic, therapeutic radiographer or optometrist) who is responsible for the diagnosis and prescribing of treatment. Under supplementary prescribing, it is also the independent prescriber who makes the diagnosis, but this must be a doctor or dentist (Department of Health 2005).

SUPPLEMENTARY PRESCRIBING AND THE CMP

Under supplementary prescribing arrangements, the supplementary prescriber will manage the care of the patient by prescribing drugs identified in a patient-specific clinical management plan (CMP). Two blank template CMPs initially developed by the Department of Health have been adopted for use by NHS Trusts. Template 1 is designed for teams who have contemporaneous access to patient records and template 2 for teams who do not. Template 2 includes two additional boxes for the prescriber to record the medication and past medical history of the patient. The template type chosen for use should reflect the supplementary prescriber's access to patient records and non-medical prescribers should use the templates endorsed by their employer.

WHAT INFORMATION MUST A CMP INCLUDE?

The CMP is a legal document, and the requirements of a CMP are set out in schedule 14 of the Human Medicines Regulations 2012. A patient-specific CMP must be prepared and agreed to by the doctor, supplementary prescriber and patient before supplementary prescribing can begin. This agreement is a voluntary partnership that can stay in place for up to 12 months. Supplementary prescribers must remember that all partners can end the agreement at any time.

SHOULD I USE INDEPENDENT OR SUPPLEMENTARY PRESCRIBING?

Supplementary prescribing is the only option for allied health profession non-medical prescribers wishing to prescribe unlicensed medicines and some controlled drugs. As outlined in Chapter 3, controlled drugs and unlicensed drugs can be prescribed by all non-medical prescribers under supplementary prescribing.

The independent prescribing of controlled drugs for some non-medical prescribers is restricted by the form of medicine and the clinical condition for which they may be prescribed. See the *British National Formulary* for details.

PRACTICE APPLICATION

Aside from these restrictions, the framework of independent and supplementary prescribing presents non-medical prescribers with a choice: prescribe independently when the prescriber is competent to diagnose, manage and prescribe treatment, or supplementary prescribing when the non-medical prescriber does not wish to or is not competent to take responsibility for the diagnosis.

PRESCRIBING IN PRACTICE

To integrate prescribing skills and knowledge, non-medical prescribers need first to visualise how they will prescribe for patients in their clinical area. Forward thinking will enable the new non-medical prescriber to prepare themselves and the practice area for when prescribing begins.

STOP AND THINK

What benefits might you, patients, colleagues and the organisation gain from you becoming a prescriber?

Prescribing education takes a generic approach and will guide non-medical prescribers to develop a broad prescribing knowledge. As the pharmacology chapters in this book show, learning is based around body systems. This might mean revisiting topics you have not considered for a long time and will certainly involve learning about new ones. Non-medical prescribers working in narrow fields of specialist practice sometimes question why such broad knowledge is necessary. Advancements in medicine and pharmacology mean that patients who present for healthcare are more often living with chronic conditions and comorbidities. This is particularly evident in older people who, because of age-related changes, are more susceptible to morbidity and mortality secondary to drug-related harm (Mortazavi et al. 2016). Drugs are used to prevent, treat and manage the symptoms of disease and as a prescriber you must be aware of how these drugs might interact with or affect the drugs you prescribe. This broad prescribing knowledge is necessary to inform your prescribing practice and help you not only to decide when to refer but also to understand why. There is a lot to learn, and a balance must be reached. You will need to think about how you can make sense of this new knowledge in the context of prescribing in your clinical area. Personal prescribing formularies are a useful way of doing this.

PERSONAL PRESCRIBING FORMULARIES

Personal prescribing formularies work by encouraging you to think about the drugs you will be prescribing in practice. This focus is a useful way to build your confidence in prescribing. Having a personal formulary and prescribing a small number of drugs increases prescriber knowledge of indications for use, dosing, contraindications and interactions. Improved knowledge has a positive outcome on effective drug therapy by enabling a concordant approach to shared decision making between patient and prescriber in the consultation (Galanter et al. 2021). Start your formulary by listing the drugs you are most likely to prescribe. The list provides a point from which you can begin to apply principles of pharmacology, consultation, law, accountability and ethics to your own prescribing practice. It is also a useful way to consider how you will integrate prescribing into your practice.

PRACTICE APPLICATION

Approach 1: Some non-medical prescribers will approach prescribing in the same way as their medical colleagues and prescribe for all patients in their care.
Approach 2: Some non-medical prescribers will consider themselves competent to prescribe for some but not all presenting conditions.
Approach 3: Some non-medical prescribers will focus on prescribing for individual patients presenting with specific conditions or comorbidities (Bowskill et al. 2013).
Whatever approach is taken, prescribing must always be within the scope of practice and individual competence.

STOP AND THINK

Which approach will you take to prescribing in your practice?
Who in your clinical team might need to be aware of your approach to prescribing?

PRESCRIBING FOR PATIENTS

For prescribers working in hospital or nursing home settings the difference between prescribing and transcribing requires clarification. As discussed in Chapter 3, prescribing is one of a number of legal routes by which a patient may receive medicines. Transcribing is, however, not prescribing.

Transcribing is the transfer of previously prescribed medicine details onto a patient-specific direction for the purposes of administration. An example of this may include the rewriting of a hospital drug chart (Rogers 2022). Policies vary from Trust to Trust and localise both who can transcribe and when transcribing can be used. Since transcribing is effectively copying information for the purposes of administration, it cannot be utilised in place of prescribing to initiate or optimise therapy (Royal Pharmaceutical Society 2019).

Those who undertake transcribing should do so in line with local policy and ensure they have the requisite skills and training. An audit trail must also exist, clearly identifying who performed the transcription (Royal Pharmaceutical Society 2019).

Prescribers in primary care settings have a different question to consider, that of repeat prescribing. Repeat prescribing is an arrangement between patient and prescriber that enables prescriptions to be regenerated at given intervals, without the requirement for consultation at each point of issue (General Medical Council 2021).

Repeat prescribing falls under the umbrella of independent prescribing, meaning there is a professional need to assess the patient and possess diagnostic competence. Prescribers engaging in this activity do so with the understanding that they are responsible and accountable for this continuation of therapy (General Medical Council 2021). As a prescriber you are responsible for the prescriptions that you sign, and this includes prescriptions initiated by doctors or other non-medical prescribers. In all instances the prescriber must ensure that the repeat prescribing criteria in Box 5.1 have been fulfilled.

BOX 5.1   CRITERIA FOR REPEAT PRESCRIBING

- Each prescription is regularly reviewed and only re-issued to meet clinical need.

- The patient/client is issued with the correct prescription.

- The correct dose is prescribed, particularly for patients whose dose varies during the course of treatment.

- The patient's condition is monitored, taking account of medicine usage and effects.

- Patients who need further examination or assessment are reviewed and do not receive repeat prescriptions without being seen by an appropriate prescriber.

- Any changes to the patient's medicines are critically reviewed and quickly incorporated into their medical record.

- A review must take place following a maximum of six prescriptions or 6 months.

_____

(Based on General Medical Council 2021)

STOP AND THINK

Under repeat prescribing, who is accountable for the diagnosis of the condition(s) for which you will prescribe medication therapy?

INTERPRETING AND APPLYING CLINICAL GUIDELINES TO PRESCRIBING

The purpose of clinical guidelines is to assist practitioners in their management of patient care and to improve patient outcomes. Guidelines are based on the most current research evidence and are associated with improved treatment outcomes and reduced mortality. They help to foster an evidence-based approach to treatment decisions, including prescribing, they educate and in some cases they champion cost-effective interventions (Graham and Harrison 2005). Clinical guidelines are also designed to standardise practice, thereby promoting continuity across a service, nationally and sometimes internationally. National guidelines are often locally devolved by way of local guidelines and regional medicine formularies. An important challenge for new prescribers is to understand how the needs of individual patients, clinical, personal or social, may necessitate divergence from or re-interpretation of guidelines.

NATIONAL GUIDELINES

One of the best recognised exponents of national guidelines in the UK is the National Institute for Health and Care Excellence (NICE). Informed by experts, carers and the public, a review of evidence takes place using literature searching. A summary of evidence is typically published, followed by a cost impact analysis (NICE 2022).

Estimation of cost-effectiveness is a key component of NICE guidelines, and this distinguishes them from many others. By using a metric called a quality-adjusted life year (QALY) NICE guidelines can quantify the cost of improving and extending patient life through intervention (NICE 2022).

It is important for prescribers to acknowledge variance across national guideline publications and recognise that evidence can be assimilated differently. To complicate things further, institutions may publish guidance documents that contradict one another, with very few national bodies having a monopoly on the evidence base. In the management of acute asthma, for example, there have been considerable differences in how NICE and the British Thoracic Society stratify therapy and define steroid potency. Over recent years, joint bodies have attempted to align these recommendations (British Thoracic Society 2017).

In certain specialist settings, NICE has a diminished influence relative to other institutions. The management of HIV, for example, is largely directed by the British Association for Sexual Health (BASHH) and the British HIV Association (BHIVA). It is therefore imperative that prescribers are familiar with the literary landscape that informs patient care in their area of prescribing practice (BHIVA 2022; BASHH 2022).

LOCAL GUIDELINES

The purpose of local guidelines is to tailor broad, national recommendations to the needs of a regional population. The reasons for doing this are multifaceted and may include one or more of the reasons outlined in Table 5.1

Table 5.1 Reasons for local guidelines

Demographics and population factors	Microbial resistance patterns in the local area will dictate the detail of antimicrobial guidelines. It is important that the agents being recommended are those to which the populous are most likely to be sensitive.
Service factors	Certain Trusts have the facilities and expertise to treat certain conditions. Other Trusts may need to transfer patients elsewhere.
Medicines supply chain	On occasion there can be regional supply chain issues that influence the availability of medication and therefore local guidance.
Variable interpretation	National guidelines often recommend drug classes rather than individual drugs. Local medicines committees have scope to conduct literature searches and make assessments about cost-effective selection.

LOCAL MEDICINES FORMULARY

A local medicines formulary endeavors to create a framework of support concerning the introduction, utilisation, withdrawal and continuation of treatment for a regional healthcare system. Decision-making groups are the arbiters of these processes, initiating exercises such as horizon scanning (for newly licensed medications), evidence and information gathering, local guideline development etc. (NICE 2014).

Medicines formularies typically denote which drugs can be prescribed within a given locality, what agents are typically first line within a drug class and details of prescribing restrictions across both primary and secondary care. Prescribers must therefore be aware of local devolution and the systems underpinning drug prescribing across the healthcare interface (Royal Pharmaceutical Council 2013).

PATIENT FACTORS

The final and arguably most important component of guideline interpretation is the integration of patient factors into decision making. National and local guidelines are created to serve the needs of a given population and standardise the delivery of care. There are instances, however, where individual circumstances and considerations require the prescriber to deviate from these recommendations (Woolf et al. 1999).

It is important that prescribers do not simply attempt to 'treat the guideline'. Patient preferences must be accounted for and how the guidance is used should be tailored to the personal circumstances and presentation of the patient. Patient factors are indeterminate and wide reaching. It is impossible to provide an exhaustive list, although some common examples have been included below:

- Swallowing capacity: May require a different formulation or route of administration.

- Previous exposure to medication: May preclude the use of certain antibiotics, for example, due to increased risk of antimicrobial resistance

- Allergy status: May preclude the use of certain drugs

- Renal impairment: May necessitate dose reduction or use of an alternative agent

- Liver impairment: May necessitate dose reduction or use of an alternative agent

- Concerns regarding adherence: May require a different formulation, route of administration, dosage regimen etc.

- Patient preference, work patterns, sleep patterns etc.

DRUGS AND DRIVING

It is important that prescribers understand their responsibility to consider drugs and driving, and to counsel patients appropriately. UK law explains that driving when unfit to do so because of legal drugs is an offence. Prescribers are advised to consult UK Government webpages, where a list of prescription medicines which can potentially impair capacity to drive safely are listed (UK Government 2024).

For those supplying or prescribing medication on this list, there is a responsibility to counsel patients on the potential sedative effects and risks posed by driving. It is, however, the responsibility of the driver to decide whether their driving proficiency has been adversely affected by taking the prescribed drug(s).

Recommended advice may include a summary of typical side effects, times of the day where the risk may be temporarily increased, the importance of adhering to and not exceeding the prescribed dose and frequency, the effect of concomitant medication, co-existing conditions and alcohol (Department for Transport 2014).

STOP AND THINK

Are there any drugs you are likely to prescribe on the government list of drugs 'likely to impair capacity' to drive safely?

COMMUNICATING PRESCRIBING DECISIONS WITHIN THE TEAM

Prescribing cannot occur in isolation – to do so could put patient safety at risk. You must be aware of, and communicate with, others who prescribe, supply or administer medicines to the patient at all times. Record keeping and communication are fundamentally important to safe and effective prescribing. Medication history along with decisions to prescribe and not to prescribe should be clearly documented in the patients' clinical record. This facilitates medicine reconciliation and provides a clear audit trail. For those working in secondary care, there is often a means of annotating the drug chart to denote medication history details. It is imperative that decisions to hold, amend or optimise therapy are also documented (Nickless and Lispcombe 2023). Prescribers have a responsibility to inform and record their prescribing activity, and you must be familiar with and act within your employer's prescribing policy.

ORGANISATIONS AND EMPLOYERS

Prescribing is part of the clinical governance framework of the organisation and each employer will consider the clinical risk of prescribing. It is here that we identify differences between employers in terms of what they will allow their non-medical prescribers to do. The law, as set out in Chapter 3, details the legal boundaries of prescribing for all healthcare professionals. Within frameworks of clinical governance, healthcare employers sometimes place restrictions on non-medical prescribing. You should access your employer's prescribing policy for guidance. Non-medical prescribers are often employed in roles which require prescribing across primary and secondary care services. These prescribing situations present a series of questions about the provision of FP10 prescription pads, access to patient records, record keeping and financial responsibility for prescribed items. If you are going to be prescribing in such a situation when qualified, you must talk to managers to address these questions before you begin to prescribe.

The most obvious restriction to prescribing is one which applies to all prescribers and is an accepted part of modern healthcare – the local prescribing formulary. Here the prescriber has an obligation to prescribe items included within the formulary, so get to know what is on the formulary. You also have an obligation from a public health perspective to prescribe within local antimicrobial guidelines. Make sure you always work with the most up-to-date guidelines and recommendations.

Integrating prescribing into your clinical practice is something that you alone can do. There is an awful lot to think about before you can use prescribing in your practice. Refer back to the questions raised in this chapter as you learn to prescribe, and prepare your team and your employer to accept you as a prescriber. There is nothing worse than successfully passing the course and not being able to prescribe because there is something stopping you that you could have prepared for in advance.

SUMMARY

- There are two types of prescribing in the UK, independent and supplementary.

- A patient-specific clinical management plan must be prepared, and an agreement signed by the independent prescriber (a doctor), the patient and supplementary prescriber before the supplementary prescriber can prescribe.

- Having a personal formulary and prescribing a small number of drugs increases prescriber knowledge of indications for use, dosing, contraindications and interactions.

- Guidelines are based on the most current research evidence and are associated with improved treatment outcomes and reduced mortality.

- Prescribers are advised to consult UK Government webpages where a list of prescription medicines which can potentially impair capacity to drive safely are listed (UK Government 2024).

- Prescribing cannot occur in isolation; to do so would put patient safety directly at risk.

- As a prescriber you must be aware of and communicate with others who prescribe, supply and administer medicines to the patient or client at all times.

ACTIVITY

1. Look carefully at the descriptions of independent and supplementary prescribing. Can you identify the differences between them?

2. What benefits might you, patients, colleagues and the organisation gain from you becoming a prescriber?

3. What approach will you take to prescribing in your practice and who in your clinical team might need to be aware of your approach to prescribing?

4. Under repeat prescribing who is accountable for the diagnosis of the condition(s) for which you prescribe medication therapy?

5. Are any of the drugs you are likely to prescribe or are listed in your personal formulary on the government list as likely to impair capacity to drive safely?

REFERENCES

BASHH (2022) *About BASHH*. https://www.bashh.org/about-bashh/about-bashh/.

BHIVA (2022) *About BHIVA*. https://www.bhiva.org/AboutBHIVA.

Bowskill, D. Timmons, S. and James, V. (2013) How do nurse prescribers integrate prescribing in practice: case studies in primary and secondary care. *J Clin Nurs* 22(13–14):2077–2086.

British Thoracic Society (2017) *BTS response to new NICE asthma guidelines*. https://www.brit-thoracic.org.uk/news/2017/bts-response-to-new-nice-asthma-guidelines/.

Department of Health (1999) *Review of Prescribing, Supply and Administration of Medicines. Final Report*. Department of Health, London.

Department of Health (2003) *Supplementary Prescribing by Nurses and Pharmacists Within the NHS in England. A Guide for Implementation*. Department of Health, London.

Department of Health (2005) *Supplementary Prescribing by Nurses, Pharmacists, Chiropodists/Podiatrists, Physiotherapists and Radiographers within the NHS in England. A Guide for Implementation*. Stationery Office, London.

Department of Health (2006) *Improving Patients' Access to Medicines: A Guide to Implementing Nurse and Pharmacist Independent Nurse and Pharmacist Independent Prescribing within the NHS in England*. Department of Health, London.

Department for Transport (2014) *Drug driving: guidance for healthcare professionals* https://www.gov.uk/government/publications/drug-driving-and-medicine-advice-for-healthcare-professionals/drug-driving-guidance-for-healthcare-professionals

Galanter, W., Equale, T., Gellad, W. et al. (2021) Personal formularies of primary care physicians across four healthcare systems. *JAMA NetW Open* 4(7):e2117038.

General Medical Council (2021) *Repeat prescribing and prescribing with repeats*. https://www.gmc-uk.org/professional-standards/professional-standards-for-doctors/good-practice-in-prescribing-and-managing-medicines-and-devices/repeat-prescribing-and-prescribing-with-repeats

Graham, I.D. and Harrison, M.B. (2005) Evaluation and adaptation of clinical practice guidelines.*Evid Based Nurs* 8(3):68–72.

Mortazavi, S.S. Shati, M., Keshtkaer, A., Malakouti, S.K., Bazargan, M., Assari, S. (2016) Defining polypharmacy in the elderly: a systematic review protocol. *BMJ Open* 6:e010989.

NICE (2014) *Developing and updating local formularies.* https://www.nice.org.uk/guidance/mpg1/chapter/Recommendations.

NICE (2022) *Assessing cost effectiveness.* https://www.nice.org.uk/process/pmg6/chapter/assessing-cost-effectiveness.

Nickless, G. and Lipscombe, M. (2023) How to perform accurate medicines reconciliation. *Pharml J.* https://pharmaceutical-journal.com/article/ld/how-to-perform-accurate-medicines-reconciliation.

Rogers, T. (2022). Understanding transcribing for medicines administration. *Specialist Pharmacy Service.* https://www.sps.nhs.uk/articles/understanding-transcribing-for-medicines-administration-in-healthcare/.

Royal Pharmaceutical Society (2013) *Medicines Optimisation:Helping patients make the most of medicines.* Royal Pharmaceutical Society. London.

Royal Pharmaceutical Society (2019) *Professional Guidance on the Administration of Medicines in Healthcare Settings.* Royal Pharmaceutical Society, London.

UK Government (2024) *Drugs and driving: the law.* https://www.gov.uk/drug-driving-law.

Woolf, S.H., Grol, R., Hutchinson, A., Eccles, M. and Grimshaw, J. (1999) Clinical guidelines: potential benefits, limitations, and harms of clinical guidelines. *BMJ* 318(7182):527–530.

FURTHER READING

General Medical Council (2022) *Good practice in prescribing and managing medicines and devices.* https://www.gmc-uk.org/ethical-guidance/ethical-guidance-for-doctors/good-practice-in-prescribing-and-managing-medicines-and-devices.

Royal Pharmaceutical Society (2024) *Professional guidance on the safe and secure handling of medicines.* https://www.rpharms.com/recognition/setting-professional-standards/safe-and-secure-handling-of-medicines/professional-guidance-on-the-safe-and-secure-handling-of-medicines (Update due Jan 23).

USEFUL WEBSITES

The Human Medicines Regulations 2012. Schedule 14. Prescription etc. by supplementary prescribers: particulars of clinical management plan.

https://www.legislation.gov.uk/uksi/2012/1916/schedule/14/made

Department of Health Northern Ireland. Prescribing by Non-Medical Healthcare Professionals.

https://www.health-ni.gov.uk/articles/pharmaceutical-non-medical-prescribing

Public Health Issues

Michael Watson and Katharine Whittingham

CHAPTER 6

LEARNING OUTCOMES

By the end of this chapter the reader should be able to:

- understand what is meant by public health

- identify the professional groups which contribute to public health

- describe where to find evidence in relation to public health

- identify health-promoting settings

- demonstrate an awareness of public health and how prescribers can contribute to key areas.

In the past, prescribers have made significant contributions to improving the public's health by prescribing medicines and providing health advice on a range of important areas, including smoking, contraception and the safe use of medicines (Neil et al. 2022). Prescribers as a group have considerable reach because they work in a number of settings, including primary care, hospitals and workplaces. In the future, prescribers' public health roles are likely to increase as governments are keen to enlist the support of key professionals to tackle pressing public health priorities.

This chapter discusses the meaning of public health and some of the different influences on health. It will also consider evidence-based approaches and priority topics, and explore how prescribers can increase their role in public health.

WHAT IS PUBLIC HEALTH?

There is a plethora of definitions of public health. However, the definition that is accepted by the Faculty of Public Health and widely used within the NHS is:

The science and art of preventing disease, prolonging life and promoting health through organised efforts of society.

Acheson (1988)

This definition is broad and includes an emphasis on prevention, the collective responsibility for health and a focus on whole populations. Public health incorporates a range of disciplines and professions, and individuals may work in or across different settings, including primary care, workplaces, schools and local communities.

For those wanting to promote health, it is crucial to understand the different types of influences on health. The main determinants of health have been classified by Dahlgren and Whitehead (1991) into five categories (Figure 6.1). These categories include both fixed factors (age, sex, hereditary factors) and potentially modifiable ones (e.g., individual lifestyle factors and working conditions). Figure 6.1 illustrates the range of different influences on health and draws attention to areas that should be targeted to produce improved health outcomes.

Although public health activities are many and varied, the Faculty of Public Health has classified them into three key domains of public health practice (Table 6.1). These domains overlap

The New Prescriber: An Integrated Approach to Medical and Non-medical Prescribing, Second Edition.
Edited by Joanne Lymn, Alison Mostyn, Roger Knaggs, Michael Randall, and Dianne Bowskill.
© 2024 John Wiley & Sons Ltd. Published 2024 by John Wiley & Sons Ltd.

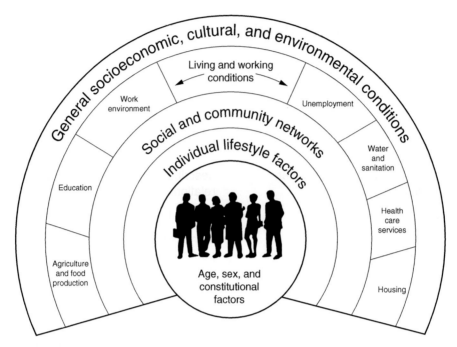

FIGURE 6.1 The main determinants of health (Dahlgren and Whitehead 1991, with permission from the author).

Table 6.1 The three domains of public health activity

Domain	Area of activity
Health improvement	Lifestyles
	Inequalities
	Education
	Housing
	Employment
	Family/community
	Surveillance and monitoring of specific diseases and risk factors
Healthcare	Clinical effectiveness
Public health: improving services	Efficiency
	Service planning
	Audit and evaluation
	Clinical governance
	Equity
Health protection	Disease and accident prevention
	Chemicals and poisons
	Radiation
	Emergency response
	Environmental health hazards

and together they provide an insight into the real breadth and complexity of the public health function. Prescribers have important roles to play in all three of the domains.

CONTRIBUTIONS TO PUBLIC HEALTH

For prescribers to make an effective contribution to public health, they must be able to identify their own public health role as well as that of others. The Centre for Workforce Intelligence (Health Education England 2021) defines the core public health workforce as all staff who engage in public health activities and identify public health and health improvement as a core part of their role. Examples include health visitors, school nurses, pharmacists, health promotion specialists, environmental health officers, and nurses working in primary and secondary care.

STOP AND THINK

What public health activities do you engage with in your role?

Although most prescribers will be part of the wider public health workforce, there will be individuals who will be integrating their prescribing skills and knowledge into their public health practice.

EFFECTIVE APPROACHES TO PROMOTING PUBLIC HEALTH PRESCRIBING

There has in the past been a dearth of information about the effectiveness of public health interventions, but public health theory provides several frameworks which can be used to guide action (Green et al. 2019; Davies and Macdowall 2006; Pencheon et al. 2006). There are, for example, theories to help identify relevant factors, theories to guide changing individual behaviour and theories to guide changing organisations and communities. In addition, the World Health Organization's Ottawa Charter provides clear direction for those wanting to develop effective interventions (World Health Organization 1986; Thompson et al. 2018).

National and global public health policies recognise the importance of striving to create the right conditions for good health and well-being to help people live better and longer. The NHS Long Term (National Health Service 2019) Plan launched in 2019 calls for improved integrated care delivery between health, social care, local government and third-sector organisations. This plan focuses on enabling everyone to get the best start in life, helping communities live well and helping people to age well. Integral to the NHS plan is a greater emphasis on prevention and public health.

Better health for all: A new vision for prevention (UK Health Security Agency 2018) sets out targets for creating a better balance between a system focused on detecting and treating illnesses, and predictive prevention public health strategies to prevent poor health. The policy advocates action to empower people to make healthier choices, to harness modern technology and to address the broader conditions that lead to health and social care needs in the first place. Importantly, the policy recognises that living well in the community also involves more than health and social care services and the important role of individuals, families, communities, employers, charities, the NHS, social care, and local and national government.

Public Health England (2017), the National Institute for Health and Care Excellence (2020) and the Royal Pharmaceutical Society (2022) outline opportunities for engagement in health-promoting interventions in primary and community pharmacy settings. Examples include advice on making healthy lifestyle changes, blood pressure monitoring, pharmacological and non-pharmacological advice for people living with long-term conditions and opportunistic support.

Recent reviews (Steed et al. 2019; Stokes et al. 2019) strengthen the evidence for community pharmacies as appropriate settings to address key public health priorities including smoking

BOX 6.1	KEY ORGANISATIONS

The Faculty of Public Health

A faculty of the Royal College of Physicians. It promotes, for the public benefit, the advancement of knowledge in the field of public health and seeks to develop public health with a view to maintaining the highest possible standards of professional competence and practice. The site has a wide range of resources and links to other organisations involved in public health. https://www.fph.org.uk/

Office for Health Improvement and Disparities

A government body focusing on the health of the nation, aiming to support everyone to live more of life in good health. There is a focus on levelling up of health disparities to break the link between background and prospects for a healthy life. https://www.gov.uk/government/organisations/office-for-health-improvement-and-disparities

National Institute for Health and Clinical Excellence (NICE)

An independent organisation responsible for providing national guidance on promoting good health and preventing and treating ill-health. Guidance is produced in three areas: public health, health technologies and clinical practice. www.nice.org.uk/

Royal Pharmaceutical Society (RPS)

The RPS has championed the profession since 1841. It supports the health and wellbeing of the population and pharmacists in particular. https://www.rpharms.com/

The Institute of Health Promotion and Education (IHPE)

The IHPE brings together all those who seek to contribute to the protection and improvement of people's health and wellbeing, and the reduction of inequalities in health. https://ihpe.org.uk/

cessation, diabetes, coronary heart disease and hypertension. Findings from these reviews suggest that community pharmacy roles can improve pharmacy users' health outcomes at a reasonable cost.

These policy and review documents are good starting points for prescribers to locate evidence-based priorities. Additionally, there are national organisations that support professionals who are seeking details about effective public health approaches (Box 6.1).

GOLD STANDARDS: HEALTH-PROMOTING SETTINGS

The World Health Organization's Ottawa Charter for Health Promotion is a seminal document of the new public health (World Health Organization 1986). The Charter was influential in guiding the development of the settings approach, which is an important cornerstone for successful public health. Prescribers need to know about the settings approach as the concept is fundamental to contemporary practice in public health, and prescribers will work in different settings.

Internationally, examples of a wide range of health-promoting settings can now be found, including:

- health-promoting schools
- health-promoting workplaces
- health-promoting prisons
- health-promoting hospitals.

The settings approach moves public health interventions away from merely focusing on individuals who are ill and towards organisations, systems and the environment, which can be used to prevent ill-health and promote health.

As the evidence indicates, the pharmacy setting provides many opportunities for promoting health. However, it is essential to differentiate between a health-promoting pharmacy and health promotion in the pharmacy. Health promotion in the pharmacy may merely involve certain aspects of health promotion carried out as part of the normal dealings with customers. In contrast, the health-promoting pharmacy enables a more comprehensive and coordinated approach. A health-promoting pharmacy will have:

- a healthy work environment
- appropriate care for clients and staff
- a strong sense of community.

KEY PRIORITY AREAS FOR PUBLIC HEALTH

The government's public health framework, All Our Health (Office for Health Improvement and Disparities 2021) is an initiative advocating health and care professionals maximise the impact they have in their working roles to improve health outcomes and reduce health inequalities. Priority topic areas in the framework include obesity, alcohol, cardiovascular disease, well-being and mental health, smoking and tobacco, and sexual and reproductive health.

STOP AND THINK

As a prescriber, will you be caring for patients/clients in any of these priority areas?

We will look at these priorities, particularly in relation to how prescribers can contribute to the key areas for public health.

- *Obesity* is a major public health challenge and is linked to significant health and well-being issues. Being obese or overweight can reduce life expectancy and increases the risk of developing conditions such as heart disease, cancer and diabetes. As issues leading to obesity are influenced by a range of causes, interventions to address this public health issue need to be mindful of biological, physiological, psychosocial, behavioral and environmental factors. Interventions can be delivered in a range of different settings, including schools, primary care, workplace and hospitals.

PRACTICE APPLICATION

Examples of activities that prescribers may be involved in include weight management clinics, lifestyle checks and advice, making healthy options more available, education campaigns and prescribing obesity drugs.

- In England there are over 10 million people who regularly consume levels of *alcohol* that are over the recommended guidelines, thus increasing their risk of developing alcohol-related diseases. Disease related to excessive alcohol intake include cancers, liver disease, heart disease, depression, stroke and pancreatitis.

PRACTICE APPLICATION

Prescribers can contribute to this key area by asking clients about alcohol intake and providing simple, brief advice and support to help them minimise harmful alcohol consumption, supervising medicines to treat alcohol withdrawal and providing advice aimed at raising awareness of the health consequences of excess alcohol

- *Cardiovascular disease* (CVD) refers to heart attacks and strokes; there are nearly 7 million people in England living with CVD. Cardiovascular disease is associated with health inequalities; people living in deprived communities are disproportionally affected and are four times more likely to die prematurely from CVD (Office for Health Improvement and Disparities 2021). Heart attacks and stroke are commonly linked to lifestyle behaviours, including smoking, diet and alcohol intake. Certain conditions make individuals at a higher risk of CVD, including atrial fibrillation, hypertension and raised cholesterol. However, a large proportion of people living with these conditions are undiagnosed, and of those with a diagnosis, a large number are not receiving optimal treatment.

PRACTICE APPLICATION

Prescribers can address this priority by ensuring optimal treatment of atrial fibrillation, hypertension and raised cholesterol. Furthermore, prescribers can offer opportunistic advice on lifestyle to reduce the risk of developing CVD.

- Evidence indicates that approximately 1 in 6 adults report a *common mental health disorder* and over 551,000 people have a severe mental health issue, for example bipolar disorder (Office for Health Improvement and Disparities 2021).

PRACTICE APPLICATION

Prescribers can support this key area by helping individuals with mental health problems to take their medicines correctly, referring individuals to appropriate agencies, helplines, websites and support groups, and by contributing to the development of health-promoting settings such as the workplace.

- In the UK *smoking* remains the leading cause of preventable illness and premature death, with over 64,000 deaths in the UK in 2019 (Office for Health Improvement and Disparities 2021). Smoking causes a wide range of illnesses, including cancer, heart disease and respiratory disease, and causes harm to others due to passive smoking.

PRACTICE APPLICATION

Prescribers can contribute through participating in NHS stop-smoking services, providing opportunistic advice, prescribing products to support quitting and participating in no smoking campaigns.

- The Framework for Sexual Health Improvement (Department of Health 2013) aims to reduce the rate of sexually transmitted infections (STIs) using evidence-based preventative interventions and treatment initiatives, reduce unwanted pregnancies by ensuring people have access to the full range of contraception and it is available in an accessible and timely manner, support women with unwanted pregnancies to make informed decisions about their options as early as possible, and continue to tackle HIV through prevention and increased access to testing to enable early diagnosis and treatment.

PRACTICE APPLICATION

Prescribers can support this priority by raising awareness of safer sex messages, providing advice and contraception (including condoms and emergency hormonal contraception) and participating in local and national campaigns.

MAKING EVERY CONTACT COUNT

The All Our Health framework encourages all health and social care professionals to maximise opportunities to work proactively to prevent illness and improve health outcomes. Prescribers are key as they work with people, families and communities to support them to make informed choices and manage their own health. This can be achieved by adopting the Making Every Contact Count (MECC) ethos.

MECC (Public Health England 2016) is a brief intervention initiative using a behavioral change approach. MECC encourages health and social care professionals to use opportunities during routine health and care interactions to have a brief or very brief discussion on health or wellbeing factors. The MECC interaction is intended to be brief (a matter of minutes) and is intended to be incorporated into existing professional clinical, care and social engagement approaches. Evidence suggests that the broad adoption of the MECC approach by people and organisations across health and care could potentially have a significant impact on the health of our population (Public Health England 2016; Thompson et al. 2018)

STOP AND THINK

How can you use the MECC approach in your role as a prescriber?

Read section 1.2.8 in the NICE guidance *Community pharmacies: promoting health and wellbeing* (www.nice.org.uk/guidance/ng102) and consider an example of MECC in relation to the points outlined.

LONG-TERM CONDITIONS

It is predicted that by 2035, two-thirds of people over 65 will be living with two or more long-term health conditions (LTCs) (Department of Health and Social Care 2023). A LTC is defined as a condition that is life limiting and cannot be cured; common LTCs are type 2 diabetes, heart disease and respiratory disease. People often have more than one LTC and therefore are prescribed multiple medications to manage their conditions, known as polypharmacy. Polypharmacy can lead to people not taking their medication as prescribed. Prescribers have a key role in medicines optimization to ensure effective management of the LTC and medication concordance, and to promote quality of life and avoid hospital admission (National Institute for Health and Care Excellence 2015). You can read more about polypharmacy and medicines optimisation in Chapter 12.

HEALTHCARE-ASSOCIATED INFECTIONS

Healthcare-associated infections can add significant time to a patient's stay in hospital and are costly to the NHS. Some infections occur due to the overprescription of general antibiotics. However, public health campaigns are now under way that not only focus on cleanliness and washing hands, but also encourage prudent prescribing of antibiotics. It is important that prescribers are up to date with the latest local antimicrobial guidelines, and that they participate in increasing public awareness on antibiotic resistance and infection control matters.

MEDICATION ERRORS

Medication errors are an important but sometimes under-recognised cause of avoidable harm to patients. Mistakes can occur at any stage, from prescribing and dispensing, through to administration and monitoring (Elliot et al. 2021). Prescribers can help to tackle this challenge by working with patients to ensure they have a better understanding of medicines, by clearly documenting medication allergies, providing opportunistic advice when appropriate and carrying out reviews.

SUMMARY

- Public health is concerned with preventing disease, prolonging life and promoting health.

- There are three main groups in the public health workforce: public health consultants and specialists, public health practitioners and the wider workforce.

- Public health encompasses a wide range of activities in different settings. Prescribers in all sectors have important roles to play.

- Key priorities for public health have been set by the government.

- Evidence-based guidance is now available to enable prescribers to make positive contributions to all domains of public health.

- There are a number of effective approaches, but the health-promoting setting is considered the gold standard.

ACTIVITY

1. What are the three domains of public health?

2. In which Canadian city was the World Health Organization's Charter for Health Promotion launched?

3. What is the name of the latest public health strategy for England?

4. What are the three criteria for a health-promoting pharmacy?

5. What is a public health initiative supporting lifestyle change called?

REFERENCES

Acheson, D. (1988) *Public Health in England.* HMSO, London.

Dahlgren, G. and Whitehead, M. (1991) *Policies and Strategies to Promote Social Equity in Health.* Institute of Future Studies, Stockholm.

Davies, M. and Macdowall, W. (eds) (2006) *Health Promotion Theory.* Open University Press, Maidenhead.

Department of Health (2013) *A Framework for Sexual Health Improvement in England.* https://www.gov.uk/government/publications/a-framework-for-sexual-health-improvement-in-england.

Department of Health and Social Care (2023) *Major conditions strategy: case for change and our strategic framework.* https://www.gov.uk/government/publications/major-conditions-strategy-case-for-change-and-our-strategic-framework/major-conditions-strategy-case-for-change and our-strategic-framework–2#chapter-1-our-nations-health.

Elliott, R., Camacho, E., Jankovic, D., Sculpher, M. and Faria, R. (2021) Economic analysis of the prevalence and clinical and economic burden of medication error in England. *BMJ Quality Safety* 30:96-105.

Green, J. Cross, R. Woodhall, J. and Tones, K. (2019) *Health Promotion. Planning and Strategies,* 4th edn. Sage, London.

Health Education England (2021) *Core public health workforce.* https://www.hee.nhs.uk/our-work/population-health/core-public-health-worksforce.

National Health Service (2019) *The NHS Long Term Plan.* https://www.longtermplan.nhs.uk/wp-content/uploads/2019/01/nhs-long-term-plan-june-2019.pdf.

National Institute for Health and Care Excellence (2015) *Medicines optimisation: the safe and effective use of medicines to enable the best possible outcomes.* https://www.nice.org.uk/guidance/ng5.

National Institute for Health and Care Excellence (2020) *Community pharmacies: promoting health and wellbeing.* https://www.nice.org.uk/guidance/qs196.

Neil, K.E., Watson, M.C. and Opare-Anoff, A. (2022) IHPE Position Statement: Safe use of medicines – promoting health. Altrincham: Institute of Health Promotion and Education. https://ihpe.org.uk/wp-content/uploads/2022/11/IHPE-Position-Statement-Pharmacy-Nov-2022.pdf.

Office for Health Improvement and Disparities (2021) *All Our Health: personalised care and population health.* https://www.gov.uk/government/collections/all-our-health-personalised-care-and-population-health.

Pencheon, D., Guest, C., Mezler, D. and Gray, M. (eds) (2006) *Oxford Handbook of Public Health Practice.* Oxford University Press, Oxford.

Public Health England (2016) *Making Every Contact Count (MECC): practical resources.* https://www.gov.uk/government/publications/making-every-contact-count-mecc-practical-resources.

Public Health England (2017) *Pharmacy: A Way Forward for Public Health. Opportunities for action through pharmacy for public health.* https://assets.publishing.service.gov.uk/government/uploads/system/uploads/attachment_data/file/643520/Pharmacy_a_way_forward_for_public_health.pdf.

Royal Pharmaceutical Society (2022) *Pharmacy 2030: a professional vision.* https://www.rpharms.com/pharmacy2030.

Steed, L., Sohanpal, R., Todd, A. et al. (2019) Community pharmacy interventions for health promotion: effects on professional practice and health outcomes (Review). *Cochrane Database of Systematic Reviews Issue 12.* Art. No.: CD011207.

Stokes, G., Rees, R., Khatwa, M. et al. (2019) Public health service provision by community pharmacies: a systematic map of evidence. EPPI-Centre, Social Science Research Unit, Institute of Education, University College London, London.

Thompson, S., Watson, M.C. and Tilford, S. (2018) The Ottawa Charter 30 years on: still an important standard for health promotion, *Int J Health Promot Educ* 56:2, 73–84.

UK Health Security Agency (2018) *Better health for all.* https://ukhsa.blog.gov.uk/2018/11/05/better-health-for-all-a-new-vision-for-prevention/.

World Health Organization (1986) *Ottawa Charter for Health Promotion.* World Health Organization, Copenhagen.

USEFUL WEBSITES

Public Health England. *All Our Health: about the framework.* https://www.gov.uk/government/publications/all-our-health-about-the-framework/all-our-health-about-the-framework.

Institute of Health Promotion and Education. https://ihpe.org.uk/.

Department of Health and Social Care. *Campaigns.* https://campaignresources.phe.gov.uk/resources/campaigns.

Pharmacology

The New Prescriber: An Integrated Approach to Medical and Non-medical Prescribing, Second Edition.
Edited by Joanne Lymn, Alison Mostyn, Roger Knaggs, Michael Randall, and Dianne Bowskill.
© 2024 John Wiley & Sons Ltd. Published 2024 by John Wiley & Sons Ltd.

SECTION INTRODUCTION

Before starting to think seriously about pharmacological concepts, it is perhaps pertinent to give some consideration to what is meant by the term 'pharmacology'.

Pharmacology is defined as:

- The branch of science relating to drugs and medicines (https://www.collinsdictionary.com/dictionary/english/pharmacology).

- 1: the science of drugs including their origin, composition, pharmacokinetics, therapeutic use and toxicology

- 2: the properties and reactions of drugs especially with relation to their therapeutic value (https://www.merriam-webster.com/dictionary/pharmacology).

As can be seen from the definitions above, pharmacology is essentially the study of how drugs act in the body to affect physiological function, so one of the main issues in terms of pharmacology and prescribing is around what constitutes a drug. A drug is:

- any synthetic, semisynthetic or natural chemical substance used in the treatment, prevention or diagnosis of disease, or for other medical reasons (https://www.dictionary.com/browse/drug)

- any substance that affects the structure or functioning of a living organism (https://www.oxfordreference.com/display/10.1093/oi/authority.20110803095731921).

It is clear, then, that the term 'drug' actually covers any substance that is taken into the body to have a specific effect. Thus, the term 'drug' encompasses a number of chemicals that may not be considered to be drugs in the conventional sense, particularly by patients, but which do impact on body function and thus have the potential to affect the action of other drugs (Figure 1).

It is important therefore that the new prescriber gathers information on all substances that the patient may be taking before making prescribing decisions.

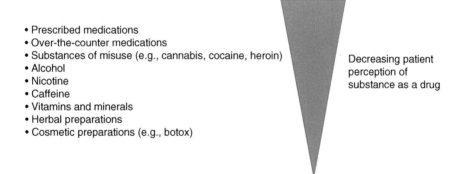

- Prescribed medications
- Over-the-counter medications
- Substances of misuse (e.g., cannabis, cocaine, heroin)
- Alcohol
- Nicotine
- Caffeine
- Vitamins and minerals
- Herbal preparations
- Cosmetic preparations (e.g., botox)

Decreasing patient perception of substance as a drug

FIGURE 1   'Drugs' which may be used by patients but may not be recognised or disclosed as such.

General Principles of Pharmacology

CHAPTER 7

Joanne Lymn and Alison Mostyn

LEARNING OUTCOMES

By the end of this chapter the reader should be able to:

- identify the main types of 'drug target' and give examples of drugs which act on each target type

- define the terms ligand, agonist, antagonist, affinity, efficacy and potency, and understand how they relate to clinical practice

- understand the difference between full and partial agonists, and give examples of each type of agonist currently used in practice

- describe the effect of both competitive and irreversible antagonists, and be able to differentiate between them and the chemical bonding involved

- understand the nature, and give examples, of non-competitive, chemical, physiological and pharmacokinetic antagonism

- understand the concept of the therapeutic index and its limitations.

HOW DO DRUGS EXERT THEIR EFFECTS ON THE BODY?

One thing that drugs have in common is that in order to affect the physiological function of the body, they need to physically interact with specific components of cells in the body. There are some exceptions to this rule, for example antacids, which are simply chemicals which act to neutralise stomach acid (Chapter 16).

Drugs also need to exert some degree of selectivity in terms of the cell types and/or cell constituents with which they interact in the body. This is obvious if we think about it: if it were not for the selectivity between the drug and its 'target' then all drugs would interact with similar cellular components and would exhibit similar effects – this is clearly not true. This selectivity is often determined by three-dimensional shape. All drugs have a specific shape and will bind to, or interact with, cellular components that have a complementary shape (Figure 7.1). This is termed the 'lock and key' hypothesis and is a useful analogy. While selectivity between locks and keys is reciprocal (each key is specific for a particular lock and each lock recognises a specific key), it is not absolute: under certain circumstances a lock can be forced open with the wrong key and a badly cut key will not be able to open its particular lock. This is true also of drugs and their targets.

Essentially, when thinking about drug 'targets' we are considering drug action at the molecular level. The immediate effects caused by the interaction between the drug and target would be considered the 'cellular' level of drug action, while the impact of the drug on tissue and body system responses would be considered the 'tissue' and 'system' levels of drug action. While the action

The New Prescriber: An Integrated Approach to Medical and Non-medical Prescribing, Second Edition.
Edited by Joanne Lymn, Alison Mostyn, Roger Knaggs, Michael Randall, and Dianne Bowskill.
© 2024 John Wiley & Sons Ltd. Published 2024 by John Wiley & Sons Ltd.

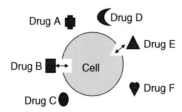

FIGURE 7.1 The importance of shape in determining the specificity of interaction between drug and cell. Only drugs B and E would be able to interact with this particular cell type and each of these would only be able to interact with a specific site on the cell.

of drugs at the 'tissue' and 'system' levels is relatively clear, it is knowledge of drug action at the 'molecular' and cellular' levels that allows us to understand, and explain, some of the most important clinical aspects of drug activity.

PRACTICE APPLICATION

Drug side effects, contraindications and interactions can often be explained by knowledge of the action of a drug at the molecular and cellular levels.

TARGET MOLECULES

The 'target' to which a drug binds in the body is almost always a protein. However, as with all good rules, there are exceptions, with the main exceptions being chemotherapeutic agents which directly interact with DNA (deoxyribonucleic acid).

The proteins to which drugs bind fall into four categories:

- receptors
- enzymes
- carrier molecules
- ion channels

Examples of commonly used drugs which act on each of these four target types are shown in Table 7.1.

RECEPTORS

Before we can really start to think about how drugs interact with receptors, we need to understand what a receptor is. A receptor is a protein which occurs naturally in the body and acts as a recognition site for the body's 'normal', or endogenous, chemical mediators, such as neurotransmitters, hormones and inflammatory mediators. The natural mediators interact with the receptor and stimulate a cellular response.

Many drugs used today are designed to be structurally similar, or mimic, these normal (endogenous) mediators so that they can act on these receptors and modulate physiological function.

STOP AND THINK

Do you think adrenaline, serotonin, histamine and dopamine interact with receptors in the body?

Table 7.1   Examples of commonly used drugs (grouped by BNF chapter) which act on each of the four categories of drug target

Receptors

Gastrointestinal system: famotidine

Cardiovascular system: bisoprolol, irbesartan

Respiratory system: salbutamol, tiotropium, montelukast, adrenaline

Central nervous system: haloperidol, clozapine, cyclizine, domperidone, ondansetron, codeine, sumatriptan, bromocriptine

Endocrine system: insulin, pioglitazone, prednisolone, ethinylestradiol, norethisterone

Eye: tropicamide, timolol

Enzymes

Cardiovascular system: ramipril, aspirin, heparin, atorvastatin

Respiratory system: roflumilast

Central nervous system: carbidopa, selegiline, donepezil

Infections: trimethoprim, rifampicin, ciprofloxacin, ritonavir, fluconazole

Carrier molecules

Gastrointestinal system: omeprazole

Cardiovascular system: digoxin, furosemide

Central nervous system: amitriptyline, citalopram

Ion channels

Cardiovascular system: amiloride, amlodipine

Central nervous system: carbamazepine, phenytoin

Receptor location

The location of a receptor is important and can determine the onset of action of a drug. Receptors are either membrane-bound, i.e. located within the cell membrane, or intracellular. Intracellular receptors (typically steroid receptors) are usually located within the nucleus. Drugs which target membrane-bound receptors, for example adrenaline, have a fast onset of action due to the ease of access to the receptor and activation of signalling molecules readily available in the cell. Drugs which target intracellular receptors, such as steroids, have a slower onset of action due to the time taken to access the receptor and the need to interact with DNA to increase or decrease the production of specific proteins. Receptor location can be clinically important, for example both adrenaline and steroids can be used in the treatment of anaphylaxis, but adrenaline works much more quickly than a steroid.

Drug–receptor interactions

Drugs which act on receptors can be divided into two classes: agonists and antagonists.

Agonists are drugs that bind to the receptor and induce the same cellular response as the normal chemical mediator. Thus, agonists produce the same response as the endogenous mediator.

Antagonists are drugs that bind to the receptor but do not produce the normal cellular response; instead, they act to block the receptor, preventing the normal mediator from binding. Thus, antagonists act to reduce or inhibit the normal physiological response.

The interaction between drugs and receptors can be divided into two components: affinity and efficacy.

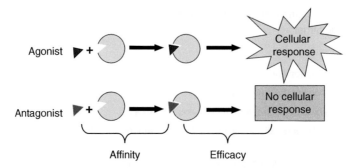

FIGURE 7.2 The agonist binds to the receptor and induces a cellular response. The antagonist binds to the receptor but does not induce a cellular response.

Affinity is the likelihood of the drug binding to the receptor. The higher the affinity of the drug for the receptor, the more likely it is to bind to that receptor.

Efficacy is the likelihood of the bound drug producing a cellular response or effect.

So, an agonist has both affinity and efficacy while an antagonist has affinity but no efficacy (Figure 7.2).

DOSE–RESPONSE CURVES

Agonism

In terms of measuring drug action, we could measure drug binding directly, but it is much more usual to measure the system/pharmacological response to the drug. For example, if we were looking at bronchodilators, we would measure the increase in peak flow and if we were looking at antihypertensives we would measure the reduction in blood pressure. Measuring system responses allows us to determine the maximal response to a drug, known as E_{max}. If we measure the biological response to different doses of drug, we can construct a dose–response curve. Dose–response curves are sigmoidal or 'S' shaped (Figure 7.3).

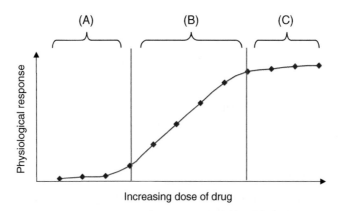

FIGURE 7.3 (A) At this end of the concentration–response curve there is only a small pharmacological response because while the drug is binding to the receptor at the molecular level. This does not occur at large enough concentrations to demonstrate a response at the system level. (B) As the concentration of drug increases, a system response becomes apparent and this part of the curve is linear. The system response increases proportionally to the dose of the drug. (C) At this stage the maximum drug response has been reached and continuing to increase the drug dose does not result in increased system response. It is at this stage that non-specific binding of the drug to other receptors may start to occur, resulting in the development of side effects.

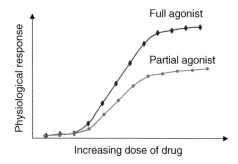

FIGURE 7.4 Comparison of the concentration–response curves of a full agonist and a partial agonist. Both dose-response curves are sigmoidal in shape. The partial agonist dose-response curve is shifted to the right of the full agonist curve. The maximal physiological response of a partial agonist is always lower than that of a full agonist and less than the maximal tissue response.

Agonists can themselves be divided into two categories:

- full agonists
- partial agonists.

A full agonist is a drug that is able to produce the maximum system response in an individual, i.e. maximum peak flow achieved using a bronchodilator. A partial agonist, on the other hand, is unable to produce a maximum system response even when all receptors are occupied.

In pharmacological terms, a partial agonist has similar affinity to, but has less efficacy than, a full agonist (Figure 7.4). While a partial agonist drug binds to the receptor, it does not always produce a cellular response; it is therefore acting as an antagonist as well as an agonist. These drugs could also be described as 'partial antagonists'. Indeed, in terms of clinical application some of the β-blockers in clinical use act as partial agonists (e.g. pindolol).

STOP AND THINK

Could a partial agonist block the effect of a full agonist?

Antagonism

An antagonist binds to a receptor in such a way as to block or prevent agonist binding. This is generally to prevent the binding of the body's natural, endogenous, mediator to the receptor and hence antagonists reduce the normal cellular/physiological response in the body.

Antagonism that involves receptor blockade can be divided into categories: competitive and irreversible.

Competitive antagonism

The binding which occurs between a drug and its target protein is generally weak and easily broken. This is known as 'reversible' binding and is important in terms of competitive antagonism, which uses easily broken hydrogen bonds. An analogy for this type of binding is the use of 'Blu-tack'© to stick something to a wall. The competitive antagonist competes with the natural

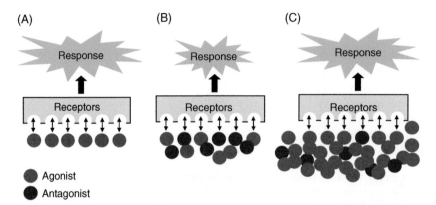

FIGURE 7.5   Visual analogy for competitive antagonism. (A) An agonist binds to receptors and produces a system response. (B) An equal concentration of competitive antagonist is added and competes with the agonist for receptor binding, reducing the level of system response. (C) An increased concentration of agonist competes with the competitive antagonist and restores the level of tissue response.

agonist for receptor binding, so agonist occupancy is reduced in the presence of a competitive antagonist. This competitive antagonism is surmountable; in other words, it can be overcome. Increasing the concentration of the agonist enough will eventually overcome the action of the competitive antagonist and restore the tissue response (Figure 7.5). In terms of a full agonist concentration–response curve, the presence of a fixed concentration of competitive antagonist acts to shift the curve to the right. The maximal tissue response, however, is not decreased, it just takes a larger dose of agonist to achieve this response (Figure 7.6).

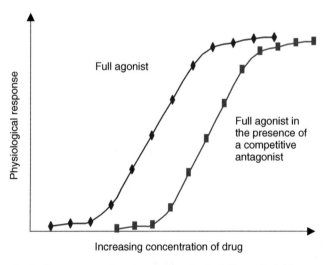

FIGURE 7.6   Difference in the concentration–response curve of a full agonist in the presence and absence of a competitive antagonist. Both dose-response curves are sigmoidal in shape. The agonist dose-response curve is shifted to the right in the presence of a competitive antagonist. The maximal physiological response of the agonist remains the same, but requires a higher concentration of agonist to produce it.

Irreversible antagonism

Unlike competitive antagonists, irreversible antagonists bind to receptors using very strong chemical bonds, known as covalent bonds. While the binding between competitive antagonists and their target proteins can be thought of as like '© Blu-tack', the binding that occurs between an irreversible antagonist and its target protein is could be thought of as a bit like using super glue. Consequently, an irreversible antagonist only dissociates from its receptor very slowly or not at all. The receptor is effectively taken out of action. This means that the addition of more agonist does not affect antagonist binding. This type of antagonism is non-surmountable (Figure 7.7). Thus, these antagonists will have a long-acting effect on the physiological processes in the body. Indeed, to increase the likelihood of agonist binding, the body would have to make new receptors, and this is a lengthy and time-consuming process. While most antagonists in clinical use are competitive and have a reversible action, there are several irreversible antagonists in clinical use (Table 7.2).

STOP AND THINK

Would irreversible antagonists have a longer or shorter duration of action than competitive antagonists?

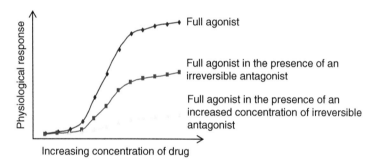

FIGURE 7.7   The maximum response of a full agonist is reduced in the presence of an irreversible antagonist.

Table 7.2   Examples of drugs in clinical use which act as agonists, competitive antagonists and irreversible antagonists

Drug action	Examples in clinical use
Agonist	Salbutamol (β_2-adrenoceptor agonist)
	Morphine (opioid receptor agonist)
	Norethisterone (progesterone receptor agonist)
Competitive antagonist	Bisoprolol (β_1-adrenoceptor antagonist)
	Famotidine (histamine H_2 receptor antagonist)
	Tiotropium (muscarinic acetylcholine receptor antagonist)
	Ondansetron ($5HT_3$ receptor antagonist)
Irreversible antagonist	Phenoxybenzamine (α-adrenoceptor antagonist)
	Candesartan (angiotensin II receptor antagonist)
	Clopidogrel (ADP receptor antagonist)

ENZYMES

An enzyme is a protein that speeds up a biological reaction without being chemically altered itself. Many reactions in the body occur only because of the action of an enzyme, and enzymes are therefore critical for maintaining mammalian homeostasis. Enzymes are specific for the type of reaction they catalyse and must interact with, or bind to, one of the substrates to catalyse the reaction. This interaction is an example of a 'lock and key' mechanism. Drugs which target enzymes inhibit their activity and they do this in several slightly different ways.

Competitive (reversible) inhibition

The drug interacts with the active site of the enzyme in a similar way to the natural substrate binding to the enzyme. Thus, the drug competes with the natural substrate for the binding site on the enzyme. This is essentially the same process as competitive antagonism, with the chemical bonds being weak and easily broken.

Irreversible inhibition

In this situation the drug binds to the enzyme using strong covalent bonds that are not easily broken. Thus, the enzyme is irreversibly inhibited in much the same way that an irreversible antagonist acts on a receptor. The action of an irreversible enzyme inhibitor is very long-lived and to overcome this inhibition, the body will need to make new enzyme.

Most drugs in clinical use act by competitive or reversible inhibition, but there are a small number of drugs which use irreversible inhibition (Table 7.3).

PRACTICE APPLICATION

Aspirin and ibuprofen both act by inhibiting the enzyme cyclooxygenase (COX) but only aspirin has an irreversible effect. It is this difference that makes aspirin, but not ibuprofen, an effective antiplatelet drug.

CARRIER PROTEINS

Ions and a number of other small molecules, such as neurotransmitters, are too polar to readily cross cell membranes and so use carrier proteins to move them across membranes (Chapter 8). The carrier proteins contain a recognition site that makes them specific for particular ions or molecules, and these recognition sites can be targeted by drugs that bind to the recognition site and prevent the interaction between the carrier protein and its specific ion/molecule. Once again, the action of drugs on these carriers can be either reversible, using weak binding forces such as hydrogen bonds, or irreversible, using covalent binding. Most drugs act reversibly or competitively on the carrier molecule, but proton-pump inhibitors act to irreversibly inhibit the proton pump.

Table 7.3 Examples of drugs in clinical use which act as reversible and irreversible enzyme inhibitors

Drug action	Examples of drugs
Reversible enzyme inhibitor	Ibuprofen, enalapril, atorvastatin, selegiline
Irreversible enzyme inhibitor	Aspirin

ION CHANNELS

Ion channels are proteins which act as gated tunnels to allow the passage of ions across membranes. These proteins can be targeted by drugs to block the ion channel, preventing the passage of ions across the membrane, as is the case with local anaesthetics. Alternatively, drugs can bind to a different area on the ion channel and modulate its activity, either by promoting channel opening, 'keeping the gate open' (e.g. benzodiazepines), or by reducing channel opening, 'shutting the gate' (e.g. dihydropyridine calcium channel inhibitors such as amlodipine).

NON-TARGET PROTEINS

It is important to remember that not all proteins which drugs bind to or interact with actually represent drug targets. Plasma proteins such as albumin actually bind to a wide range of drugs but do not represent drug targets. Plasma proteins are not drug targets for two reasons:

- they bind many different drug types and do not therefore exhibit any specificity

- binding of a drug to a plasma protein does not directly produce a system change in the body.

This is not to say that binding to plasma proteins is unimportant: plasma protein binding can have profound effects on drug action within the body and we will discuss this further in Chapters 8 and 9.

DRUG ANTAGONISM

There are a number of forms of drug antagonism, other than antagonism by receptor blockade, which also impact on clinical practice.

NON-COMPETITIVE ANTAGONISM

This type of antagonism refers to the situation where the antagonist blocks the activity of the agonist without competing for a binding site. The antagonist does not interact at receptor level, so agonist binding occurs normally. Instead, the antagonist acts to inhibit part of the cellular response to the agonist or acts on a different component of the target (allosteric antagonism) (Figure 7.8). Examples of drugs which act as non-competitive antagonists include calcium channel blockers such as nifedipine. Normally the binding of noradrenaline or angiotensin II to their specific receptors results in increased calcium concentration and leads to smooth muscle contraction. Calcium channel blockers do not interfere with the agonist (such as noradrenaline or angiotensin II) binding to its receptor, but instead prevent calcium entering the cell and therefore inhibit cell contraction.

CHEMICAL ANTAGONISM

A chemical antagonist binds to a drug in solution, either in gastric fluid or in plasma, to produce a complex that has no activity. An example of a drug which acts as a chemical antagonist is protamine,

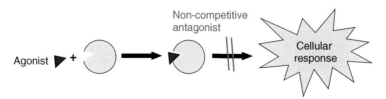

FIGURE 7.8   Site of action of a non-competitive antagonist.

which binds to heparin in the plasma and forms an inactive complex. The activity of heparin in the plasma is then lost. Protamine is used as an antidote to overanticoagulation with heparin.

PHARMACOKINETIC ANTAGONISM

This refers to the situation where the antagonist reduces the activity of the drug by modulating the pharmacokinetic processes. This can occur in several ways.

- The antagonist reduces the absorption of the active drug from the GI tract.
- The antagonist increases the metabolism of the active drug in the liver.
- The antagonist increases the rate of excretion of the active drug from the body.

An example of a drug that acts as a pharmacokinetic antagonist is rifampicin, which speeds up the metabolism of a number of other drugs, thus reducing their activity. These types of interactions are very important in the clinical context (further information is given in Chapters 9 and 12).

PHYSIOLOGICAL ANTAGONISM

This refers to the situation where the physiological antagonist has the opposite effect to another drug in the body. Thus, the activities of both the physiological antagonist and the drug are effectively cancelled out.

Physiological antagonism occurs more frequently in patients who are taking large numbers of drugs (polypharmacy), such as the elderly.

THERAPEUTIC INDEX

Rather than measuring a drug's value purely in terms of the desired response, a more appropriate measure of drug activity takes into account both wanted and unwanted effects. The therapeutic index (TI) is such a measure, considering both beneficial and toxic effects. The TI can be defined as the median toxic dose of a drug (the dose which produces unwanted effects in 50% of the population) divided by the median effective dose (the dose which produces a therapeutic effect in 50% of people):

$$TI = \frac{\text{median toxic dose}}{\text{median effective dose}} \qquad TI = \frac{TD_{50}}{ED_{50}}$$

If the median toxic dose is much larger than the median effective dose, then the drug will have a wide TI and hence a large safety margin. Drugs that have a narrow TI need to be monitored regularly to ensure that toxicity does not develop.

PRACTICE APPLICATION

Most drugs in clinical practice have a wide TI. However, some drugs, including warfarin, phenytoin and theophylline, have a narrow TI and their levels in the body need to be monitored.

SUMMARY

- Drugs generally need to interact with target molecules to exert an effect.
- Drug targets are generally one of the following types of proteins: receptors, enzymes, ion channels, carrier molecules.

• Receptors are recognition sites for the body's natural chemical mediators.

• Agonists bind to receptors and induce a physiological response while antagonists bind to receptors but do not produce a response.

• Affinity is the likelihood of a drug binding to a receptor while efficacy is the likelihood of this binding resulting in a physiological response.

• Potency describes the product of a drug's affinity and efficacy.

• Partial agonists always give a submaximal response even when all receptor sites are bound.

• Competitive antagonism is surmountable, can be overcome and involves weak binding such as hydrogen bonds; irreversible antagonism involves strong covalent bonds, is not surmountable so cannot be overcome.

• Non-competitive antagonism does not compete for the same receptor binding site but instead acts on the cellular response induced by the agonist or binds to a different site on the receptor.

• Chemical antagonism is the combination of an antagonist and a drug in solution resulting in the production of an inactive complex.

• Pharmacokinetic antagonists act to reduce drug absorption or increase drug metabolism or excretion.

• Physiological antagonism can be the result of polypharmacy.

• The therapeutic index is a measure of the safety of a drug.

ACTIVITY

1. Which of the following is not a drug target?

    (a) Receptor

    (b) Carrier protein

    (c) Lipid

    (d) Enzyme

2. Which of the following statements about partial agonists is true?

    (a) They can achieve a maximal response.

    (b) They have similar efficacy to a full agonist.

    (c) The dose–response curve of a partial agonist is shifted to the left of the dose–response curve of a full agonist.

    (d) They have a similar affinity to a full agonist.

3. Which of the following drugs acts as an irreversible receptor antagonist?

    (a) Salbutamol

    (b) Bisoprolol

    (c) Atorvastatin

    (d) Candesartan

4. Which of the following forms of drug antagonism describes the action of protamine on heparin?

    (a) Receptor blockade

    (b) Non-competitive antagonism

    (c) Chemical antagonism

    (d) Pharmacokinetic antagonism

5. Which of the following drugs acts to irreversibly inhibit enzyme activity?

    (a) Aspirin

    (b) Ibuprofen

    (c) Atorvastatin

    (d) Ramipril

6. Which of the following statements is correct?

    (a) Agonists mimic the body's normal physiological response.

    (b) Agonists have affinity but no efficacy.

    (c) Irreversible antagonists use hydrogen binding.

    (d) Antagonists have similar efficacy to agonists.

REUSABLE LEARNING OBJECTS

Targets for drug action. https://www.nottingham.ac.uk/helmopen/rlos/pharmacology/pharmacodynamics/actions/drug-targets/

An introduction to receptor pharmacology. https://www.nottingham.ac.uk/helmopen/rlos/pharmacology/pharmacodynamics/receptors/intro-receptor/

Action of drugs that target enzymes. https://www.nottingham.ac.uk/helmopen/rlos/pharmacology/pharmacodynamics/actions/drugenzymes/

Action of drugs that target carriers. https://www.nottingham.ac.uk/helmopen/rlos/pharmacology/pharmacodynamics/actions/carriers/

Action of drugs that target ion channels. https://www.nottingham.ac.uk/helmopen/rlos/pharmacology/pharmacodynamics/actions/ion-channels/

FURTHER READING

Birkett, D.J. (2002) *Pharmacokinetics Made Easy*, 2nd edn. McGraw-Hill, Australia.

British National Formulary (online). London, BMJ Group and Pharmaceutical Press. https://bnf.nice.org.uk/about/frequently-asked-questions-for-the-bnf-and-bnf for-children-general/

McGavock, H. (2015) *How Drugs Work. Basic Pharmacology for Healthcare Professionals*, 4th edn. Radcliffe Publishing, Oxford.

Neal, M.J. (2020) *Medical Pharmacology at a glance*, 9th edn. Wiley-Blackwell, Oxford.

Page, C.P., Curtis, M.J., Walker, M. and Hoffman, B. (2006) *Integrated Pharmacology*, 3rd edn. Mosby, London.

Ritter, J.M., Flower, R., Henderson, G. et al. (2023) *Rang and Dale's Pharmacology*, 10th edn. Elsevier, Amsterdam.

Smith, H.J. and Williams H. (2006) *Introduction to the Principles of Drug Design and Action*, 4th edn. CRC Press

Pharmacokinetics 1: Absorption and Distribution

CHAPTER 8

Joanne Lymn and Alison Mostyn

LEARNING OUTCOMES

By the end of this chapter the reader should be able to:

- define the terms absorption and distribution, and differentiate between them

- describe the mechanisms used by drug molecules to cross cell membranes

- understand the importance of physiochemical properties on drug behaviour

- understand the influence of environmental pH on lipid solubility and drug absorption

- understand the nature of plasma protein binding and its effect on drug distribution, and give examples which impact clinical practice

- describe the concept of the volume of distribution and consider its impact on clinical practice.

Pharmacokinetics can be defined as 'what the body does to a drug' or, perhaps more specifically, how the body handles a drug. Pharmacokinetics can be divided into four separate processes:

Absorption
Distribution
Metabolism
Excretion

The first letter of each of these processes has been highlighted in bold because you may see the acronym ADME referred to in drug literature or other textbooks. ADME refers to the processes of absorption, distribution, metabolism and excretion.

This chapter is going to concentrate on the first two of these processes: absorption and distribution.

In Chapter 7 we described how drugs need to be present at an adequate concentration at the target to exert a pharmacological effect. It is the processes of absorption and distribution that are key to ensuring that this occurs.

HOW DO DRUGS GET INTO THE BODY?

Almost all drugs need to cross cell membranes to get into the body. For example, drugs which are given orally will need to cross the membranes of the cells in the gastrointestinal (GI) tract, while drugs administered by transdermal patch will need to cross the membranes of skin cells to reach the bloodstream.

The New Prescriber: An Integrated Approach to Medical and Non-medical Prescribing, Second Edition.
Edited by Joanne Lymn, Alison Mostyn, Roger Knaggs, Michael Randall, and Dianne Bowskill.
© 2024 John Wiley & Sons Ltd. Published 2024 by John Wiley & Sons Ltd.

STOP AND THINK

Not all routes of administration require drug absorption to occur. Why do you think the intravenous and inhaled routes do not strictly require drug absorption to occur?

CELL MEMBRANES

If you remember some basic biology, you will recall that cell membranes consist of a lipid bilayer or two layers of lipid molecules. Each lipid molecule consists of a polar, or water-loving, head and a non-polar, or water-hating, tail (Figure 8.1). The majority of the lipids contained in mammalian cell membranes are cholesterol, phospholipids and glycolipids. Perhaps the most interesting thing about lipid bilayers is that they will form spontaneously in aqueous solutions as the lipid molecules will automatically arrange themselves so that the hydrocarbon tails are facing away from the aqueous environment.

MECHANISMS OF CROSSING CELL MEMBRANES

Now that we know why drugs need to cross cell membranes, we need to turn our attention to how they do it. There are two main mechanisms by which drugs can cross cell membranes:

1. diffusion directly through lipid

2. combination with a carrier protein.

Diffusion through lipid

This is exactly what it says it is: the drug literally diffuses through the membrane from an area of high concentration to an area of lower concentration. The ability of drugs to use this mechanism is dependent on their chemical nature. So, what do we mean when we say that a drug's ability to diffuse through lipid depends on its chemical nature? Essentially, it means that 'like dissolves in like', i.e. non-polar substances dissolve freely in non-polar solvents. Lipids are non-polar so non-polar substances will dissolve freely in lipids. In Figure 8.1 we show that cell membranes consist of a lipid bilayer so non-polar substances will diffuse freely across cell membranes, while polar or charged molecules will not (Figure 8.2).

Examples of 'like dissolves in like' are common in general life, particularly in relation to cooking. If you add a few drops of red food dye to a pan of water, they dissolve completely, making the water pink. On the other hand, when cooking pasta, you might add a few drops of oil to the pan of water, but this does not dissolve in the water no matter how hard you try, it remains in small, discrete globules which are easily visible in the water. If you added a few drops of olive oil to a pan of vegetable oil, however, it would dissolve completely. So, in terms of pharmacokinetics,

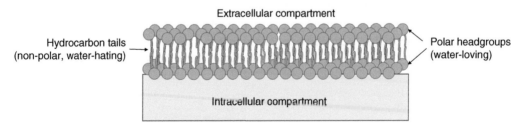

FIGURE 8.1   The lipid bilayer that makes up the cell plasma membrane.

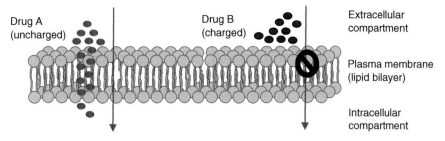

FIGURE 8.2 Diffusion through a lipid.

Table 8.1 Terms used to describe lipid solubility

Lipid soluble	Nonpolar
	Unionised
	Lipophilic
	Hydrophobic
	Uncharged
Water soluble	Polar
	Ionised
	Lipophobic
	Hydrophilic
	Charged

the most important chemical factor that determines a drug's ability to diffuse across cell membranes is its lipid solubility.

STOP AND THINK

Is high lipid solubility good for drug absorption?

There are a number of terms which are often used interchangeably to describe a drug's lipid solubility (Table 8.1) and it is important to be aware of all these terms and what they mean.

Acid–base relationships and lipid solubility

In reality, many drugs are weak acids or weak bases, which means they exist as a mixture of non-polar and polar forms. The ratio of non-polar to polar forms is defined by the pKa of the drug, which is the pH at which the drug exists at a 50:50 equilibrium between the non-polar (unionised) and polar (ionised) forms. Remember, only the non-polar form is lipid soluble and hence only this form will readily diffuse across cell membranes.

A basic knowledge of acids and bases is important for pharmacology because the pH of the environment the drug is in will affect the amount of drug in the non-polar, lipid-soluble form, thus affecting the extent and rate at which it is able to cross membranes. This has an impact on both absorption and excretion (Chapter 9). Weak acids in solution are able to give up a hydrogen ion (H^+) and become ionised (negatively charged), while weak bases are able to accept a hydrogen ion and become ionised (positively charged). On the other hand, strong acids, like the hydrochloric acid in the stomach, are permanently ionised and exist as H^+ and Cl^-.

pH refers to the acidity or alkalinity of a solution, or the number of free hydrogen ions (H^+); the higher the concentration of H^+, the lower the pH, or the more acidic the solution. A change in the pH of the environment from the pKa of the weak acid or base (as might occur with the movement of drug from the stomach to the intestine) will substantially affect the proportion of the non-polar (unionised) form. A change of 1 pH unit below the pKa of a weak acid will result in 90% of the drug being unionised while a change of 2 pH units below the pKa will result in 99% of the drug being unionised. Similarly, a change of 1 pH unit above the pKa of a weak base will result in 90% of the drug being ionised and a change of 2 pH units will result in 99% being ionised.

In an acid environment like the stomach, there are plenty of free H^+ ions and hence there is no need for a weak acid to give up its own H^+. Thus drugs which are weak acids tend to exist in the unionised (non-polar) form in the stomach and can start to be absorbed across the stomach membranes.

Drugs which are weak bases, however, will be more inclined to accept H^+ from the plentiful supply in the stomach acid and will as a result exist mainly in the ionised (polar) form and will not start to be absorbed until further down the GI tract when the pH of the environment is more favourable.

It might be simpler just to consider acidic drugs as unionised in acidic conditions while basic drugs are unionised in basic conditions and ionised in acidic conditions (Table 8.2). Hence, 'like with like favours absorption'.

PRACTICE APPLICATION

If you know the pKa of a drug and the pH of the environment, you can work out its exact degree of ionisation using simple calculators available on the internet.

Examples of common drugs that are acidic and basic in chemical nature are identified in Table 8.3.

Table 8.2 Key facts concerning the degree of ionisation of drugs that are weak acids and weak bases

	Weak acids	Weak bases
Acid environment (e.g., stomach)	Unionised	
Basic environment (e.g., gut)		Unionised

Table 8.3 Examples of commonly used drugs that are either acidic or basic in nature

Acidic drugs	Basic drugs
Aspirin	Caffeine
Phenytoin	Theophylline
Warfarin	Morphine
Methotrexate	Pethidine
Zidovudine	Erythromycin
Penicillin V	Amphetamine
Tetracycline	Propranolol
Levodopa	Trimethoprim

Use of a carrier molecule

In this case the drug will bind to (interact with) the carrier protein on the outer surface of the plasma membrane. This interaction between drug and carrier protein leads to a conformational change, or change in the shape, of the carrier protein, resulting in the protein essentially flipping over so that the drug binding site is located on the inner surface of the plasma membrane. The drug is then released from the carrier protein into the intracellular compartment. This release of drug again causes a conformational change in the protein so that it flips back to its original position and is thus ready to bind to and carry another drug molecule across the membrane (Figure 8.3).

Since this method of crossing cell membranes requires the drug to interact with the carrier protein at a specific binding site, it can show saturation kinetics at high drug concentrations. Essentially, the rate of absorption across the cell membrane is determined by the number of available carrier molecules.

It may be easier to understand what is meant by saturation using visualisation. If, for example, the cell membrane contains 10 carrier molecules and there are five drug molecules, then these will all be carried across the cell membrane within a specific time period. Similarly, if there are 10 drug molecules then these could all be carried across the cell membrane within the same time period; this would appear to increase the rate of absorption of the drug. However, if the number of drug molecules increases to 30, the rate of absorption remains constant, or saturated, because there is a fixed number of carrier molecules that can only carry a fixed number of drug molecules within a fixed time period (Figure 8.4). A drug that exhibits 'saturable' absorption is gabapentin.

PRACTICE APPLICATION

Carrier molecules can act as drug targets (Chapter 7). Drugs can bind to carrier molecules, thus preventing other drugs from using these carrier molecules.

For example, probenicid used to be given with penicillin to prolong its action: probenicid binds to the carrier molecules in the kidney tubule, thus preventing penicillin from binding. In this way the excretion of penicillin from the body was delayed and hence it remained active in the body for longer.

Carrier molecules are important:

• in the GI tract: levodopa (a drug used to treat Parkinson's disease) and fluorouracil (an anticancer drug) both use carrier molecules to cross the intestinal mucosa

• in the biliary tract: a considerable number of drugs and metabolites of drugs are transported from the liver into the bile using carrier proteins

• at the blood–brain barrier: levodopa is carried across the blood–brain barrier

• in the renal tubule: acidic and basic carrier proteins exist in the kidney and act to carry drugs into the renal tubule.

DRUG ABSORPTION

Absorption is defined as the passage of the drug from its site of administration into the plasma. Drug absorption is essential for almost all drugs, except those given intravenously and inhaled respiratory drugs. This is because drugs given intravenously enter the plasma directly and therefore bypass the need to cross cell membranes, while anti-asthma drugs given by the inhaled route are delivered directly to the cells in the airways on which they will act. A small number of drugs do not need to be absorbed to exert their clinical effect, for example vancomycin is not well-absorbed orally, but can be used to treat infections within the GI tract.

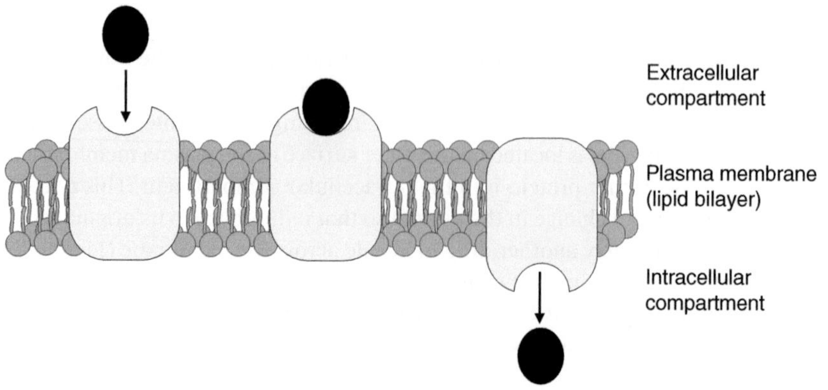

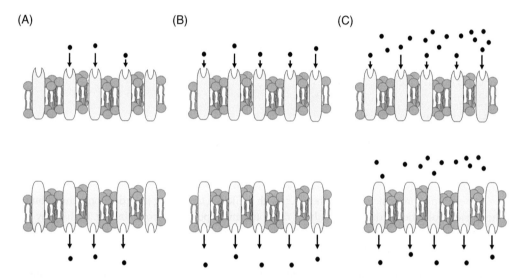

FIGURE 8.3 A drug crossing a cell membrane using a carrier molecule.

Extracellular
compartment

Plasma membrane
(lipid bilayer)

Intracellular
compartment

(A)   (B)   (C)

FIGURE 8.4 Saturation of a carrier protein and its impact on drug absorption. (A) Complete drug absorption occurs. (B) Complete drug absorption occurs (rate appears to increase). (C) Carriers are saturated and the rate of absorption remains fixed.

While drug absorption can start in the stomach (specifically weak acids), most absorption occurs in the small intestine. This is because the small intestine has a much larger surface area due to the villi and microvilli of the ileum (~200 m² compared to 1 m² in the stomach), and also because drugs tend to be in the intestine for a much longer period of time compared to the stomach. Drug absorption can be reduced in individuals suffering from diarrhoea as the length of time within the intestine is reduced. Conversely, constipation, which can occur with advancing age as well as a side effect of certain drugs, for example codeine, can increase the opportunities for drug absorption.

Most drugs are administered orally and are influenced by factors such as age and disease, which affect GI function. The absorption of drugs from other routes can also be affected by several factors (Chapter 10).

DRUG DISTRIBUTION

Drug distribution refers to the specific localisation of drugs within the body. Once drugs have been absorbed into the plasma, they are carried around the body in the bloodstream prior to reaching their specific site of action. Drugs can be distributed within several different compartments of the body, including:

- plasma
- interstitial fluid (fluid which surrounds the cells)
- transcellular fluid (e.g., digestive secretions, cerebrospinal fluid)
- intracellular fluid (fluid contained in the cells)
- adipose tissue (fat)

The relative proportions of these drug compartments are shown in Figure 8.5.

Drug distribution exhibits a number of patterns depending on which of these compartments the drug localises in, and may be classified as follows:

- remains within the vascular system
- distributes in body water
- concentrates in specific tissues
- distributes throughout body water and tissues.

These distribution patterns in turn are dependent on:

- plasma protein binding
- accumulation in tissues.

PLASMA PROTEIN BINDING

As discussed previously in this chapter, many drugs exist as weak acids or bases consisting of a mixture of ionised and unionised forms. While the unionised form is good for absorption, passing readily through the plasma membranes, it is relatively insoluble in the aqueous environment of the plasma and needs to bind to plasma proteins in order to move around the body in the plasma.

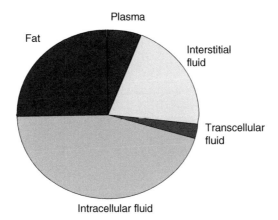

FIGURE 8.5   The relative proportions of drug compartments in the body.

Table 8.4 Examples of drugs that bind to the plasma proteins albumin and acid-glycoprotein

Albumin	Acid-glycoprotein
Aspirin	Propranolol
Warfarin	Lidocaine
Indometacin	Diazepam
Phenytoin	Chlorpromazine
Diazepam	

It is important to remember that plasma proteins do not represent drug targets as they do not show specificity in terms of their binding nor does drug binding to them induce a physiological response; they are essentially a transport system.

The major plasma proteins are albumin, acid-glycoprotein and β-globulin, with albumin being arguably the most important of these. Examples of drugs bound to plasma proteins are shown in Table 8.4.

Drugs bind readily and reversibly to plasma proteins according to the following equation:

$$\text{unbound drug} + \text{free plasma protein} \leftrightarrow \text{plasma protein} - \text{drug complex}$$

It is important to be aware that only the unbound, or free, drug is available to act on its specific drug target and exert a pharmacological effect. As the unbound drug passes into the tissues, there is a corresponding release of plasma protein-bound drug. The extent of plasma protein binding is different for individual drugs (Table 8.5) but may be as high as 99%, in which case the fraction of free, unbound drug available to have a pharmacological effect will only be 1%.

It is possible, therefore, that a reduction in the concentration of plasma proteins in the body (e.g., hypoalbuminaemia) can affect the activity of highly plasma protein-bound drugs such as warfarin and phenytoin (Figure 8.6). Hypoalbuminaemia can occur in patients suffering from cirrhosis, nephritic syndrome, severe burns, chronic inflammation and malnutrition.

Plasma protein binding may also be affected by competition between drugs. Albumin has two major drug-binding sites (site I and site II) which bind acidic drugs. Drugs which bind to the same site will compete with each other for the binding site, resulting in drug displacement.

Table 8.5 Examples of drugs across the range of plasma protein concentrations

Drug	Plasma protein binding (%)
Warfarin	99
Diazepam	96
Propranolol	90
Phenytoin	87
Fentanyl	80
Theophylline	40
Digoxin	30
Gentamicin	<10

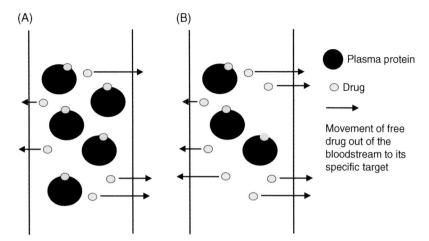

FIGURE 8.6 (A) A normal plasma protein concentration with 50% of drug free and able to leave the bloodstream to reach its specific target. (B) A reduced plasma protein concentration but the same drug dose; in this situation 70% of the drug is free and available to act on its target.

Warfarin and non-steroidal anti-inflammatory drug (NSAIDs) both bind to site I and the NSAIDs will displace warfarin from the albumin binding site, resulting in an increase in the free warfarin concentration. This is one reason why NSAIDs should not be used in patients taking warfarin.

STOP AND THINK

What is the likely pattern of distribution for drugs which are very tightly bound to plasma proteins or are very large in size?

Accumulation in tissues

Most drugs exert their effects in body tissues and the degree of accumulation of drugs in the tissues depends on the lipid solubility of the drug. As discussed previously, the more lipid soluble a drug is, the more readily it will cross plasma membranes. Drugs which can cross cell membranes often tend to be distributed throughout body fluids and tissues. Some highly lipid-soluble drugs such as the benzodiazepines can accumulate in body fat. Remember, body fat is a highly non-polar body compartment. Obese individuals may experience a longer duration of action of highly lipophilic drugs, such as benzodiazepines due to increased adipose tissue.

Blood flow to the tissue

In just the same way that blood flow impacts drug absorption, it also affects drug distribution. Drugs will distribute to the most highly vascularised tissue, such as the heart, lungs and brain, first. This is followed by tissues which have a moderate blood flow, such as muscle, and then lastly tissues such as fat which have a low blood supply. Benzodiazepines take some time to accumulate in body fat because of the low blood flow to this area, hence accumulation only occurs following chronic use of these drugs. However, this low blood supply also means that these drugs are only slowly released from fat stores once drug administration has ceased.

Specific drug accumulation

Some drugs have a high affinity for particular areas of the body and will accumulate in these areas. For example, tetracycline has a high affinity for calcium and consequently accumulates in areas of the body that have high levels of calcium such as bones and teeth.

PRACTICE APPLICATION

Accumulation of tetracycline in developing teeth results in discolouration which is permanent and may affect bone growth. This is why we do not give tetracycline to children or pregnant women.

Similarly, the drug chloroquine is used to prevent malaria and for the treatment of rheumatoid arthritis and systemic lupus erythematosus. It has, however, been shown to have a high affinity for melanin-containing tissues and can accumulate in the retina of the eye, causing retinopathy. The prevalence of hydroxycholoroquine retinopathy can be up to 50% after 20 years of therapy. The Royal College of Ophthalmologists has issued guidelines for screening to prevent ocular toxicity for patients on long-term treatment.

VOLUME OF DISTRIBUTION

The volume of distribution (Vd) is defined as the total volume of plasma that would be required to contain the total body content of the drug at the same concentration at which it is present in the plasma. This is not a real volume but rather represents a theoretical volume and describes the ability of the drug to distribute throughout body tissues. Consequently, it is referred to as the apparent volume of distribution. It is measured in litres and can be calculated from the following equation:

$$Vd(apparent) = \frac{\text{amount of drug in the body}}{\text{plasma drug concentration}}$$

Drugs that are retained within the plasma, because of either their size or their protein binding, will have a Vd similar to that of the circulating volume, and drugs which distribute throughout body tissues will have a Vd similar to that of total body water. However, drugs which have high affinity for specific peripheral tissues may show very low plasma concentrations and hence will have a Vd that is much larger than that of the circulating volume (Figure 8.7). In general, then, lipid-soluble drugs will tend to have a larger Vd than more water-soluble polar drugs.

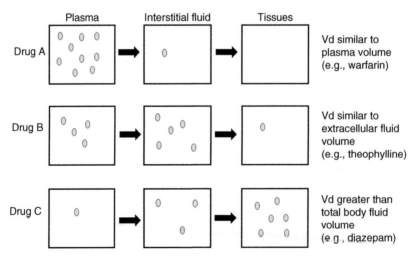

FIGURE 8.7 Different patterns of drug distribution in the body and examples of each.

The Vd is important clinically:

- in calculating the loading dose of drugs

- in overdose: drugs with a small Vd could be treated by dialysis as they are relatively contained within the plasma while drugs with a larger Vd cannot as these have left the plasma compartment and are distributed throughout body tissues.

STOP AND THINK

Why is it that overdoses of digoxin (Vd 500 l) and nortriptyline (Vd 1500 l) cannot be managed by dialysis?

SUMMARY

- Lipid-soluble drugs are readily absorbed.

- Most drugs are weak acids or weak bases and exist in a mixture of charged and uncharged forms.

- Environmental pH will affect the proportion of charged forms of weak acids and bases.

- The rate of absorption of polar drugs which use carrier molecules is saturable.

- Absorption of oral drugs occurs in the intestine and is influenced by gastric motility.

- Drug absorption is not required for drugs given intravenously or for inhaled respiratory drugs.

- Many drugs are carried around the body bound to plasma proteins.

- Plasma proteins are not drug targets.

- Only free drugs that are not bound to plasma protein can exert a pharmacological effect.

- Drug distribution is affected by plasma protein binding, lipid solubility and blood flow.

- Drugs are distributed to the brain, heart and lungs first and adipose tissue last.

- Drugs that are very large or with a high affinity for plasma proteins will remain within the plasma.

- Lipid-soluble drugs will distribute more readily to tissues and show a larger Vd than polar drugs.

- Vd is important for calculating loading dose.

ACTIVITY

1. The passage of a drug molecule across a lipid membrane is influenced by the:

     - lipid solubility of the drug   True/False

     - route of administration   True/False

     - degree of ionisation of the molecule   True/False

     - pH of the surrounding medium   True/False

     - presence of carrier molecules   True/False

2. With regard to drug absorption, which of the following statements are correct?

     - Drug absorption is required for drugs given by all routes. True/False

- The rate and extent of absorption following oral administration are dependent on the pH of the gut.   True/False

- Drug absorption always starts in the stomach.   True/False

- Drug absorption is unaffected by the lipid solubility of a drug.   True/False

- The rate of absorption of very polar drugs may depend on carrier molecules.   True/False

3. With regard to plasma protein binding, which of the following statements are correct?

- Drugs bound to plasma proteins readily cross cell membranes.   True/False

- Albumin, acid-glycoprotein and β-globulin are all plasma proteins.   True/False

- Plasma protein concentrations can be reduced in severe malnutrition.   True/False

- Plasma proteins are important drug targets   True/False

- Plasma protein binding can restrict the pattern of drug distribution.   True/False

4. With regard to the volume of distribution, which of the following statements are correct?

- It represents the total volume of the body.   True/False

- It is generally larger for lipid-soluble compared to polar drugs.   True/False

- It is important for calculating a loading dose.   True/False

- It is not affected by the size of the drug or its plasma protein binding.   True/False

- It describes the ability of a drug to distribute throughout body tissues.   True/False

---

USEFUL WEBSITES

British National Formulary (online). BMJ Group and Pharmaceutical Press, London. https://bnf.nice.org.uk/.

Hydroxychloroquine and Chloroquine Retinopathy Monitoring Guideline and Recommendations 2020. https://www.rcophth.ac.uk/resources-listing/2609/

REUSABLE LEARNING OBJECTS

Acids, alkalis and bases: an introduction. https://www.nottingham.ac.uk/nursing/sonet/rlos/science/acid_base_intro/index.html

Acids, alkalis and bases: further application. https://www.nottingham.ac.uk/nursing/sonet/rlos/science/acid_base_further_app/

Concentration gradients. https://www.nottingham.ac.uk/nursing/sonet/rlos/bioproc/gradients/index.html

Plasma proteins and drug distribution. https://www.nottingham.ac.uk/nursing/sonet/rlos/bioproc/plasma_proteins/index.html

Volume of distribution. https://www.nottingham.ac.uk/nursing/sonet/rlos/bioproc/vd/

FURTHER READING

Abelow, B. (1998) *Understanding Acid-Base.* Lippincott, Williams and Wilkins, Philadelphia.

Birkett, D.J. (2010) *Pharmacokinetics made Easy*, 2nd edn. McGraw-Hill, London and Sydney.

Lindup, W.E. and Orme, M.C.L.E. (1981) Plasma protein drug binding. *BMJ* 282:212–214.

McFadden, R. (2019) *Introducing pharmacology for nursing and healthcare*, 3rd edn. Routledge.

Ritter, J.M., Flower, R., Henderson, G., et al. (2023) *Rang and Dale's Pharmacology*, 10th edn. Elsevier, Amsterdam.

Smith, H.J. (2006) *Smith and Williams' Introduction to the Principles of Drug Design and Action*, 4th edn. Taylor and Francis, Boca Raton.

CHAPTER 9

Pharmacokinetics 2: Metabolism and Excretion

Joanne Lymn and Alison Mostyn

LEARNING OBJECTIVES

By the end of this chapter the reader should be able to:

- understand the terms metabolism and excretion, and differentiate between them

- understand the nature and relevance of drug metabolism, with particular reference to inducers and inhibitors, pharmacogenetics, active metabolites, toxic metabolites, pro-drugs and link to clinical practice

- understand the concepts of first-pass metabolism and bioavailability, and how they are related

- describe how drug metabolism may be affected by age and disease

- understand the fundamental processes involved in drug excretion via the kidneys

- understand how renal drug excretion can be affected by physiochemical properties, pH, age and disease

- understand the nature of biliary excretion and the importance of enterohepatic recycling and link to clinical practice

- understand the concept of drug clearance and link to clinical practice

- understand the concept of half-life and link to clinical practice.

DRUG ELIMINATION

Drug elimination is the loss of drug from the body and comprises two processes: metabolism and excretion. Metabolism is defined as the enzymatic conversion of one drug entity to another, while excretion is the removal of the drug from the body, most commonly via the kidney. It is important to recognise that the definition of metabolism is not concerned with inactivating drugs. Drug metabolism is often referred to in textbooks as being 'detoxification'; this is not entirely accurate as drug metabolism does not always result in pharmacological inactivation, as we shall see later.

DRUG METABOLISM

In Chapter 8 we defined lipid solubility as the key determinant of a drug's ability to cross cell membranes and stated that lipid solubility was good for absorption. However, drugs cannot distinguish between the cell membranes of the gastrointestinal (GI) tract and the renal tubules, so lipid-soluble drugs are readily reabsorbed from the tubules back into the circulation. Consequently, lipid-soluble drugs are not excreted efficiently by the kidneys. Lipid solubility is therefore good for drug absorption

The New Prescriber: An Integrated Approach to Medical and Non-medical Prescribing, Second Edition.
Edited by Joanne Lymn, Alison Mostyn, Roger Knaggs, Michael Randall, and Dianne Bowskill.
© 2024 John Wiley & Sons Ltd. Published 2024 by John Wiley & Sons Ltd.

but bad for drug excretion. Hence the purpose of metabolism is to make drugs more polar and less lipophilic, thereby enhancing the body's ability to excrete them.

Drug metabolism occurs primarily in the liver, although some can occur in the gut, lungs and plasma. Drug metabolism in the gut wall is important for oral drugs and we will discuss this in more detail later in the chapter. Above we defined metabolism as the enzymatic conversion of one chemical entity to another; the most important enzyme system involved is called the cytochrome P450 system. Drug metabolism can be divided into two different phases, simply called phase I metabolism and phase II metabolism. These two phases can occur singly or sequentially (phase I followed by phase II). Both of these types of reaction reduce lipid solubility, thereby increasing excretion efficiency.

Phase I drug metabolism reactions can be divided into three types of chemical reactions:

- oxidation

- reduction

- hydrolysis.

The cytochrome P450 family of enzymes are involved in phase I oxidation and reduction reactions. The key point to remember about phase I metabolism is that while it reduces lipid solubility, it does not necessarily result in inactivation of the drug.

Phase II drug metabolism involves the process of conjugation, which means the attachment of a polar chemical group (glucuronyl, methyl, acetyl, sulphate or glutathione) to the drug or phase I metabolite. Unlike phase I metabolism, while phase II metabolism reduces lipid solubility it almost always results in drug inactivation (Figure 9.1).

CYTOCHROME P450 ENZYME SYSTEM

Location

The cytochrome P450 enzymes are located in the smooth endoplasmic reticulum of liver cells (hepatocytes) and the gut wall. This represents the ideal location since for drugs to reach these enzymes, they must cross the cell membrane and find their way to the endoplasmic reticulum.

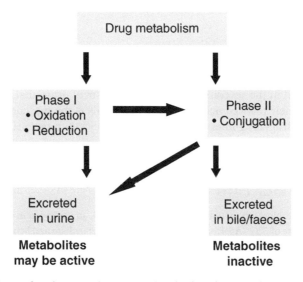

FIGURE 9.1 The phases of, and enzymatic processes involved in, drug metabolism.

Table 9.1   Examples of drugs that are substrates for individual cytochrome P450 enzymes

CYP1A2	CYP2C19	CYP2C9	CYP2D6	CYP3A4
Amitriptyline	Amitriptyline	Amitriptyline	Amitriptyline	Amlodipine
Clozapine	Citalopram	Diclofenac	Carvedilol	Clarithromycin
Olanzapine	Diazepam	Fluoxetine	Fluoxetine	Diazepam
Paracetamol	Lansoprazole	Ibuprofen	Lidocaine	Domperidone
Propranolol	Omeprazole	Losartan	Metoclopramide	Fentanyl
Theophylline	Phenytoin	Ondansetron	Paroxetine	Lidocaine
Verapamil	Propranolol	Phenytoin	Propranolol	Nifedipine
Warfarin	Warfarin	Tramadol	Timolol	Ondansetron
		Warfarin		Propranolol
				Simvastatin

Drugs in blue are metabolised by more than one isoform of cytochrome P450. A more complete list of cytochrome P450 enzymes and their drug substrates can be found at https://drug-interactions.medicine.iu.edu/Home.aspx.

Only lipid-soluble drugs will be able to do this easily. Drug metabolism is more important for lipid-soluble drugs because without metabolism they will not be excreted efficiently, so where better to house the metabolising enzymes than this highly membranous structure within the cells?

Activity

The cytochrome P450 group of enzymes is a large superfamily of related enzymes that are involved in the metabolism of drugs, steroids and carcinogens. While there are around 74 families of cytochrome P450, there are only three main families involved in human drug metabolism. These are referred to as CYP1, CYP2 and CYP3. Each family contains a number of individual enzymes that are represented by the addition of a further letter and number, for example CYP1A2, CYP2C9, CYP2D6 and CYP3A4. Each of these individual enzymes has distinct drug substrate specificities, although there may be some overlap in these specificities with more than one enzyme acting on the same substrate but at different rates (Table 9.1).

Inducers

The activity of specific cytochrome P450 enzymes can be induced, or sped up, by a variety of drugs, foodstuffs and herbal supplements. This is hugely important because induction of a cytochrome P450 enzyme will result in the speeding up of the metabolism of drugs that are substrates of that enzyme, resulting in their reduced activity (Figure 9.2). This is the mechanism that underlies a number of important drug–drug interactions. Examples of cytochrome P450 inducers are shown in Table 9.2.

PRACTICE APPLICATION

Rifampicin speeds up (induces) the activity of CYP3A4. Oestradiol, an oestrogen in combined oral contraceptive pills, is a substrate of CYP3A4. Rifampicin speeds up the metabolism and hence reduces the activity of oestradiol, leading to possible contraceptive failure. This is the reason why the dose of oral contraceptive may be increased along with the use of additional contraceptive precautions in women taking a short course of rifampicin.

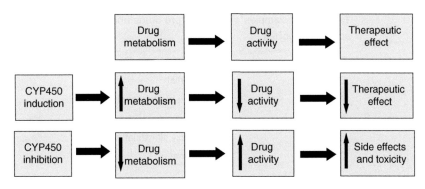

FIGURE 9.2   Possible effects of cytochrome P450 induction and inhibition on the metabolism and activity of substrate drugs.

Table 9.2   Examples of drugs, foodstuffs and herbal supplements that either induce or inhibit cytochrome P450 activity

	Cytochrome P450 inducers	Cytochrome P450 inhibitors
Drugs	Rifampicin (CYP2B6, CYP2C8, CYP2C19, CYP2C9, CYP3A4)	Fluconazole (CYP2C9, CYP3A4)
	Carbamazepine (CYP2C19, CYP3A4)	Fluoxetine (CYP2C19, CYP2D6)
		Erythromycin (CYP3A4)
	Phenytoin (CYP3A4)	Cimetidine (CYP1A2, CYP2C19, CYP2D6)
	Glucocorticoids (CYP3A4)	
Foods	Leafy green vegetables (CYP1A2)	Grapefruit juice (CYP3A4)
	Cigarette smoke (CYP1A2)	Cranberry juice (CYP3A4)
	Ethanol (CYP2E1)	Licorice
Herbals	St John's wort (CYP3A4)	St John's wort (CYP2D6, CYP2C9, CYP2C19)
	Valerian (a component of herbal Nytol) (CYP3A4)	Gingko (CYP2C9)
		Ginseng (CYP2D6, CYP2C19)
	Gingko (CYP1A2)	Echinacea (CYP3A4)

Inhibitors

The activity of specific cytochrome P450 enzymes can be inhibited or reduced by a variety of drugs, foodstuffs and herbal supplements. This is hugely important because inhibition of a cytochrome P450 enzyme will result in the metabolism of drugs that are substrates of that isoform being reduced, resulting in increased drug activity and possible side effects or toxicity (Figure 9.2). This mechanism underlies a number of important drug–drug interactions. Examples of cytochrome P450 inhibitors are shown in Table 9.2.

PRACTICE APPLICATION

Grapefruit juice inhibits CYP3A4 activity, reducing the metabolism of simvastatin, which is a substrate of this enzyme. This results in an increase in the activity of simvastatin and the side effect profile, particularly muscle effects. This is why concomitant use of simvastatin and grapefruit juice should be avoided.

Table 9.3 Examples of common pro-drugs and their active metabolites

Pro-drug	Active metabolite
Enalapril	Enalaprilat
Abacavir	Carbovir monophosphate
Famciclovir	Penciclovir
Simvastatin	6-hydroxy simvastatin acid
Codeine	Morphine

PRO-DRUGS

A pro-drug is a drug administered in an inactive form that only becomes active following metabolism. This is an ideal drug design as it allows the inactive parent drug to be administered in a lipid-soluble form that would be readily absorbed. The active metabolite is then released following metabolism, at which point the drug is also more polar in nature and therefore more readily excretable (Table 9.3).

PHARMACOGENETICS

Pharmacogenetics can be defined as clinically important hereditary variation in the response to drugs. The large number of cytochrome P450 enzymes makes genetic variation in these enzymes almost inevitable and this genetic variation can be important therapeutically. Genetic variations in, or polymorphisms of, specific cytochrome P450 enzymes can result in patients being either slow (poor) metabolisers (their CYP450 enzyme is less effective than the norm) or fast (extensive or ultra-rapid) metabolisers (their CYP450 enzyme is more efficient than the norm). For slow metabolisers this may result in increased drug activity within the body and possible side effects/toxicity while for fast (extensive) metabolisers there may be a lack of therapeutic effect. The most important cytochrome P450 enzymes in terms of clinical impact of polymorphisms are CYP2C9, CYP2C19 and CYP2D6, and these polymorphisms are more common in specific ethnic groups (Table 9.4), making ethnicity an important issue for safe and effective prescribing.

Table 9.4 Examples of polymorphisms in cytochrome P450 isoforms, prevalence in different ethnic groups and clinical impact

CYP isoform	Polymorphism	Drugs affected
CYP2C9	PM 11% Caucasians 0% Asians	Increased activity of warfarin, candesartan, losartan, diclofenac, ibuprofen, fluvastatin and phenytoin
CYP2C19	PM 20% Asians	Increased activity of proton-pump inhibitors and some antidepressants (citalopram, amitriptyline)
	EM 18% Ethiopians	Decreased activity of proton-pump inhibitors and some antidepressants (citalopram, amitriptyline)
CYP2D6	PM 8% Caucasians	Increased activity of tramadol, venlafaxine and metoprolol, reduced codeine clinical effect
	UM 28% North Africans	Lack of therapeutic effect of tramadol, venlafaxine and metoprolol, increased codeine clinical effect

PM, poor metaboliser; EM, extensive metaboliser; UM, ultra-rapid metaboliser.

Perhaps one of the best examples of the effect of genetic polymorphisms on clinical therapeutics is that of debrisoquine, which was previously used in the treatment of essential hypertension. The use of debrisoquine resulted in excessive hypotension in a number of patients and this was related to their lack of ability to metabolise the drug. The enzyme involved in debrisoquine metabolism is CYP2D6 and studies suggest that up to 8% of Caucasians have this 'poor metaboliser' polymorphism, which impacted greatly on the clinical use of this drug, resulting in it falling out of favour (Caldwell, 2004).

STOP AND THINK

Would you use the same dose of proton pump inhibitor for Caucasian, Asian and Ethiopian patients?

ACTIVE AND TOXIC METABOLITES

As mentioned earlier in the chapter, phase I metabolism does not always inactivate drugs. There are several drugs, including diazepam, morphine, imipramine, verapamil and propranolol, which, following phase I metabolism, exhibit active metabolites. This means that the pharmacological activity is retained even after the parent drug has disappeared from the plasma.

STOP AND THINK

Why should drugs with active metabolites be used with caution in the elderly and/or patients with renal failure?

Phase I drug metabolites can also be toxic. The most important example of a drug with a toxic metabolite is paracetamol. The majority (95%) of paracetamol undergoes phase II metabolism to an inactive metabolite. The remainder (5%) undergoes phase I metabolism and results in the production of the toxic metabolite *N*-acetyl-*p*-benzo-quinoneimine (NAPQI). Under normal circumstances this is not a problem as the NAPQI rapidly undergoes phase II metabolism, being conjugated to glutathione, which inactivates it. In overdose situations problems arise because the liver's store of glutathione becomes depleted and can no longer inactivate the NAPQI (Figure 9.3).

FIRST-PASS METABOLISM AND BIOAVAILABILITY

First-pass metabolism (sometimes called presystemic metabolism) is defined as the metabolism of the drug that occurs in the gut wall and the liver prior to that drug reaching the systemic circulation and only affects drugs that are given orally. Orally administered drugs are absorbed through the GI tract and enter the hepatic portal system, passing through the liver prior to entering the systemic circulation (Figure 9.4).

Bioavailability is defined as the proportion of administered drug that is available in the systemic circulation. Bioavailability is therefore affected by the degree of both drug absorption and first-pass metabolism. Drugs which undergo high first-pass metabolism have low bioavailability and drugs which undergo little or no first-pass metabolism exhibit high bioavailability.

The percentage bioavailability of a drug is important in determining the dose required in relation to the route of administration. Drugs that are given intravenously are defined as having 100% bioavailability because the entire drug dose is delivered directly into the systemic

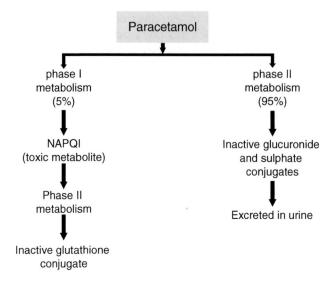

FIGURE 9.3 The metabolism of paracetamol and production of toxic metabolite. NAPQI, *N*-acetyl-*p*-benzo-quinoneimine.

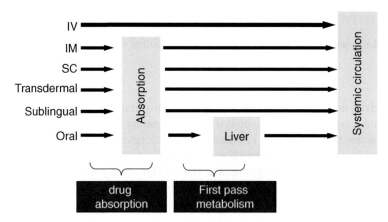

FIGURE 9.4 Changes in absorption and first-pass metabolism affect different routes of drug administration. IV, intravenous; IM, intramuscular; SC, subcutaneous.

circulation, thus avoiding problems with absorption and first-pass metabolism. If the oral bioavailability of a drug is only 20% then you would need to administer five times the dose of the same drug given intravenously to ensure similar drug levels within the systemic circulation. An example of a drug that requires a much higher dose when given orally compared to intravenously is morphine.

The degree of first-pass metabolism that occurs between individuals for the dose of drug can be very variable and this can result in wide variations in the oral bioavailability of the drug. The use of other drugs or dietary supplements that impact cytochrome P450 enzymes will result in altered bioavailability.

First-pass metabolism can also be affected by age and disease, which again will result in changes in oral bioavailability and unpredictability in terms of therapeutic effects.

FACTORS AFFECTING DRUG METABOLISM

Age

Both liver size and hepatic blood flow decrease with increasing age. There is an additional decline in the activity of cytochrome P450 enzymes in the liver with age. The effect of these changes is to reduce drug metabolism, which will result in increased drug activity within the body. Furthermore, changes in liver function will also act to reduce first-pass metabolism, which could lead to increased bioavailability of certain oral drugs.

The activity of cytochrome P450 enzymes is reduced in neonates, resulting in decreased drug metabolism. Conversely, the activity of cytochrome P450 enzymes in children is often greater than that of adults, resulting in increased drug metabolism and possible loss of therapeutic effect. More detail on this will be provided in Chapter 11.

Disease

A number of diseases can affect drug metabolism. Most obviously, diseases affecting the liver, such as cirrhosis, alcoholic liver disease and carcinoma, impact drug metabolism through a reduction in functional hepatocytes. This seems to result in a decrease in the activity of the cytochrome P450 enzymes involved in phase I metabolism but not in the activity of the conjugating enzymes involved in phase II metabolism. Infectious diseases can also result in the reduction of cytochrome P450 enzyme activity and decrease drug metabolism. Similarly, diseases that result in decreased blood flow to the liver, such as heart failure and shock, will necessarily result in reduced drug metabolism.

DRUG EXCRETION

The two main routes of drug excretion are via the kidneys (in the urine) and via the biliary system (in the faeces).

RENAL EXCRETION

The rate at which individual drugs are excreted by the kidneys is highly variable but is essentially determined by the rates of glomerular filtration, tubular secretion and passive diffusion as depicted in the following equation:

$$\text{renal excretion} = \text{glomerular filtration} + \text{tubular secretion} - \text{passive diffusion}$$

Glomerular filtration

About 20% of renal blood flow passes through the glomerulus of the kidney and the leaky nature of the glomerular capillaries results in plasma diffusing through the capillary walls into the renal tubule. This is known as the glomerular filtrate and contains not just plasma but free, unbound drugs, which are contained within that plasma. Drugs that are bound to plasma proteins cannot diffuse through the glomerular capillaries because of their size. Very large drugs such as heparin will similarly be retained within the bloodstream as they will also be too big to pass through the glomerular capillaries.

Tubular secretion

The remaining 80% of the renal blood flow passes through to the peritubular capillaries of the proximal tubule. Here there are two major carrier systems that carry drugs from the bloodstream into the renal tubule: the acidic carrier system, which carries weak acids (e.g., furosemide, indometacin, thiazide diuretics, penicillin) into the renal tubule, and the basic carrier system, which carries weak bases (e.g., amiloride, dopamine, pethidine) into the renal tubule.

These carrier systems can operate against a gradient and consequently represent the most efficient mechanism of renal excretion. They can reduce drug concentrations in the plasma to almost zero. However, they are subject to competitive inhibition, which may lead to drug interactions and unwanted effects. As mentioned previously (Chapter 8), penicillin and probenecid both compete for the acidic carrier. The presence of probenecid reduces the renal excretion of penicillin, prolonging its activity in the body, and probenecid was given with penicillin for this very reason. On the other hand, both uric acid and thiazide diuretics compete for this acidic carrier system. This can result in reduced renal excretion of uric acid and is the mechanism underlying the possible side effect of gout in patients taking thiazide diuretics.

Passive diffusion

The nature of the kidney is such that most of the plasma filtered through the glomerular capillaries is reabsorbed as it passes through the renal tubule. As plasma is reabsorbed, the concentration gradient between drug in the renal tubule and unbound drug in the plasma changes and drugs that are lipid soluble will be reabsorbed across the membranes of the renal tubule into the plasma. As a result, very lipid-soluble drugs are only slowly excreted by the kidneys while polar, water-soluble drugs cannot readily cross membranes and are retained in the tubule.

FACTORS AFFECTING RENAL DRUG EXCRETION

pH of the environment

Just as drug absorption can be affected by local pH, so can renal drug excretion. Essentially the concept remains the same: alteration of the pH changes the proportion of drug in the unionised, lipid-soluble form. While in Chapter 8 we were interested in increasing the concentration of the lipid-soluble form to enhance drug absorption, in terms of renal excretion it is important to reduce the concentration of the lipid-soluble form, thus reducing passive diffusion and enhancing excretion.

Modulation of urinary pH has been used to promote drug excretion in overdose situations (Table 9.5).

STOP AND THINK

Why do you think aspirin overdose is sometimes treated by alkalinisation of the urine?

Age

Both renal mass and renal perfusion are reduced with increasing age. This decreased blood flow through the kidneys and reduction in the number of functional nephrons results in decreased renal excretion of drugs. Similarly, both glomerular filtration and tubular secretion are reduced with increasing age, which also reduces renal excretion of drug.

Table 9.5 Effect of modulation of urinary pH on the renal excretion of weak acids and bases

	Weak acids	Weak bases
Acidic urine	Reabsorbed into the bloodstream	Excreted
Alkaline urine	Excreted	Reabsorbed into the bloodstream

Disease

Reduced renal blood flow, as can be seen in shock, will reduce the delivery of drug to the kidney and hence result in reduced renal excretion. Similarly, renal disease will result in reduced renal mass, thus reducing drug excretion, and may require a reduction in drug dosage in patients, particularly for drugs that are excreted unchanged, for example metformin, or have active metabolites, for example morphine.

BILIARY EXCRETION

Biliary excretion is the major route of excretion for large, ionised molecules, particularly glucuronide and sulphate conjugates. These phase II metabolites are transferred from hepatocytes to the bile by non-specific carrier systems that can be competitively inhibited in a manner similar to that seen in the renal tubule. Negatively charged drugs/metabolites compete with other negatively charged drugs/metabolites, while positively charged drugs/metabolites compete with other positively charged drugs/metabolites.

Drugs are then delivered by the biliary system to the small intestine, where they may be excreted in the faeces or undergo enterohepatic recycling.

Enterohepatic recycling

Drugs that have been conjugated in phase II metabolism are often transferred into the bile and delivered to the small intestine as described above. Bacteria within the small intestine can then hydrolyse some of the conjugate, releasing the original free drug. A portion of this free (unconjugated) drug can then be reabsorbed through the membranes of the GI tract and returned to the liver and systemic circulation prior to being re-metabolised and re-excreted as a conjugate (Figure 9.5). This recirculation of drug can occur many times before the drug is finally eliminated from the body and creates a reservoir of drug.

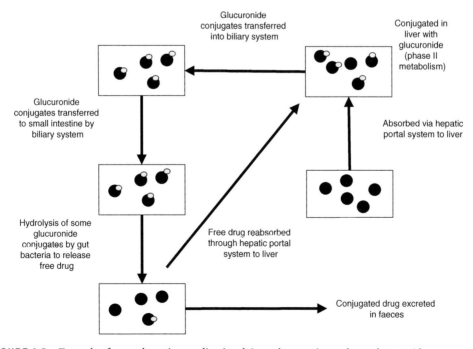

FIGURE 9.5   Example of enterohepatic recycling involving a drug conjugated to a glucuronide.

This recycling is important for a number of prescribed drugs, including rifampicin, morphine and benzodiazepines.

DRUG CLEARANCE

Drug clearance is defined as the rate of drug elimination divided by the plasma concentration. Drug clearance is concerned with the rate at which the active parent drug is removed from the body and consists of both metabolism and excretion. Metabolic or hepatic clearance is the conversion of the active parent drug to a metabolite, while renal clearance is the removal of the drug by the kidneys.

The relative importance of hepatic and renal clearance depends on the nature of the individual drug. Drugs that are highly lipid soluble will probably undergo extensive hepatic clearance while for drugs that are polar in nature, renal clearance will be more important. The main determinants of renal clearance are the rate of active tubular secretion and the rate of passive diffusion. Drugs that undergo mainly renal clearance should be used with care in patients whose renal function may be impaired. Examples of drugs which undergo mainly renal clearance are shown in Table 9.6.

HALF-LIFE

Half-life ($t_{1/2}$) is defined as the time taken for the peak plasma concentration of the drug to fall by half (Figure 9.6) and for most drugs this remains constant regardless of the dose of drug administered. Half-life is dependent on the clearance of the drug and its volume of distribution. If a drug is rapidly cleared by either hepatic or renal clearance, then the half-life of the drug will be short.

Table 9.6 Examples of drugs that undergo mainly renal clearance

Drug
Gentamicin
Furosemide
Atenolol
Benzylpenicillin
Cimetidine
Digoxin

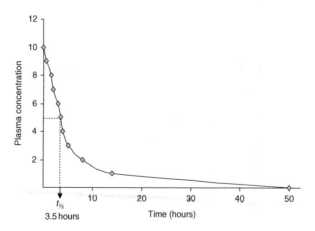

FIGURE 9.6 The change in concentration of drug in plasma with time and a determination of half-life.

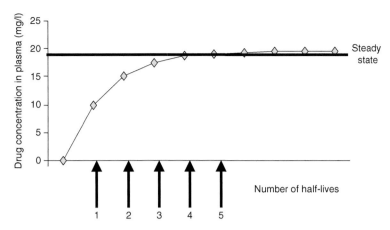

FIGURE 9.7   Concentration of drug in plasma. The half-life of the drug is 2 hours and steady state is reached after five half-lives (10 hours).

However, if the drug is only slowly cleared from the body, then the half-life will be longer. Similarly, drugs which have a very large volume of distribution are likely to have a longer half-life than drugs with a small volume of distribution.

Anything that reduces clearance, such as increasing age or disease, will increase the half-life of a drug and anything that increases clearance, such as cytochrome P450 induction, will decrease drug half-life. Similarly, changes in the volume of distribution of a drug, as might be seen in the elderly, will affect half-life. Half-life is important in determining the time interval between drug doses and the time taken for drug concentrations to reach steady state in the plasma. Drugs such as ibuprofen ($t_{1/2}$ = 2 hours) which have short half-lives need to be given frequently whereas drugs such as ethosuximide ($t_{1/2}$ = 50 hours) which have long half-lives need only be given once daily. Steady state is reached when the plasma drug concentration does not drop below therapeutic levels between doses; this usually takes three to five half-lives to be achieved (Figure 9.7).

SUMMARY

- The purpose of drug metabolism is to make drugs more polar and therefore easier to excrete.
- The cytochrome P450 superfamily of enzymes is important in phase I metabolism while phase II metabolism involves conjugation.
- Phase I metabolism can result in the production of active and/or toxic metabolites.
- Pro-drugs are inactive until they are metabolised.
- Genetic variation can impact drug metabolism and hence drug activity.
- Cytochrome P450 enzyme activity can be both induced (sped up) and inhibited (slowed down) by other drugs, dietary components and herbal preparations.
- First-pass metabolism is the metabolism of oral drugs in the gut wall and liver prior to reaching the systemic circulation.
- Bioavailability is the percentage of administered drug that is available in the systemic circulation.
- Renal excretion consists of glomerular filtration, tubular secretion and passive diffusion.
- Renal excretion is affected by local pH, age and disease.
- Biliary excretion is common for drugs that are conjugated either to glucuronide or sulphate.

- Enterohepatic recycling of glucuronide conjugates creates a reservoir of drug.
- Drug clearance involves both hepatic and renal clearance.
- Half-life is the time taken for the plasma concentration of the drug to drop by half.

ACTIVITY

1. Which of the following statements regarding drug metabolism are correct?

    It is increased in children compared to adults.   True/False

    It is decreased by rifampicin.   True/False

    It is decreased by grapefruit juice.   True/False

    It is decreased in elderly patients.   True/False

    It is more important for lipid-soluble drugs.   True/False

2. Which of the following statements regarding first-pass metabolism are correct?

    It affects bioavailability.   True/False

    It affects drugs given SC and IM.   True/False

    It never affects drugs administered IV.   True/False

    It occurs prior to the drug entering the systemic circulation.   True/False

    It can be reduced in elderly patients.   True/False

3. Which of the following statements regarding passive diffusion of drug in the renal tubule are correct?

    It depends on the pH of the urine.   True/False

    It depends on the rate of glomerular filtration.   True/False

    It depends on the degree of plasma protein binding.   True/False

    It depends on the age of the patient.   True/False

    It depends on the lipid solubility of the drug.   True/False

4. Which of the following statements regarding biliary excretion and enterohaptic recycling are correct?

    It affects drugs that undergo only phase I metabolism.   True/False

    It can be disrupted by broad-spectrum antibiotics.   True/False

    It results in drug excretion in the faeces.   True/False

    It is more important for unionised molecules.   True/False

5. Which of the following statements regarding half-life are correct?

    It determines the time to reach steady state.   True/False

    It increases with increasing drug clearance.   True/False

    It is longer in drugs with a large volume of distribution.   True/False

    It determines the dosing schedule of drugs.   True/False

    It can be affected by increasing age.   True/False

FURTHER READING

Bank, P.C.D., Swen, J.J. and Guchelaar, H.-J. (2018) Implementation of pharmacogenomics in everyday clinical settings. *Adv Pharmacol* 83:219–246.

Birkett, D.J. (2010) *Pharmacokinetics made Easy*, 2nd edn. McGraw-Hill, London and Sydney.

Caldwell, J. (2004) Pharmacogenetics and individual variation in the range of amino acid adequacy: the biological aspects. *J Nutr* 134:1600S–1604S.

Frye, R.F., Zgheib, N.K., Matzke, G.R., *et al.* (2006) Liver disease selectively modulates cytochrome P450-mediated metabolism. *Clin Pharmacol Ther* 80(2):235–245.

Lauschke, V.M., Milani, L. and Ingelman-Sundberg, M. (2018) Pharmacogenomic biomarkers for improved drug therapy—recent progress and future developments. *AAPS J* 20:4.

Matalová, P., Urbánek, K. and Anzenbacher, P. (2016) Specific features of pharmacokinetics in children. Drug Metab Rev 48:70–79.

McFadden, R. (2019) *Introducing Pharmacology for Nursing and Healthcare*, 3rd edn. Routledge.

Ritter, J.M., Flower, R.J., Henderson, G. et al. (2023) *Rang and Dale's Pharmacology*, 10th edn. Elsevier, London.

Shi, S. and Klotz, U. (2011) Age-related changes in pharmacokinetics. *Curr Drug Metab* 12(7):601–610.

Smith, H.J. (2006) *Smith and Williams' Introduction to the Principles of Drug Design and Action*, 4th edn. Taylor and Francis, Boca Raton.

Waring, R.H., Harris, R.M. and Mitchell, S.C. (2017) Drug metabolism in the elderly: A multifactorial problem? *Maturitas* 100:27–32.

USEFUL WEBSITES

British National Formulary (online). BMJ Group and Pharmaceutical Press, London. http://www.medicines complete.com.

Flockhart, D.A., Thacker, D., McDonald, C. and Desta, Z. The Flockhart Cytochrome P450 Drug–Drug Interaction Table. Division of Clinical Pharmacology, Indiana University School of Medicine (updated 2021). https://drug-interactions.medicine. iu.edu/Home.aspx

REUSABLE LEARNING OBJECTS

Half-life of drugs. https://www.nottingham.ac.uk/ nursing/sonet/rlos/bioproc/halflife/index.html

Kidney anatomy. https://www.nottingham.ac.uk/nursing/ sonet/rlos/bioproc/kidneyanatomy/index.html

Physiology of the kidneys. https://www.nottingham. ac.uk/nursing/sonet/rlos/bioproc/kidneyphysiology/ index.html

Liver anatomy. https://www.nottingham.ac.uk/nursing/ sonet/rlos/bioproc/liveranatomy/index.html

Physiology of the liver. https://www.nottingham.ac.uk/ nursing/sonet/rlos/bioproc/liverphysiology/index. html

The kidneys and drug excretion. https://www.notting ham.ac.uk/nursing/sonet/rlos/bioproc/kidneydrug/ index.html

The liver and drug metabolism. https://www.notting ham.ac.uk/nursing/sonet/rlos/bioproc/liverdrug/ index.html

Understanding first-pass metabolism. https://www. nottingham.ac.uk/nursing/sonet/rlos/bioproc/ metabolism/default.html

Introduction to drug clearance. https://www.notting ham.ac.uk/nursing/sonet/rlos/bioproc/clearance1/ index.html

CHAPTER 10

Routes of Administration

Joanne Lymn and Roger Knaggs

LEARNING OBJECTIVES

By the end of this chapter the reader should be able to:

- identify routes of drug administration and give examples of drugs that use each route

- distinguish between routes used for local and systemic drug effects, and between enteral and parenteral routes of administration

- describe the potential barriers to drug absorption from the oral route

- explain why first-pass metabolism and gastric instability may lead to drugs being given via the sublingual administration route

- describe how the rectal, transdermal, ocular and inhalation routes can result in both local and systemic drug action

- discuss the differences in rate of absorption and bioavailability, and advantages of the different parenteral routes of drug administration.

The route of administration of a drug refers to the path by which the drug enters the body. The route chosen depends on both the ultimate site of action of the drug and its physical and chemical characteristics. Examples of different routes of administration are shown in Table 10.1.

One way of classifying routes of administration is to think about whether the drug will have a local or systemic effect on the body.

LOCAL VERSUS SYSTEMIC DRUG EFFECT

Drugs given to exert a local effect are often thought of as having a topical route of administration, in that they are applied directly to the site of action. In its simplest form this refers to creams and ointments that are applied directly to the skin for local effect, eyedrops that are instilled directly into the eyes and eardrops that are instilled directly into the ears. There are, however, some complexities to this topical/local effect, including the use of the inhaled route for a respiratory effect and the use of oral vancomycin to treat *Clostridiodies difficile* infection.

Drugs given to have a systemic effect on the body will need to enter the body to have an effect at a more distant site of action. They will therefore need to undergo some or all pharmacokinetic processes to exert their therapeutic effect. The actual route of administration chosen will largely be determined by the intended therapeutic indication and speed of onset required (whether an emergency or not). Drugs can have both local and systemic effects on the body and the route of administration chosen is in part determined by the effect required (Table 10.2).

Drugs that are administered for a systemic effect in the body can be further divided into those given by enteral and parenteral routes of administration. Roughly speaking drugs given by enteral routes use the digestive system, including the mouth, stomach, intestine and rectum, whilst parenteral routes bypass the digestive system (Table 10.3).

The New Prescriber: An Integrated Approach to Medical and Non-medical Prescribing, Second Edition.
Edited by Joanne Lymn, Alison Mostyn, Roger Knaggs, Michael Randall, and Dianne Bowskill.
© 2024 John Wiley & Sons Ltd. Published 2024 by John Wiley & Sons Ltd.

Table 10.1 Examples of different routes of drug administration

Oral	Ocular	Inhalation
Subcutaneous	Intramuscular	Intravenous
Rectal	Sublingual	Transdermal

Table 10.2 Routes of administration available and whether they are routinely used for local or systemic drug effect

Local drug effect	Systemic drug effect
Oral (vancomycin)	Oral
Rectal	Sublingual
Topical creams and ointments	Rectal (not always reliable)
Ocular	Transdermal
Inhalation for respiratory diseases	Subcutaneous injection
	Intramuscular injection
	Intravenous injection

Table 10.3 Examples of enteral and parenteral routes of drug administration

Enteral routes of administration	Parenteral routes of administration
Oral	Subcutaneous injection
Rectal	Intramuscular injection
Sublingual	Intravenous injection
	Transdermal

Drug absorption from parenteral routes is generally more rapid and predictable than via the oral route, and avoids first-pass metabolism and gastric instability.

This chapter will highlight different routes of administration for drugs, and discuss why the different routes of administration are available for drugs and why the route chosen may be determined by the pharmacokinetics of the drug.

ORAL ADMINISTRATION

Oral administration is probably the easiest and most convenient route of drug administration for most people. Drugs can be administered as solids or solutions, making this a suitable route for most people, including children and older people. Oral administration is, however, the most complex route of administration in terms of presenting the greatest number of barriers to the drug prior to reaching the systemic circulation. Ideally, drugs should be relatively stable in the acidic environment of the stomach and should be lipid soluble to be effectively absorbed from the gastrointestinal (GI) tract. Highly polar acids and bases are only absorbed slowly and incompletely, with much of the drug being eliminated in the faeces. After absorption from the GI tract, the drug travels to the liver via the portal circulation and may undergo substantial first-pass metabolism, thus reducing the amount of active drug reaching the circulation.

STOP AND THINK

Why is phenoxymethylpenicillin but not benzylpenicillin given by the oral route?

EXCIPIENTS AND BULKING AGENTS

Excipients and binding agents are added to the active ingredient in tablets and can contribute to the taste of some oral drug formulations, although sometimes this can be overcome by using a sugar or film coating. Flavourings can be added to liquid preparations to make them more palatable to children, but the use of sugar in these preparations is now discouraged to reduce the possibility of dental caries. Similarly, it is not wise to make drugs too palatable for children as this may encourage overuse. Some drugs (e.g., phenoxymethylpenicillin, penicillin V) are relatively unstable in solution and have to be stored in powder form prior to use; some also have to be kept refrigerated until the course is finished. Another potential concern is the use of lactose as a bulking agent, which may cause issues for people with coeliac disease.

PRACTICE APPLICATION

People may be allergic to the excipients, such as colourings, added to the drug and not necessarily to the drug itself.

FACTORS AFFECTING ABSORPTION OF ORALLY ADMINISTERED DRUGS

Rate of gastric emptying

After oral administration most drug absorption occurs in the intestine, particularly the small intestine, rather than the stomach and hence the rate at which drug is delivered to the intestine will affect the rate of absorption.

Drugs taken after meals are usually more slowly absorbed because movement to the small intestine is delayed. Intake of fluid with orally administered drugs can increase the rate of gastric emptying and hence speed up the rate of drug absorption. Some drugs (e.g., morphine) can themselves cause gastric stasis and are therefore often given by other routes.

PRACTICE APPLICATION

Metoclopramide (an antiemetic) is often prescribed in combination with analgesic medicines for the treatment of migraine. In addition to treating the nausea often associated with migraine, metoclopramide acts on the stomach muscle to speed up the emptying of the stomach and thus the passage of the analgesic into the intestine, thereby increasing its rate of absorption.

Disease

Drug absorption can be affected by diseases that affect the available surface area of the GI tract. Inflammatory bowel disease, bowel cancer and coeliac disease can all affect absorption of drugs due to damage to the intestinal wall. This may reduce drug absorption through reduced surface area. Sometimes this may paradoxically result in increased drug absorption because it is thought that the damaged mucosa becomes quite leaky, which allows drug molecules to pass through more quickly.

Transit time in GI tract

In Chapter 8 we established that the majority of drug absorption occurs in the intestine, even for weak acids that start to be absorbed from the stomach. Consequently, the length of time the drug is in the intestine is important for absorption. Normal transit time in the intestine can be anything between 4 and 10 hours, but most drugs are absorbed relatively rapidly, within an hour.

PRACTICE APPLICATION

Patients with severe diarrhoea may have significantly reduced drug absorption after oral administration simply because drugs taken orally pass through the GI tract so quickly.

Presence of other substances in the GI tract

The absorption of drugs from the GI tract can be affected by the presence of other drugs or ions. Tetracycline antibiotics such as tetracycline, oxytetracycline and demeclocycline should not be given with milk because these drugs bind to the calcium ions in the milk to form large insoluble complexes that cannot be readily absorbed across the GI tract, reducing the absorption of the antibiotic.

Similarly, tetracycline should not be given with antacids as it binds to the magnesium, aluminium or calcium ions contained in the antacid. This results in the production of large insoluble complexes, leading to reduced absorption. Antacids will also act to alter the pH of the local environment, thus affecting the amount of drug in the unionised form and impacting drug absorption.

STOP AND THINK

The interaction between antacids and tetracycline is an example of which form of drug antagonism?

SUBLINGUAL ADMINISTRATION

Drugs are administered by the sublingual route when a rapid response is required, particularly when the drug is either unstable at gastric pH or rapidly metabolised by the liver. Drugs absorbed from the mouth pass straight into the systemic circulation without entering the hepatic portal system and so escape the effects of first-pass metabolism. The degree of first-pass metabolism that occurs with a drug may be a determining factor in the route of administration. For example, glyceryl trinitrate (GTN) undergoes very high first-pass metabolism, with around 99% of the dose when administered orally being metabolised on its first pass through the liver and only 1% reaching the systemic circulation. It is for this reason that GTN is usually administered sublingually or transdermally; drug absorption from both of these routes enters the systemic circulation directly, thus avoiding the first-pass effect.

RECTAL ADMINISTRATION

Administration of drugs via the rectum can be used for local or systemic effects. Rectal administration may be an alternative for patients who are vomiting or unable to swallow. Diazepam can be administered rectally to children in status epilepticus where intravenous access is difficult. While the surface area for absorption is small, the rectal mucosa is well supplied with blood vessels, making drug absorption into the systemic circulation from this route possible. Unfortunately, however, blood flow is variable, making drug absorption erratic and consequently rectal absorption gives more variable plasma concentrations than oral administration.

TRANSDERMAL ADMINISTRATION

Drugs administered by the transdermal route may have a local topical effect on the skin or a systemic effect (Table 10.4). Absorption from the skin is primarily dependent on the lipid solubility of the drug, with only very lipid-soluble drugs being able to penetrate this tough outer body layer for a systemic effect. These drugs can be delivered by transdermal patch whereas drugs applied to the skin as creams, lotions, ointments or gels generally have a local effect on the skin itself.

Transdermal patches are being increasingly used (e.g., oestrogen in hormone replacement therapy and nicotine in cigarette addiction withdrawal). This produces a steady rate of delivery and avoids first-pass metabolism. Development costs are large and hence patch formulations tend to be expensive and are only suitable for very lipid-soluble drugs that are active in small quantities. The integrity of the skin is probably the most important factor in the absorption of these drugs as the dermis is well supplied with blood vessels and a break in the skin will allow topical drugs to be taken into the systemic circulation.

OCULAR ADMINISTRATION

Administration of drugs to the eye relies on absorption through the epithelium of the conjunctival sac. Often it is possible to have desirable local effects without causing systemic side effects (e.g., dorzolamide lowers ocular pressure in glaucoma but avoids the acidosis caused by oral administration), but systemic effects can occur (e.g., timolol, a beta-blocker, used for glaucoma can result in bronchospasm in asthmatic patients).

INHALATION

Drugs used for their effects on the lung are given by inhalation. This allows high local concentrations in the lungs to be obtained with minimal systemic effects. Importantly, drug delivery by inhalation can avoid the first-pass metabolism effects seen when these drugs are given orally. However, beta$_2$-adrenoceptor agonists (e.g., salbutamol) used in high concentrations can be absorbed into the systemic circulation and induce side effects. Muscarinic antagonists such as ipratropium have a quaternary ammonium ion that makes them both highly charged and large in size, thus they are poorly absorbed across membranes and do not generally enter the systemic circulation.

STOP AND THINK

Why is the dose of salbutamol given by inhalation in the microgram range while the dose of oral salbutamol is in the milligram range?

Particles of solid or liquid droplets inhaled are deposited in the lungs by impaction. Only a proportion of inhaled drug reaches the lower respiratory tract, with the majority being deposited in the mouth and pharynx. This drug will then be swallowed, potentially being absorbed into the systemic circulation and resulting in side effects. It is possible to increase the proportion of a dose that reaches the required site. Patient education on correct use of an inhaler includes synchronising the operation of the spray during inhalation and teaching the patient to hold their breath after administration. Use of a spacer device also increases the amount of drug deposited in the lower airways.

INTRAMUSCULAR INJECTION

Intramuscular administration generally results in reliable plasma concentrations being attained. The rate of absorption following intramuscular administration depends on local blood flow and the site of injection. If a drug is distributed throughout a large volume of muscle, the rate of absorption is increased. Dispersion of drug within tissue can be enhanced by massage of the injection site. Transport away from the muscle depends on local blood flow. Blood flow is greater in muscles of the upper arm than in the gluteal mass or thigh. Muscle blood flow is not constant and increases with exercise, and can decrease in shock and heart failure.

The pH of the injected solution can also greatly affect drug absorption. The pH changes gradually from its initial value to that of interstitial (tissue) fluid (pH 7.4). According to the pH partition hypothesis (Chapter 8), drugs are more rapidly absorbed when a significant proportion of the drug exists as the free unionised molecule.

SUBCUTANEOUS INJECTION

Absorption following subcutaneous injection is influenced by the same factors that determine intramuscular injections. Absorption of drugs via these routes is dependent on the blood flow to these areas. However, as cutaneous blood flow is lower than in muscle so subcutaneous absorption will tend to be slower and consequently drugs given by intramuscular injection generally have a faster onset of action than drugs given subcutaneously simply because muscle is more highly perfused than subcutaneous tissues.

The major advantage of this route of administration is that it is possible to teach patients how to undertake subcutaneous injections safely and hence this route is suitable if self-administration is required (e.g., regular insulin injections for diabetes mellitus). The main disadvantage of subcutaneous injection is that the volume that can be injected is smaller than for intramuscular injection. As with intramuscular injection, drugs given by the subcutaneous route will show a slower rate of absorption in patients suffering from hypovolaemic shock as the blood flow to these areas is reduced to protect essential organs.

INTRAVENOUS INJECTION

Injection directly into a vein is the fastest and most reliable route of administration to give a highly predictable plasma concentration. Intravenous administration does not exhibit the same variability of absorption as other routes of administration. As with other parenteral routes of administration, intravenous injection avoids first-pass metabolism effects and also avoids problems associated with drug instability at gastric pH.

STOP AND THINK

What is the bioavailability of drugs administered intravenously?

Intravenous administration is useful for drugs that are not absorbed from the GI tract because of size or being very polar in nature or too irritant to be given by other routes. However, if given too quickly, plasma concentrations may rise at such a rate that normal mechanisms of distribution and excretion are saturated, resulting in toxicity and side effects. Given that intravenous administration requires cannulation of a vein, it is not suitable for routine self-administration.

SUMMARY

- Drugs can be administered for local or systemic effects.

- Oral administration is the most convenient enteral route for drugs that have a systemic effect.

- Parenteral routes include subcutaneous, intramuscular and intravenous injections and have a faster onset of action than the enteral route.

- The rate of drug absorption from the oral route can be decreased by gastric stasis, bowel disease and diarrhoea.

- Interaction with other drugs or foodstuffs in the gastrointestinal tract can reduce absorption from the oral route.

- Sublingual drug administration avoids first-pass metabolism and problems associated with gastric instability.

- Systemic absorption from the rectal route is erratic and may result in variable plasma drug concentrations and response.

- Only drugs that are very lipid soluble and have a high potency can be given transdermally for a systemic effect.

- Ocular administration and inhalation can be used for local drug action in the eye and the lungs, respectively.

- While the use of the ocular and inhalational routes reduces the likelihood of systemic side effects, it does not prevent them.

- Drug absorption from the intramuscular and subcutaneous route is dependent on local blood flow. Intravenous drug administration avoids the variability in absorption associated with other routes but can result in side effects and toxicity.

ACTIVITY

1. Which of the following routes are routinely used to give systemic effects?

Oral	True/False
Intravenous	True/False
Inhalation	True/False
Ocular	True/False
Transdermal	True/False

2. Which of the following routes are routinely used for parenteral administration?

Oral	True/False
Subcutaneous	True/False
Intramuscular	True/False
Rectal	True/False
Sublingual	True/False

3. Drug absorption from the oral route can be decreased by which of the following?

Diarrhoea	True/False
Use of metoclopramide	True/False
Gastric stasis	True/False
Antacids	True/False
Taking with food	True/False

4. Which of the following routes of drug administration avoid first-pass metabolism?

Inhaled	True/False
Oral	True/False
Sublingual	True/False
Transdermal	True/False
Intramuscular	True/False

5. Which of the following statements concerning intramuscular drug administration are correct?

Results in 100% bioavailability	True/False
Is affected by blood flow	True/False
Is unaffected by shock	True/False
Is used to produce systemic effects	True/False
Is dependent on the pH of the injected solution	True/False

FURTHER READING

Al Hanbali, O.A., Khan, H.M.S., Sarfraz, M., Arafat, M., Ijaz, S. and Hameed, A. (2019) Transdermal patches: Design and current approaches to painless drug delivery. *Acta Pharm* 69(2):197–215.

Cates, C.J., Welsh, E.J. and Rowe, B.H. (2013) Holding chambers (spacers) versus nebulisers for beta-agonist treatment of acute asthma. *Cochrane Database Syst Rev.* https://www.cochranelibrary.com/cdsr/doi/10.1002/14651858.CD000052.pub3/full.

Eadala, P., Waud, J.P. and Matthews, S.B., et al. (2009) Quantifying the 'hidden' lactose in drugs used for the treatment of gastro-intestinal conditions. *Aliment Pharmacol Ther* 29:677–687.

Irving, P.M., Shanahan, F. and Rampton, D.S. (2008) Drug interactions in inflammatory bowel disease. *Am J Gastroenterol* 103:207–219.

Lam, J.K.W., Cheung, C.C.K., Chow, M.Y.T., et al. (2020) Transmucosal drug administration as an alternative route in palliative and end-of-life care during the COVID-19 pandemic. *Adv Drug Deliv Rev* 160:234–243.

Lavorini, F., Magnan, A., Dubus, J.C., et al. (2007) Effect of incorrect use of dry powder inhalers on management of patients with asthma and COPD. *Respir Med* 102:593–604.

Page, C.P., Hoffman, B., Curtis, M. and Walker, M. (2006) *Integrated Pharmacology*, 3rd edn. Mosby, London.

Ritter, J.M., Flower, R., Henderson, G., et al. (2023) *Rang and Dale's Pharmacology*, 10th edn. Elsevier, Amsterdam.

Roberts-Thomson, P.J., Chan, A., Kupa, A., et al. (1984) Urticaria and angio-oedema. *Med J Aust* 1:S34–S37.

Vertzoni, M., Augustijns, P., Grimm, P., et al. (2019) Impact of regional differences along the gastrointestinal tract of healthy adults on oral drug absorption: An UNGAP review. *Eur J Pharm Sci* 134:153–175.

Wilson, C.G. and Washington, N. (1989) *Physiological Pharmaceutics. Biological Barriers to Drug Absorption.* Ellis Horwood, Chichester.

CHAPTER 11

Variations in Drug Handling

Michael Randall

LEARNING OUTCOMES

By the end of this chapter the reader should be able to:

- understand and explain the pharmacokinetic differences in response to drugs from birth to old age

- understand the pharmacodynamic differences in response to drugs in the elderly

- understand the implications for drug dose and choice in neonates, and paediatric and elderly patients

- understand the reasons for the differences in response to drugs in those patients with renal or hepatic impairment

- understand the implications for drug dose and choice in patients with renal or hepatic impairment

- understand the importance of pharmacogenetics.

WHY IS THERE VARIABILITY?

There is a saying 'no two people are alike'; this is true in many ways, including the way different people respond to drugs. This is because of differences in their biological and chemical make-up.

Although individuals vary widely in their response to drugs, there are broad themes that apply to different groups of people, with variations across different age groups, genetics and ethnicity. There are also differences in the way people with renal and hepatic impairment respond to drugs.

PHARMACOKINETIC VARIABILITY WITH AGE

NEONATES

It is important to remember that neonates exhibit variability in their ability to handle drugs that are specific to them. Neonates are not 'young children' and it is important to remember this when calculating drug dosages for neonates. Preterm neonates are particularly unique, as they may be born with immature body systems and therefore have reduced ability to handle drugs. There are specific reference texts giving dosage advice for neonatal patients and the *British National Formulary for Children* (BNF-C) often gives separate doses for neonates.

Absorption

Enteral drug absorption is erratic in the neonate because the stomach does not always empty effectively. In an ill neonate there may be no enteral absorption. In a preterm neonate of 28 weeks or less, the skin is very thin and acts as a poor barrier to water loss, and there is increased absorption

The New Prescriber: An Integrated Approach to Medical and Non-medical Prescribing, Second Edition.
Edited by Joanne Lymn, Alison Mostyn, Roger Knaggs, Michael Randall, and Dianne Bowskill.
© 2024 John Wiley & Sons Ltd. Published 2024 by John Wiley & Sons Ltd.

of topical agents and anything else that comes into contact with the skin, for example skin cleansers which contain alcohol. Neonates have small muscle bulk, so the intramuscular route is generally avoided.

PRACTICE APPLICATION

The most reliable routes of absorption in the neonate are intravenous, inhaled (if direct action in the lung is required), rectal and buccal.

Distribution

Distribution into fat- or water-based tissue is affected by the amount of fat or water tissue available. Neonates have variable amounts of fat tissue. Preterm neonates of 29 weeks or less and those who have not been able to grow fully in the uterus may have little body fat. Term neonates still have proportionally higher amounts of body water than adults. This affects the distribution of lipid-soluble drugs, for example diazepam, where the volume of distribution is decreased in neonates with a smaller proportion of body fat. Practically, this means the drug is less likely to accumulate in the body fat, and the elimination half-life of the drug may be decreased, requiring lower doses or longer dose intervals. Conversely, neonates born to diabetic mothers may have a larger than average amount of body fat. Practically, this means the drug accumulates in the body fat, creating a 'reservoir' and the elimination half-life of the drug may be increased.

STOP AND THINK

Why might benzodiazepine withdrawal be a problem in a neonate born to a benzodiazepine-addicted mother with diabetes?

Protein binding of the drug to albumin in the plasma is also affected in the neonate, as preterm neonates born at 27 weeks or less have albumin concentrations that are only two-thirds of those seen in adults. This reduces the proportion of each dose which is bound to plasma albumin and hence increases the proportion of free, unbound drug that can then act on the target sites. An example of a drug affected by this is furosemide and practically it means lower doses are required.

Metabolism

At birth many enzyme systems involved in drug metabolism are not completely mature, therefore the metabolism of most drugs is reduced.

Phase I metabolising enzymes (cytochrome P450 enzymes) generally reach adult capacity around the age of 6 months although the enzymes involved in phase II conjugation reactions take longer to reach adult levels, with glucuronidation pathways not reaching adult levels until around 3 years of age. It is this lack of conjugating activity that can result in grey baby syndrome following the use of chloramphenicol in neonates. Chloramphenicol is metabolized in the liver by glucuronidation, but the neonatal liver is unable to metabolise chloramphenicol effectively and so chloramphenicol accumulates in the body and can reach toxic levels (Cummings et al. 2022). Some neonates are born with hyperbilirubinaemia, where there are high levels of unconjugated bilirubin in the blood. As bilirubin competes for binding sites involved in the metabolism of drugs in the liver, the metabolism of some drugs may be reduced, resulting in longer half-lives.

Excretion

Neonates have reduced renal function, which will cause slow elimination of most drugs, therefore half-lives are longer and dose intervals should be extended or doses reduced. For drugs that have a narrow therapeutic index, close monitoring of plasma drug levels should be carried out.

PRACTICE APPLICATION

Gentamicin, an antibiotic commonly used in neonates, is usually dosed at 24- or 36-hour intervals.

PAEDIATRICS

As with neonates, it is important to remember when calculating drug dosages that children are not 'small adults'. Their body systems may still be immature, which affects their ability to handle drugs. The standard reference source for drug doses in children is the BNF-C.

Absorption

Very young children have a reduced concentration of gastric acid and reduced gut motility when compared to older children. This results in longer dissolution times of some solid dosage forms that need gastric acid to be absorbed and increased time in the stomach for absorption. On balance, a longer absorption time has a greater clinical effect, increasing the peak plasma levels of some drugs. Older children have similar oral absorption rates to adults. As in neonates, topical absorption of drugs is dependent on skin thickness, and younger children have relatively thin skin, leading to increased absorption of drugs and other agents by the topical route. Absorption from inhaled drugs is similar to that in adults, provided the child has an adequate inhaler technique.

Distribution

Children under the age of 1 year still have proportionally higher amounts of body water than adults. This affects distribution in a similar way to neonates. Protein binding of drugs in young children is reduced, again due to low albumin levels.

Metabolism

The immaturity of enzyme systems involved in metabolism is corrected as children get older and, due to the relative increase in hepatic blood flow and liver size in children compared to adults, these systems actually function more efficiently. When looked at in terms of doses in milligrams per kilogram (mg/kg), children require a higher dose of theophylline than adults, as the metabolism is more efficient in children until their enzyme systems are fully mature.

Excretion

In young children the kidneys are still immature, resulting in lower rates of glomerular filtration and tubular secretion (glomerular filtration rates do not reach adult levels until 6 months of age, while tubular secretion does not reach adult levels until around 8 months of age). Practically this increases the half-life of renally cleared drugs, for example gentamicin. However, once children reach about 8 months old, kidney function is mature and the excretion of renally cleared drugs is comparable to that of adults.

PRACTICE APPLICATION

Doses for children are usually in mg/kg, divided into age categories. This takes into account the pharmacokinetic differences in different age groups.

ELDERLY

As adults grow older changes occur in their body composition and ability to handle drugs. There are no specific reference texts for dosing of drugs in the elderly, but the *British National Formulary* (BNF) sometimes lists dosing schedules for the elderly alongside those for adults.

Absorption

Older people have a reduced concentration of gastric acid, so their gastric fluid is less acidic than in younger adults, which may increase the dissolution time of drugs in the stomach. Gastric emptying is delayed as peristalsis slows and can result in drugs being present in the stomach for longer. These factors have a counteracting effect on each other when it comes to drug absorption. There is also reduced blood flow to the gastrointestinal (GI) tract, which in theory reduces the amount of drug carried away from the GI area to the rest of the body. In practice, there is no real change in drug absorption as a person gets older.

Distribution

The balance of body water to body fat changes as a person gets older, with an increase in the body fat. This affects the distribution of water- and lipid-soluble drugs. There is also a reduction in muscle mass. Benzodiazepines (e.g., diazepam) are lipid soluble, and so they deposit into the increased body fat to create reservoirs. This increases the length of time the drug is in the body to exert an effect, and so longer dosing intervals are needed. Digoxin is highly bound to muscle and therefore it has a reduced volume of distribution due to reduced lean body mass. This leads to increased plasma concentrations after a standard dose. There is also a lower concentration of plasma proteins, including albumin, in the elderly. This means there are fewer plasma proteins for drugs to bind to, for example warfarin, resulting in a higher proportion of the drug dose being 'free' and able to exert an effect. These distribution effects are usually only important when starting a drug or increasing the dose, as once steady state is achieved the body will balance the effect of distribution with metabolism and elimination.

Metabolism

Metabolism of drugs is generally reduced because of reduced hepatic blood flow and a reduced liver mass and functioning liver cells. There may also be altered first-pass metabolism as liver function is reduced. Drugs which are pro-drugs and need converting by the liver to their active forms are less effective. Drugs which are not pro-drugs but undergo first-pass metabolism, for example nifedipine, will undergo less metabolism, so higher plasma concentrations are available to exert a therapeutic effect. As patients age, their hepatic metabolism may be reduced and in the case of diazepam, the plasma half-life increases by approximately an hour for each year of ageing.

As the elderly usually have concomitant medical conditions and exact liver function is hard to measure, it is hard to predict the exact effect on the metabolism of specific drugs.

Excretion

The glomerular filtration rate declines by about 1% per year from the age of 40, so the effects of excretion can be seen in adults from a relatively early age. Estimated glomerular filtration rate (eGFR) (Chapter 19) is often reported as standard and this, once recalculated to take into account body surface area, is used to measure renal function when deciding on the degree of renal failure a patient has. The more traditional creatinine clearance (CrCl), calculated using the Cockcroft–Gault equation (Box 11.1), is also used to calculate and quantify renal function for drug dosing. The Cockcroft–Gault equation is not completely accurate for the older patient, although age and weight are factors in it. Older people have less muscle mass, as discussed earlier, and so produce less

BOX 11.1 COCKCROFT GAULT EQUATION

Cockcroft-Gault equation

$$CrCl = \frac{(140 - age)\,(weight)\,(sex\ factor)}{serum\ creatinine}$$

Sex factor: males = 1.23, females = 1.04

creatinine from muscle breakdown. They may therefore have artificially low creatinine levels, and therefore a lower CrCl than their actual renal function.

Renal function is often adversely affected in the short term by dehydration and urinary tract infections, so in general drug doses for newly started drugs are not altered until the patient is fully hydrated and CrCl is re-measured. Drugs the patient has been on for some time with no problem may need their doses decreasing in the short term if the patient develops an infection to avoid toxicity, for example digoxin. Drugs may also affect renal function, for example non-steroidal anti-inflammatory drugs (NSAIDs), so caution is needed when using these drugs at all in the elderly.

STOP AND THINK

Why is the BNF dose of imidapril in the elderly listed as initially 2.5 mg, maximum 10 mg daily?

PHARMACODYNAMIC VARIABILITY

Pharmacodynamic changes can be described as changes in the responsiveness of the organs of the body that cause the changes in the effect of the drugs.

ELDERLY

The elderly can show either an increased or decreased effect of the drug when compared to younger adults (Table 11.1).

Table 11.1 Pharmacodynamic changes in the elderly

Drug class	Pharmacodynamic change	Effect	Action taken
Benzodiazepines	Increased affinity or increased numbers of benzodiazepine binding sites	Increased sensitivity to therapeutic and side effects	Use lower doses and short-acting drugs, e.g., lorazepam
β-blockers	Fall in the responsiveness of beta receptors	Reduced sensitivity to therapeutic effects Heart failure	Avoid monotherapy and use other drug classes where possible
	Reduced cardiac reserves		Avoid non-selective β-blockers, use cardio-selective ones with caution
Anticholinergics	Reduced number of cholinergic neurones	Increased sensitivity to side effects, e.g., confusion	Avoid where possible
Tricyclics, phenothiazines and levo-dopa	Reduced responsiveness of baro-receptors to blood pressure changes	Greater risk of falls due to postural hypotension	Avoid where possible, monitor postural hypotension if drug is used

LIVER FAILURE

A patient with impaired hepatic function will have limited ability to metabolise drugs. The drug plasma level then builds up and becomes toxic. To avoid this, the dosing interval is usually extended and sometimes the dose will need to be decreased. Some drugs undergo first-pass metabolism in the liver to become active. Their bioavailability will be decreased and doses may have to be increased. Other drugs undergo extensive first-pass metabolism and their bioavailability will be increased, with more drug available to have an effect. Doses may have to be decreased.

Drugs interact with the liver in three basic ways. They can either induce or inhibit liver enzymes, and therefore affect the metabolism of themselves and other drugs, and they can cause drug-induced liver disease, in which case their metabolism can be affected as described above and careful drug choice in liver disease is necessary.

Inducing or inhibiting liver enzymes

Some drugs are metabolised by enzyme systems in the liver. The main system involved is the cytochrome P450 system (Chapter 9), although others are involved too. Drugs can have an effect on a patient's liver enzymes. They can either induce their activity (make them work more) or inhibit their activity (make them work less) to have an effect on the metabolism of the drug, other hepatically metabolised drugs and anything else metabolised by the enzyme. A drug that inhibits enzymes will also inhibit its own metabolism along with other things. If one of these enzyme-inducing or -inhibiting drugs is prescribed, you will need to consider their effect on the other drugs prescribed and may need to alter the drugs used or change doses. It is important to slowly increase the doses of enzyme-inducing drugs until the target dose is reached.

STOP AND THINK

Phenytoin is an enzyme inducer. What effect might be seen if phenytoin is added to the prescription of a patient who used the oral contraceptive pill?

Drug-induced liver disease

Drugs can cause actual liver disease or they can change a patient's liver function test results without causing overt illness. An example of this is rifampicin, commonly used to treat tuberculosis, which can cause a benign rise in liver function tests, but sometimes liver impairment.

Drug choice in liver disease

It is hard to quantify a patient's degree of liver failure and therefore predict their response to drug doses. When prescribing from a class of drugs, those with shorter half-lives are preferable to those with longer half-lives. Patients with liver failure may develop hepatic encephalopathy, which is a complication typified by a reduced level of consciousness and confusion. Drugs that have side effects of drowsiness or confusion should be avoided in these patients to allow prompt diagnosis of encephalopathy and to prevent worsening of the drowsiness. The symptoms of liver failure include fluid retention, especially ascites and an increased risk of GI bleeds. Drugs that can cause fluid retention or GI bleeds should be avoided in liver failure, for example NSAIDs.

STOP AND THINK

Sulphonylureas, used to treat diabetes, have varying half-lives. The symptoms of hypoglycaemia include drowsiness. Which is the better drug to treat diabetes in liver disease: gliclazide (short half-life) or glibenclamide (long half-life)?

Some patients with liver failure also develop kidney failure as a result of portal hypertension. Extra care is needed in these patients to avoid worsening both their kidney and liver failure.

RENAL IMPAIRMENT

It is possible to quantify kidney failure using the patient's serum creatinine to estimate GFR, as discussed earlier. There are many reference sources that give information on drug doses in the varying degrees of kidney failure, and the drug-specific details in each monograph of the BNF are the simplest.

A patient with impaired renal function will have limited ability to excrete renally cleared drugs. The drug plasma level then builds up and becomes toxic. To avoid this, the dosing interval is usually extended and sometimes the dose needs to be decreased. As with liver failure, drugs with shorter half-lives are preferable to those with longer half-lives in the same class. Drugs that act on the kidney will have reduced efficacy, for example thiazide diuretics and nitrofurantoin. Alternatives should be used. As a general rule, drugs that can cause or worsen kidney failure should be avoided. If the patient is on dialysis, either haemodialysis or peritoneal dialysis, the drug dose and choice may be affected. There are specialist reference sources which give advice in these situations.

PHARMACOGENETICS

This is an emerging area of therapy, where genetic variations in metabolic enzymes and receptors lead to pharmacokinetic and pharmacodynamic differences between individuals.

Pharmacokinetic variations

A common cause of the pharmacogenetic variation is via single nucleotide polymorphisms, where a single mutation in the genetic code leads to amino acid substitutions in the relevant protein. This was first identified in the 1970s when some patients (1–3%) were poor metabolisers of the old antihypertensive debrisoquine and became severely hypotensive due to impaired metabolism. Subsequent to this observation, the metabolic difference has been ascribed to genetic isoforms of CYP2D6, with patients being either poor metabolisers, wild type or ultra-rapid metabolisers (due to multiple copies of the gene). Patients who are poor metabolisers will have prolonged half-lives of active drugs such as debrisoquine, hence the hypotensive effect, but have reduced ability to activate pro-drugs such as codeine. In the case of the latter, poor metabolisers have impaired ability to activate codeine to morphine and so codeine has little or no activity in these patients. There are ethnicity differences in terms of CYP polymorphisms that can impact how well people respond to certain drugs (McGraw and Waller 2012), an example of this is that patients of Chinese origin have a high prevalence of different CYPD2 genotypes and are less likely to benefit from codeine.

The antiplatelet drug clopidogrel requires metabolic activation via CYP2C19. Due to genetic differences around 4–30% of patients are resistant to clopidogrel because of the CYP2C19*C allele, but patients with CYP2C19*17 have increased bioactivation and so are at increased risk of bleeding.

Many antipsychotic and antidepressant drugs are metabolized by CYP2C19 or CYP2D6 enzymes, of which there are different alleles present in different ethnic groups that can influence the effectiveness of these drugs. For example, 31.6% of Europeans are CYP2C19 ultrarapid metabolisers, meaning drugs metabolized by CYP2C19 may be less effective in this group. On the other hand, 14.2% of East Asians are CYP2C19 poor metabolisers so drugs may be more effective in this population (Milosavljević et al. 2021).

Pharmacodynamic variations

Drug receptors may also show genetic variations that can affect drug–receptor interactions, desensitization and disease progression. For example, genetic variations in the β_1-adrenoceptor are associated with differences in risk factors for heart failure and in the response to β-blocker treatment (Liu et al. 2012). In the treatment of asthma, variations in the β_2-adrenoceptor are associated with increased responsiveness to long-acting β_2-adrenoceptor agonists.

Pharmacogenetics and adverse drug reactions

Pharmacogenetic variation can also increase the risk of adverse events. In the case of simvastatin, the OATP1B1 transporter is encoded by SLCO1B1 and effluxes simvastatin to remove it from the circulation. However, in patients with the SLCO1B1*5 variant there is loss of function, with impaired efflux of simvastatin, leading to increased plasma concentrations and increasing the risk of myopathy.

Another example is Stevens-Johnson syndrome, which is a severe dermatological reaction to certain drugs and in the case of carbamazepine is associated with the HLA-B*15:02 allele. This allele is rare in Europeans but more prevalent in Han Chinese and Thai populations, thus these patient groups should be screened for this allele prior to treatment.

SUMMARY

Neonates, particularly very preterm neonates, have different pharmacokinetics and require different dosing schedules from children.

- Drug distribution in the tissues of the neonate is variable and can affect the half-lives of both water- and lipid-soluble drugs.

- Neonates have a reduced concentration of plasma albumin, which affects the distribution of protein-bound drugs.

- Due to immaturity of kidney and liver cells, neonates have impaired metabolism and elimination. This tends to increase the half-life of drugs.

- Older children have more mature body systems than younger children.

- Doses for children are usually in mg/kg, divided into age categories. This takes into account the pharmacokinetic differences in different age groups.

- The proportion of body water to body fat changes in the elderly, resulting in changes in the distribution of both water- and lipid-soluble drugs.

- The elderly have a reduced concentration of plasma albumin, which affects the distribution of protein-bound drugs.

- The function of liver and kidney cells deteriorates with age, which affects ability to metabolise and eliminate drugs.

- The elderly also undergo pharmacodynamic changes in the way they handle drugs. This is due to changes in responsiveness of the organs of the body, which cause the changes in effect of the drugs.

- Drugs whose side effects mimic the symptoms of liver failure should be avoided in patients with liver failure.

- Patients with liver failure will have reduced liver enzyme induction or inhibition, which may affect the interaction of drugs with each other.

- Kidney failure can be quantified using the estimated glomerular filtration rate (eGFR) but calculated creatinine clearance (CrCl) from the Cockcroft–Gault equation may also be used when working out drug doses.

- Drugs which act directly on the kidney may have a reduced effect in kidney failure and should be avoided.

- Drugs which can worsen kidney failure should be avoided in patients with pre-existing kidney failure.

- Genetic variations in metabolic pathways can influence plasma half-lives and impaired activations of pro-drugs.

- Genetic variations in target proteins can influence adverse drug reactions and the responses to pharmacotherapy.

ACTIVITY

1. Which of the following statements regarding drug dosing in neonatal patients are correct?

   - The skin is more permeable to agents.   True/False
   - Body systems are mature.   True/False
   - Plasma albumin concentration is reduced.   True/False
   - Gentamicin dose intervals are increased.   True/False
   - Therapeutic drug monitoring is not performed.   True/False

2. Which of the following statements regarding drug dosing in children are correct?

   - The skin is more permeable to agents.   True/False
   - Young children have a higher amount of body water than adults.   True/False
   - Doses of albumin-bound drugs may need altering.   True/False
   - The adult BNF can be used for children's doses.   True/False
   - Children's doses are usually quoted in mg/kg.   True/False

3. Which of the following statements regarding drug dosing in the elderly are correct?

   - Generally lower doses are used.   True/False
   - Generally shorter dosage intervals are used.   True/False
   - Renal function improves with age.   True/False
   - Lower loading doses of warfarin are used.   True/False
   - Short-acting benzodiazepines are preferred.   True/False

4. Which of the following statements regarding drug dosing in renal impairment are correct?

   - No dose amendments are required.   True/False
   - Renal function cannot be easily categorised.   True/False

- NSAIDs are drugs of choice. True/False

- Drug dose is not affected by dialysis. True/False

- Generally longer dosage intervals are used. True/False

5. Which of the following statements regarding drug dosing in liver impairment are correct?

- NSAIDs are drugs of choice. True/False

- Degree of liver impairment can be calculated. True/False

- Long-acting drugs are preferred. True/False

- Drugs which cause drowsiness are preferred. True/False

- Enzyme activity can be affected by drugs. True/False

REFERENCES

Cummings, E.D., Kong, E.L and Edens, M.A. (2022) Gray baby syndrome. In: *StatPearls* [Internet]. StatPearls Publishing, Treasure Island, FL. PMID: 28846297.

Liu, W.-N., Fu, K.-L., Gao, H.-Y., et al. (2012) β1 adrenergic receptor polymorphisms and heart failure: A meta-analysis on susceptibility to β-blocker therapy and prognosis. *PLoS One* 7(7):e27659.

McGraw, J.E. and Waller, D. (2012) Cytochrome P450 variations in different ethnic populations. *Expert Opin Drug Metab Toxicol* 8(3):371–382.

Milosavljević, F., Bukvić, N., Pavlović, Z., et al. (2021) Association of CYP2C19 and CYP2D6 poor and intermediate metabolizer status with antidepressant and antipsychotic exposure. A systematic review and meta-analysis *JAMA Psych* 78(3):270–280.

FURTHER READING

Armour, D. and Cairns, C. (2002) *Medicines in the Elderly*. Pharmaceutical Press, London.

British National Formulary (online). BMJ Group and Pharmaceutical Press, London. https://bnf.nice.org.uk/.

British National Formulary for Children (online). BMJ Group and Pharmaceutical Press, London. https://bnfc.nice.org.uk/.

Corsonello, A., Pedone, C., Corica, F., et al., Gruppo Italiano di Farmacovigilanza nell'Anziano (GIFA) Investigators (2005) Concealed renal insufficiency and adverse drug reactions in elderly hospitalized patients. *Arch Intern Med* 165:790–795.

Kanneh, A. (2002) Paediatric pharmacological principles: an update. Part 2. Pharmacokinetics: absorption and distribution. *Paediatr Nurs* 14(9):39–43.

Kanneh, A. (2002) Paediatric pharmacological principles: an update. Part 3. Pharmacokinetics: metabolism and excretion. *Paediatr Nurs* 14(10):39–43.

Lichtman, S.M. (2007) Pharmacokinetics and pharmacodynamics in the elderly. *Clin Adv Hematol Oncol* 5:181–182.

Peters, S. (2007) Part IV: Genetic variations on beta2-adrenergic receptors: long-acting and short-acting beta2-agonists and therapeutic response. *Curr Med Res Opin* Suppl 3:S29–S36.

Ritter, J.M., Flower, R., Henderson, G., et al. (2023) *Rang and Dale's Pharmacology*, 10th edn. Elsevier, Amsterdam.

Ritter, J.M., Lewis, L.D., Mant, T.G.K. and Ferro, A (2008) *A Textbook of Clinical Pharmacology*, 5th edn. Hodder Arnold, London.

Turnheim, K. (2003) When drug therapy gets old: pharmacokinetics and pharmacodynamics in the elderly. *Exp Gerontol* 38:843–853.

Whittlesea, C. and Hodson, K (2018) *Clinical Pharmacy and Therapeutics*, 6th edn. Elsevier Health Sciences, Edinburgh.

Waller, D.G., Sampson, A.P. and Hitchings, A.W. (2021) *Medical Pharmacology and Therapeutics*, 6th edn. Elsevier, Edinburgh.

Winter, M. (2004) *Basic Clinical Pharmacokinetics*, 4th edn, Lippincott, Williams and Wilkins, Philadelphia.

CHAPTER 12

Polypharmacy and Medicines Optimisation

Daniel Shipley

LEARNING OUTCOMES

By the end of this chapter the reader should be able to:

- define the terms 'polypharmacy' and 'medicines optimisation'

- appreciate the clinical significance and personal burden of polypharmacy

- appreciate why certain patient/client groups are at greater risk of/from polypharmacy

- identify commonly used drugs that are particularly problematic with regard to polypharmacy

- understand the role of medicines optimisation in the prevention and resolution of polypharmacy

- discuss the utility of medicines optimisation strategies/toolkits.

WHAT IS POLYPHARMACY?

Definitions of polypharmacy exist based on the number of medications present. In a systematic review conducted by Masnoon et al. (2017), polypharmacy was deemed to be present when five or more daily medications were in situ. This is counterbalanced by the World Health Organization (WHO), which implores clinicians to place their focus on evidence-based practice rather than a numerical value (Antimisiaris and Cutler 2017).

Polypharmacy is, in essence, a term that refers to the use of multiple drugs by an individual. Over the years, the word has acquired a negative connotation, but both appropriate and problematic examples of polypharmacy are seen in clinical practice.

Appropriate polypharmacy can be classified as an optimised combination of medication that helps to maintain the individual's quality of life and minimise harm. The appropriateness of this combination is underpinned by patient-centred care, regular review and evidenced-based practice.

Problematic polypharmacy is typically an inappropriate drug combination where the intended benefit is not realised. The collection of agents is unlikely to be evidence-based, potentially comprising interactions, a high pill burden and a proliferation of adverse drug reactions (ADRs) (Chapter 13). In many cases, the side effects themselves are treated with medication and the patient struggles to adhere to the regimen.

From a UK perspective, polypharmacy is a growing concern. National Health Service (NHS) England prescribing data have shown a 46.8% increase in the number of items dispensed between 2006 and 2016 (Royal Pharmaceutical Society 2022). A study in 2018 illustrated a quadrupling in the number of people exposed to polypharmacy, i.e., five or more medications, over the last 20 years (Gao et al. 2018). On a macro level, polypharmacy could be seen as an inevitable by-product of an expanding and aging population contending with multiple long-term conditions. By 2039, the

The New Prescriber: An Integrated Approach to Medical and Non-medical Prescribing, Second Edition.
Edited by Joanne Lymn, Alison Mostyn, Roger Knaggs, Michael Randall, and Dianne Bowskill.
© 2024 John Wiley & Sons Ltd. Published 2024 by John Wiley & Sons Ltd.

anticipated life expectancy in the United Kingdom for men and women will be 93 and 96 years, respectively. This essentially means that a growing number of people will spend a significant proportion of their life contending with ailing health and the medication associated with that.

The causes of polypharmacy are numerous and multifaceted. Loosely speaking, they can be divided into (a) the behaviours of individuals, namely healthcare professionals and patients, and (b) an aging population contending with multiple comorbidities. From a healthcare professional point of view, the proliferation of problematic polypharmacy typically has its roots in a reactive, often paternalistic, approach to medication prescribing and review. This prescribing pattern is sometimes referred to as a 'cascade', i.e. a sequence of events involving misdiagnosis, suboptimal monitoring/review, and the misinterpretation of an ADR as a new medical complaint.

PRACTICE APPLICATION

The relationship that exists between practitioner and patient undoubtedly influences the incidence of polypharmacy. Shared decision making and patient-centred care are thought to promote several positive outcomes, namely medication adherence, prudent service use and engagement with review. Passive or paternalistic receipt of medical care, meanwhile, has the propensity to generate polypharmacy.

WHICH PATIENT GROUPS ARE MOST IMPACTED?

OLDER PATIENTS AND MULTIMORBIDITY

Chronic diseases are more prevalent in older people and in many instances several morbidities co-present. It is common therefore to see the management of multiple ailments being treated by numerous pharmacological interventions. This challenge is further complicated by pharmacokinetic changes secondary to either older age or disease.

For example, if we focus on the inevitable age-related decline in renal function, we can conclude that drugs predominantly excreted by the kidney are more likely to accumulate (Chapter 11). These excretory mechanisms will not eliminate the drug as they ordinarily should. This may lead to an increased prevalence of side effects, which could be misconstrued as a new medical condition, prompting the initiation of further medication. By prolonging the half-life of a drug, exposure will increase and so will the likelihood of interactions with concomitant medication.

STOP AND THINK

Can you think of any other physiological changes in the older person that may affect the performance of medication?

PATIENTS WITH POOR ADHERENCE

Adherence is a measure of how well the patient's relationship with therapy synchronises with clinician recommendations (NICE 2022). A report from the WHO indicated that only half of medication prescribed globally is used as directed (Brown and Bussell 2011). It is fair therefore to conclude that many patients are not realising the full impact of their intended treatment.

Without properly establishing the extent of an individual's adherence, clinicians can erroneously assume that treatment failure has occurred. This can potentially lead to the prescribing of additional medication, an increased pill burden and the propensity for both interactions and ADRs.

Adherence to medication is subject to several variables, including personality traits, cultural beliefs and mental health. For example, older adults emanating from the far east of Asia typically have a deep trust and even a reliance on physicians, seeing them as figures of authority. In addition, the link between mental health challenges and poor medication adherence has long been established with a range of cognitive, behavioural, practical and medication contributing factors.

PATIENTS WITH LEARNING DISABILITIES, AUTISM OR A DUAL DIAGNOSIS

People with intellectual disabilities (IDs) are often prescribed medication to treat mental health conditions and behavioural issues such as aggression. In many instances off-label prescribing occurs and the rationale for use is poorly documented. This can negatively affect a clinician's capacity to review. The drugs employed are often psychotropic, many of which can cause significant side effects, such as weight gain, type 2 diabetes and fatigue.

Whilst the life expectancy of those with IDs is significantly lower than that of the general population, advancing age and multimorbidities underline a highly vulnerable, often maligned population who may struggle to communicate their challenges. Three major enquiries (spearheaded by Public Health England, the Care Quality Commission and NHS Improving Quality) identified 35,000 people with IDs in UK being medicated for severe mental illness without clinical justification. In many cases, administration of psychotropic drugs proceeded for many years without review and the requisite liaison with carers and family members.

NHS England have attempted to raise awareness of this issue through an initiative called Stopping over medication of people with a learning disability (STOMP). This project involves healthcare institutions around the country working collaboratively to evoke cultural change amongst clinicians (NHS England 2022).

DURING DISCHARGE AND ADMISSION

When patients are discharged back into the community or admitted to hospital, they encounter a healthcare interface. During these transitions, the likelihood of medication errors can increase. In some instances, this can result in polypharmacy, invariably due to a breakdown in communication between healthcare providers. Two processes fraught with complication include medicines reconciliation and discharge planning.

Medicines reconciliation is not simply a process of ensuring that regular medication is charted on a drug card, but also clearly documenting the reasons why certain agents have been held, stopped or amended. A key component of discharge planning meanwhile is ensuring that changes to a patient's medication are communicated to clinicians in primary care. If either of these two processes falter, there is a strong possibility that medication could be erroneously introduced or continued.

PATIENTS WHO HAVE BEEN HISTORICALLY UNDER-REPRESENTED IN DRUG TRIALS

Women receiving medication are statistically more likely to experience ADRs compared to men. The reasons are multifaceted and, in some instances, not entirely clear. From a physiological point of view, female patients tend to have a lower glomerular filtration rate compared to their male counterparts and a faster rate of age-related decline. In addition, a higher incidence of chronic kidney disease is observed in Black, Hispanic and Asian populations relative to White.

These examples illustrate how ethnicity, gender and genetic variability influence the kinetic performance of a drug within a given population (Chapter 11). This is further complicated due to the under-representation of women and certain ethnic groups in drug trials. Given the fact that dosing regimens are typically underpinned by population kinetics, there is a strong possibility that certain populations are being overmedicated. The inextricable link between ADRs and polypharmacy is likely to yield a higher pill burden in these groups.

STOP AND THINK

Can you explain the link between genetic polymorphism and hepatic drug metabolism?

WHAT ARE THE IMPLICATIONS FOR HEALTHCARE SERVICES?

Working on the premise that polypharmacy can potentially lead to more ADRs and interactions, we can conclude that the extreme ramifications of this could lead to hospitalisation. A prospective analysis conducted in 2022 found that 16.5% of medical admissions to Liverpool University Hospital Foundation Trust were due to ADRs. The study was conducted over a 1-month period (Osanlou et al. 2022)

Assessment tools generated by the research group graded 18.4% and 21.1% of ADRs as either 'avoidable' or 'possibly avoidable', respectively. The average length of stay was 6.1 days, generating a direct cost of £490,716 to the Trust. Based on admission data from other care facilities around the United Kingdom, the projected yearly cost to the NHS in England was £2.21 billion (Osanlou et al. 2022).

WHICH DRUGS ARE MOST PROBLEMATIC?

Providing a list of problematic drugs is almost impossible because the severity of risk is very much dependent on the context and the individual. Most tools that identify points of intervention are typically divided by condition, for example β blockers in asthma or antiplatelets (rather than anti-coagulants) in atrial fibrillation.

It is possible, however, to identify drugs that are frequent polypharmacy protagonists. One such example is proton pump inhibitors (PPIs) such as omeprazole and lansoprazole (Chapter 16). A contributor to their inappropriate use includes off-label, undocumented reasons for prescribing, leading to inappropriate continuation and absence of review.

This can be problematic, particularly in older patients, where long exposure to PPIs is associated with an increased risk of bone fracture, *Clostridium difficile* infections and interstitial nephritis. Furthermore, omeprazole can act as a mild CYP450 enzyme inhibitor, moderately increasing exposure to concomitant medication that shares the same metabolic pathway.

Polypharmacy in some instances can exist beyond the control of a non-medical prescriber. PPIs such as esomeprazole have become available to buy in supermarkets over recent years. Whilst the availability of drugs outside of a prescription has several potential benefits, licence reclassification can reduce the opportunity for medication review.

General Sales List medicines can also be problematic. Inappropriate and long-term administration of ibuprofen, for example, is fraught with complications given that non-steroidal anti-inflammatory drugs are a major cause of adverse renal effects, gastrointestinal complications, worsening heart failure and significant interactions with other medication.

STOP AND THINK

What other drugs have you encountered that are implicated in polypharmacy or simply increase pill burden?

MEDICINES OPTIMISATION

Medicines optimisation is an approach that aims to maximise the intended benefit of medication to a given individual. In many ways, medicines optimisation could be characterised as a preventative strategy to tackle the proliferation of inappropriate polypharmacy. The goals of medicines optimisation are outlined in Box 12.1.

BOX 12.1	THE GOALS OF MEDICINES OPTIMISATION (NHS ENGLAND 2023)

To help patients:

- improve their outcomes
- take medicines correctly

- avoid taking unnecessary medicines
- reduce wastage of medicines
- improve medicines safety

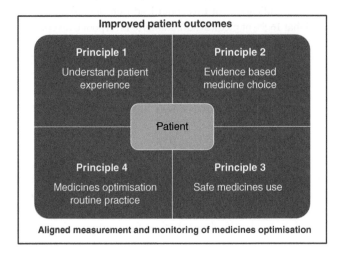

FIGURE 12.1   Medicines optimisation based on the NHS England medicines optimisation model (NHS England 2023).

NHS England has proposed four principles that healthcare professionals should embrace to embed medicines optimisation in their practice. The principles, understanding the patient experience, evidence-based medicine choice, medicines optimisation as routine practice and safe medicines use, are considered from a patient perspective, as shown in Figure 12.1. None of these principles are effective in isolation and they must be combined (NHS England 2023). A consistent approach to monitoring and follow-up across the healthcare service, together with robust communication, facilitates a culture where medicines optimisation is ingrained. A patient-centred approach should sit at the heart of this process.

PRINCIPLE 1: AIM TO UNDERSTAND THE PATIENT'S EXPERIENCE

To successfully optimise medicine use, clinicians need to cultivate a concordant relationship with their patients. Reaching a shared agreement with the service user about therapeutic goals is associated with desirable outcomes, including medication adherence and follow up. This can only be achieved if the patient's relationship with the medication is fully understood by the prescriber. Simple examples include patient working patterns, dexterity and previous experiences with therapy.

PRINCIPLE 2: EVIDENCE-BASED CHOICE OF MEDICINES

Desirable outcomes for individuals, patient populations and the wider healthcare service can be obtained by following evidence-based literature and selecting cost-effective treatments. Equally, this approach can promote the deprescribing of inappropriate medicines. Possessing knowledge and being sympathetic towards patient-specific factors means that clinical guidelines can be appropriately tailored to the needs of the individual.

PRINCIPLE 3: ENSURE MEDICINES USE IS AS SAFE AS POSSIBLE

'Safe use of medication' is a broad term that encapsulates minimising unwanted effects and interactions along with improving the systems and processes supporting patient care. Several desirable by-products can be realised by avoiding harm, namely improved patient–clinician dynamics, safe disposal of medication and reduced hospital admissions. Appropriate and consistent lines of communication between healthcare professions are integral to these outcomes.

PRINCIPLE 4: MAKE MEDICINES OPTIMISATION PART OF ROUTINE PRACTICE

To be effective and yield consistently beneficial outcomes, medicines optimisation needs to be culturally embedded across an organisation. As service users engage with different healthcare providers, it is important that documentation and discussion take place to promote continuity. By understanding the patient's journey across various interfaces, clinicians are in a better position to signpost, safety net and communicate.

IMPLEMENTATION STRATEGIES

Whilst the Royal Pharmaceutical Society has neatly defined medicines optimisation (Royal Pharmaceutical Society 2013), the practicalities of designing or enacting strategies to facilitate this across a healthcare service can be found elsewhere. The following recommendations, whilst not exhaustive, have been made by the National Institute for Health and Care Excellence (NICE 2015).

(A) SYSTEMS WHICH HELP IDENTIFY AND REPORT PATIENT SAFETY INCIDENTS

Recording and reporting medication safety incidents is essential for root-cause analysis and the review of ineffectual or unsafe practice. This ambition can only be realised if an organisation champions transparency and frames incident reporting as an opportunity for learning. Reporting (and acting on) safety concerns is a mainstay of medicines optimisation, enabling Trusts to introduce supportive interventions. These may include the use of prescribing technology, i.e., automated safety alerts, interaction notifications etc. Studies have shown that clinical decisions support software can significantly decrease errors related to medication (Scott et al. 2011).

(B) COMMUNICATION STRATEGIES WHEN TRANSFERRING PATIENT CARE

It is important for prescribers to remember that the interfaces of patient care can increase the propensity for prescribing errors, polypharmacy and cost-inefficiencies. When patients are being transferred from one care setting to another, it is important that accurate information is shared with the new care provider. This information naturally needs to be received and acted on.

Various systems exist across the NHS that are designed to improve the quality of information sharing, many of which are computer enabled. A study by Mehta et al. (2017) demonstrated a statistically significant improvement ($P < 0.001$) in both the completeness and proportion of discharge summaries following the introduction of an electronic hospital communication system.

As with any process, however, the quality of digital delivery is reliant on human input. This was underlined in a 2014 study which evaluated adherence to National Prescribing Centre guidance for discharge communication. Despite the advent of computerised systems, a mere 48.9% of documentation was compliant with how changes to therapy should be recorded (Hammad et al. 2014).

(C) MEDICINES RECONCILIATION

Medicines reconciliation goes hand in hand with optimised communication when transferring a patient from one care setting to another. Medicines reconciliation is a process which ensures that prescribed medication synchronises with pre-admission/discharge practice. A key component of this process is therefore taking an accurate medication history.

This definition of medicines reconciliation, however, is simplistic. The need to hold, amend and refine medication invariably occurs at the interface, meaning that medicines reconciliation should also involve robust communication of changes.

MEDICINES OPTIMISATION TOOLKITS AND DEPRESCRIBING

Several tools have been devised to aid approaches to medicines optimisation. The STOPP/START criteria, for example, places emphasis on the initiation and de-prescribing of medication that is typically omitted or poorly reviewed in the elderly. STOPP stands for Screening Tool of Older Persons' potentially inappropriate Prescriptions. START meanwhile is an acronym for Screening Tool to Alert to Right Treatment (O'Mahony 2020).

PRACTICE APPLICATION

The acceptability of the STOPP/START tool in clinical practice is subject to debate and different levels of success. Several variables can influence its impact, namely the working dynamics between prescriber and pharmacist, inter-individual differences (i.e., clinical knowledge) and integration of the tool within digital prescribing platforms.

A less prescriptive tool which focuses on consultation approach rather than simply the scrutiny of drug combinations is called NO TEARS (see Box 12.2).

The purpose of this strategy is to provide clinicians with a consultation aid that lends itself to a broad range of clinical areas. By design NO TEARS is intended to be flexible, enabling the clinician to tailor it to their individual consultation style. The major limitation is the absence of definite, clinical recommendations (Lewis 2004).

STOP AND THINK

The STOPP criteria recommends that angiotensin-converting enzyme inhibitors should be reviewed in hyperkalaemia. Use the *British National Formulary* to identify why this might be the case.

| BOX 12.2 | NO TEARS MEDICINES OPTIMISATION TOOL (LEWIS 2004) |

Need and indication
Open questions
Tests and monitoring
Evidence and guidelines
Adverse events
Risk reduction or prevention
Simplification and switches

SUMMARY

- The word 'polypharmacy' describes a situation where multiple drugs are being administered to an individual. Both appropriate and inappropriate examples of polypharmacy are possible.

- Polypharmacy invariably occurs due to a prescribing pattern, sometimes referred to as a 'cascade', i.e., a sequence of events involving misdiagnosis, suboptimal monitoring/review and the misinterpretation of an adverse drug reaction as a new medical complaint.

- Polypharmacy is commonly seen in the older person, where age-related changed in physiology can increase the likelihood of adverse drug reactions and interactions.

- Suboptimal adherence to medication can increase the proliferation of polypharmacy because the desired therapeutic impact of medication is not fully realised. This can lead to the initiation of further agents.

- An initiative called STOMP, championed by NHS England, has been introduced to minimise polypharmacy those with disabilities, a patient group which has been historically overmedicated and infrequently reviewed.

- Healthcare interfaces, for example discharge and admission, can invariably present scenarios where medication errors occur. During patient transfer it is important that communication and documentation processes are robust.

- When treating individuals based on clinical guidelines, it is important to recognise that certain patient groups have been underrepresented in clinical drug trials, and personalisation of care may be necessary.

- Polypharmacy and the associated complications (e.g., adverse drug reactions, side-effect-related admissions etc.) are of considerable cost to the NHS.

- Certain drugs are more common culprits of polypharmacy than others, but the individual's relationship with these agents is an important variable.

- Medicines optimisation is an approach that aims to maximise the intended benefit of medication to a given individual. It is a strategy that can both prevent and rectify issues synonymous with polypharmacy.

- Medicines optimisation comprises four principles: aim to understand the patient's experience, evidence-based choice of medicines, ensure medicines use is as safe as possible and make medicines optimisation part of routine practice.

- For medicines optimisation to be possible, medicines reconciliation must be undertaken, a process that ensures that prescribed medication synchronises with pre-admission/discharge practice.

- Various tools exist that facilitate medicines optimisation, such as the STOPP/START criteria and NO TEARS. These instruments are not a substitute for patient-centred care and sound clinical reasoning.

ACTIVITY

1. Polypharmacy can be both appropriate and problematic.   True/False

2. Reduced kidney function can decrease the half-life of medication, thereby increasing the likelihood of adverse effects.   True/False

3. STOMP is a national project helping to stop the overmedication of people with a learning disability, autism or a dual diagnosis. True/False

4. Patient discharge is an example of a healthcare interface where the propensity for polypharmacy and/or medication errors increases. True/False

5. Caucasian patients are more likely to have kidney failure compared to Black African or Black Caribbean patients. True/False

6. Drugs implicated in polypharmacy are almost exclusively prescription-only medicines. True/False

7. Proton pump inhibitors (e.g., omeprazole) can cause drug interactions due to being mild enzyme inducers. True/False

8. The process of medicines optimisation comprises four key principles. True/False

9. Medicines reconciliation is a process that ensures that prescribed medication synchronises with pre-admission/discharge practice. True/False

10. The STOPP/START criteria are an example of a medicine optimisation tool. True/False

REFERENCES

Antimisiaris, D. and Cutler, T. (2017) Managing polypharmacy in the 15-minute office visit. *Prim Care* 44(3):413–428.

Brown, M.T. and Bussell, J.K. (2011) Medication adherence: WHO cares? *Mayo Clin Proc* 86(4):304–314.

Gao, L., Maidment, I., Matthews, F.E., Robinson, L., Brayne, C., Medical Research Council Cognitive Function and Ageing Study (2018) Medication usage change in older people (65+) in England over 20 years: findings from CFAS I and CFAS II. *Age Ageing* 47(2):220–225.

Hammad, E.A., Wright, D.J., Walton, C., Nunney, I. and Bhattacharya, D. (2014) Adherence to UK national guidance for discharge information: an audit in primary care. *Br J Clin Pharmacol* 78(6):1453–1464.

Lewis, T. (2004) Using the NO TEARS tool for medication review. *BMJ* 329(7463):434.

Masnoon, N., Shakib, S., Kalisch-Ellett, L. and Caughey, G.E. (2017) What is polypharmacy? A systematic review of definitions. *BMC Geriatr* 17(1):230.

Mehta, R.L., Baxendale, B., Roth, K., et al. (2017) Assessing the impact of the introduction of an electronic hospital discharge system on the completeness and timeliness of discharge communication: a before and after study. *BMC Health Serv Res* 17(624) https://doi.org/10.1186/s12913-017-2579-3.

NHS England (2022) Stopping over medication of people with a learning disability, autism or both (STOMP).

Improving Health. https://www.england.nhs.uk/learning-disabilities/improving-health/stomp/ (accessed 16 December 2022).

NHS England (2023) Medicines optimisation. https://www.england.nhs.uk/medicines-2/medicines-optimisation/ (accessed 31 January 2023).

NICE (2015) Medicines optimisation: the safe and effective use of medicines to enable the best possible outcomes. https://www.nice.org.uk/guidance/ng5 (accessed 1 Febraury 2023).

NICE (2022) Medicines adherence: involving patients in decisions about prescribed medicines and supporting adherence. https://www.nice.org.uk/guidance/cg76. (accessed 15 December 2022).

O'Mahony, D. (2020) STOPP/START criteria for potentially inappropriate medications/potential prescribing omissions in older people: origin and progress. *Expert Rev Clin Pharmacol* 13(1):15–22.

Osanlou, R., Walker, L., Hughes, D.A., Burnside, G. and Pirmohamed, M. (2022) Adverse drug reactions, multimorbidity and polypharmacy: a prospective analysis of 1 month of medical admissions. *BMJ Open* 12(7):e055551.

Royal Pharmaceutical Society (2013) Medicines Optimisation: Helping patients to make the most of medicines. https://www.nhs.uk/aboutNHSChoices/professionals/healthandcareprofessionals/your-pages/Documents/rps-medicines-optimisation.pdf (accessed 1 Febraury 2023).

Royal Pharmaceutical Society (2022) Polypharmacy: Getting our medicines right. https://www.rpharms.com/recognition/setting-professional-standards/polypharmacy-getting-our-medicines-right. (accessed 13 December 2022).

Scott, G.P., Shah, P., Wyatt, J.C., Makubate, B. and Cross, F.W. (2011) Making electronic prescribing alerts more effective: scenario-based experimental study in junior doctors. *J Am Med Inform Assoc* 18(6):789–798.

GUIDANCE

NHS England (2022) Stopping over medication of people with a learning disability, autism or both (STOMP). Improving Health. https://www.england.nhs.uk/learning-disabilities/improving-health/stomp/ (accessed 16 December 2022).

NHS England (2023) Medicines optimisation. https://www.england.nhs.uk/medicines-2/medicines-optimisation/ (accessed 31 January 2023).

NICE (2015) Medicines optimisation: the safe and effective use of medicines to enable the best possible outcomes. https://www.nice.org.uk/guidance/ng5 (accessed 1 Febraury 2023).

NICE (2022) Medicines adherence: involving patients in decisions about prescribed medicines and supporting adherence. https://www.nice.org.uk/guidance/cg76. (accessed 15 December 2022).

Royal Pharmaceutical Society (2013) Medicines Optimisation: Helping patients to make the most of medicines. https://www.nhs.uk/aboutNHSChoices/professionals/healthandcareprofessionals/your-pages/Documents/rps-medicines-optimisation.pdf (accessed 1 Febraury 2023).

Royal Pharmaceutical Society (2022) Polypharmacy: Getting our medicines right. https://www.rpharms.com/recognition/setting-professional-standards/polypharmacy-getting-our-medicines-right. (accessed 13 December 2022).

CHAPTER 13

Adverse Drug Reactions and Interactions

Alison Mostyn and Daniel Shipley

LEARNING OUTCOMES

By the end of this chapter the reader should be able to:

- describe the differences between type A and type B adverse drug reactions

- understand which patient groups are more susceptible to adverse drug reactions

- understand the different mechanisms of common adverse drug reactions

- identify and manage possible adverse drug reactions

- understand which adverse drug reactions must be reported to the MHRA using the Yellow Card system

- understand the different mechanisms of common drug and food interactions

- identify and manage drug–drug and drug–food interactions.

ADVERSE DRUG REACTIONS: SOME DEFINITIONS

An adverse drug reaction (ADR) is any undesirable effect of a drug that is not an anticipated therapeutic effect occurring during clinical use. The World Health Organization (WHO) definition of an adverse drug reaction is 'a response to a drug which is noxious, unintended and occurs at doses used in man for prophylaxis, diagnosis or therapy'. The UK Commission on Human Medicines defines an ADR as 'an unwanted or harmful reaction experienced after the administration of the drug or combination of drugs under normal conditions of use and suspected to be related to the drug'. Patients often call ADRs 'side effects'.

CLASSIFICATION OF ADRs

ADRs are usually classified into two types: A and B. Type A reactions are exaggerated (*A*ugmented) responses to the normal pharmacological action of the drug given at a therapeutic dose. These reactions are usually dose dependent: the higher the dose, the more likely a type A reaction is to occur. An example of this occurs with glicazide, where too high a dose can cause hypoglycaemia. This can be managed by reducing the dose.

Type B reactions are *B*izarre effects that are not predictable according to the drug's pharmacological action, and occur at any dose. An example of this is malignant hyperthermia after anaesthesia. These reactions can result in severe illness and death. Table 13.1 highlights other differences between these types of reactions.

SUSCEPTIBLE PATIENT GROUPS

There are certain patient groups that are particularly susceptible to ADRs (Table 13.2).

The New Prescriber: An Integrated Approach to Medical and Non-medical Prescribing, Second Edition.
Edited by Joanne Lymn, Alison Mostyn, Roger Knaggs, Michael Randall, and Dianne Bowskill.
© 2024 John Wiley & Sons Ltd. Published 2024 by John Wiley & Sons Ltd.

Table 13.1 Characteristics of type A and type B adverse drug reactions (adapted from Whittlesea and Hodson 2018)

	Type A (augmented response)	Type B (bizarre response)
Pharmacologically predictable	Yes	No
Dose-dependent	Yes	No
Incidence	High	Low
Time of occurrence	Soon after first dose or dose increase	Variable, can be months or even years into (or after) treatment
Morbidity	High	Low
Mortality	Low	High
Management	Dose reduction	Stop drug
Rechallenge	Yes, with caution	No

Table 13.2 Susceptible patient groups

Patient group	Reason
Polypharmacy	Multiple disease states and multiple drugs combine to cause interactions and ADRs
Elderly	Often have polypharmacy, also altered pharmacokinetics and pharmacodynamics
Young children	Altered pharmacokinetics and pharmacodynamics, also unlicensed and off-label use of drugs
Gender	Women are at greater risk of ADRs than men due to altered pharmacokinetics and pharmacodynamics
Concomitant disease	Multiple disease states and multiple drugs combine to cause interactions and ADRs Also altered pharmacokinetics
Race and genetics	Altered pharmacokinetics and pharmacodynamics

ADR, adverse drug reaction.

PRACTICE APPLICATION

Patients with liver failure who take a loop diuretic, for example furosemide, are prone to the ADR of hypokalaemia (low serum potassium). Such patients may be given a combination of a loop diuretic and a potassium-sparing diuretic, for example amiloride, in the form of co-amilofruse. The amiloride does not have a large diuretic effect but it does prevent loss of potassium ions, as an ADR.

MECHANISMS OF ADRS AND EXAMPLES

PHARMACEUTICAL CAUSES

ADRs can occur due to drug formulation, release characteristics from the dosage form and alterations in the amount of drug in the dosage form. A common example of this is symptoms of opioid overdose in heroin users when a particularly pure preparation of heroin is circulating on the streets. Another example is pain following too rapid administration of clarithromycin injection; this is due to the excipients in the injection form.

Poor formulations of drugs (e.g., the use of diethylene glycol as a solvent, which caused many deaths in the USA in the 1930s) can cause ADRs. Nowadays it is less likely for excipients to cause ADRs as they are strictly tested. The warnings associated with enoxaparin injection used in pregnant women, due to a toxic excipient, show that mistakes can still be made, even when strict quality control processes are in place. The increasing availability of fake or counterfeit drugs in the UK may see an increase in ADRs due to poor quality control and the use of banned excipients.

PHARMACOKINETIC CAUSES

Changes in pharmacokinetic parameters will cause changes in the concentration of drug at its site of action. Any increase in concentration of the drug may cause a type A ADR as there will effectively be an increased dose of the drug available to act on the target receptors. Elimination and metabolism are the main pharmacokinetic stages where changes can lead to ADRs.

Examples of metabolism ADRs include those associated with the cytochrome P450 enzyme system (see Chapter 9). This enzyme system metabolises many drugs and changes in the activity of the cytochrome P450 enzyme system, usually due to genetic differences, can result in impaired metabolism of certain drugs, leading to an increase in plasma levels and type A ADRs. There are also many drug interactions via this system, which will be discussed later in the chapter. A drug commonly affected by this is warfarin. Other enzyme systems are affected by genetics and some drugs which produce ADRs via this method include isoniazid, hydralazine, paracetamol and oestrogens.

Examples of elimination ADRs include when a patient has renal impairment that leads to reduced elimination of the drug, and therefore a type A ADR, for example with digoxin and gentamicin. Doses of renally cleared drugs must be reduced in patients with renal impairment (Chapter 19).

PHARMACODYNAMIC CAUSES

Glucose-6-phosphate dehydrogenase (G6PD) deficiency is a common cause of ADRs in a small group of patients. G6PD is an enzyme required to maintain the stability of red blood cells and there are some patients who have an inherited deficiency of this enzyme. These patients are at risk of haemolysis when exposed to certain drugs, for example sulphonamides and nitrofurantoin, and these drugs should be avoided in patients with G6PD deficiency. There is a specific section in the *British National Formulary* (BNF) listing which drugs should be avoided. There are other genetic enzyme deficiencies and changes which can cause apparently idiosyncratic or bizarre (type B) ADRs.

Malignant hyperthermia is a type B ADR following administration of certain general anaesthetics and muscle relaxants. It is thought to be due to an abnormal release of calcium following administration of these drugs and occurs, unpredictably, in a few patients only. Another type B ADR due to pharmacodynamic causes is cholestatic jaundice, which can be caused by many drugs, including oral contraceptives and some antibiotics, including flucloxacillin. This is an unpredictable reaction that is not always reversible on withdrawal of the drug and can occur some weeks after the causative drug has been stopped.

STOP AND THINK

Patients who undergo gastrointestinal surgery may be given a dose of co-amoxiclav as a prophylactic antibiotic. Both co-amoxiclav and anaesthetic agents can cause cholestatic jaundice. How would you establish which drug caused the ADR?

There are also immunological reactions, sometimes known as hypersensitivity reactions. These are classed as type B reactions and include symptoms of a typical allergic reaction, blood dyscrasias, serum sickness, vasculitis, Stevens-Johnson syndrome and contact dermatitis. These reactions usually have no relation to the pharmacological effects of the drug, can be seen at very small doses if rechallenge is undertaken, usually disappear on withdrawal of the drug and sometimes occur as a delayed response after the first dose of the drug. Some drugs can cause an ADR on withdrawal of the drug, for example rapid withdrawal of β-blockers, corticosteroids and benzodiazepines.

IDENTIFICATION AND MANAGEMENT OF ADRs

Patients who present with an ADR will often consider the ADR as a new symptom. They will not realise that their symptom is an ADR. It is up to you as a prescriber to identify a suspected ADR to a specific drug and then manage it accordingly.

The first step in identifying an ADR is to take a thorough history from the patient. Include questions about the length of treatment of the drugs they are on, whether they have been treated with drugs in the same class before, how long they have had the symptoms, whether they are worse or better in relation to doses of drugs and questions to exclude a non-ADR reason for the symptoms.

For type A reactions, you will usually be able to discover a clear time association between starting a new drug or increasing a dose and the onset of the symptoms. The summary of product characteristics (SPC) for the drug will list all the adverse reactions seen during the clinical trials for the suspected drug and maybe reactions seen during post-marketing surveillance. However, if you strongly suspect a symptom is associated with a particular drug, and this is not listed in the SPC, you could be observing a new ADR to that drug.

PRACTICE APPLICATION

A patient on many antihypertensives who presents with dizziness should have their blood pressure monitored as part of the patient assessment. If their blood pressure is low, the patient is experiencing a type A reaction to their antihypertensives and the medication should be optimised.

For type B reactions, it is usually harder to make an association between drugs and symptoms, and these are usually diagnosed at the end of a process of eliminating other possible diagnoses.

The management of ADRs involves making a risk/benefit decision, in conjunction with the patient if possible, about what the risks are in stopping the drug or continuing with it and suffering the ADR. Some patients will prefer to continue with a drug if they are seeing a benefit and put up with the inconvenience of a minor ADR.

STOP AND THINK

If you are taking a loop diuretic for heart failure, and experiencing the ADR of increased frequency of urination, would you want to continue with the diuretic?

If the ADR is serious, then the drug would usually be stopped. This is one of those rare situations where drugs can be abruptly stopped without tapering the dose down, for example β-blockers. Sometimes a drug from the same class will not have the same side-effect profile and can be substituted. However, other ADRs are class effects and so a drug from a different class must be used.

Some ADRs resolve on their own once the causative drug is stopped, although other ADRs may take longer to resolve and the patient may prefer to take another drug to treat the ADR whilst they wait for the symptoms to subside. This is particularly the case with skin reactions, which can take some time to settle and may be treated with steroid creams or oral steroids.

Occasionally an ADR can be predicted, and if the drug is necessary then prophylactic drugs to treat the ADR symptoms can be given. An example of this is antiemetics given alongside emetogenic chemotherapy or a proton-pump inhibitor given to prevent the gastrointestinal (GI) side effects of non-steroidal anti-inflammatory drugs (NSAIDs).

It is important to remember to record any suspected ADRs and action taken documented in the shared medical notes to prevent other prescribers using the same drug in the future.

YELLOW CARD SCHEME

If an ADR to a particular drug is noticed, it is important for the wider health community that the ADR is recorded nationally. The Medicines and Healthcare products Regulatory Agency (MHRA) is a government agency that ensures that all UK medicines, amongst other things, are of an acceptable standard in terms of safety, quality, performance and effectiveness. The MHRA and the Commission on Human Medicines, another government committee, run the Yellow Card scheme in the UK for reporting suspected ADRs to drugs, blood products, vaccines, herbal products and radiation contrast media. Anyone suspecting an ADR, including a patient, can complete a Yellow Card and send it to the MHRA. Yellow Cards can be found in the back of the BNF, and online at the MHRA website. The MHRA collates the information sent on the Yellow Card reports and uses this information to produce monthly drug safety updates and maintain a database of all Yellow Card reports for all drugs. Table 13.3 gives details of the types of ADRs that the MHRA is interested in receiving Yellow Cards for. The general motto is, if in doubt, report it.

Table 13.3 Types of ADRs to be reported to the Medicines and Healthcare products Regulatory Agency via the Yellow Card system

Type	Report
Drug type	
New (black triangle in BNF)	All suspected ADRs
Herbal medicines	All suspected ADRs
Older drugs	Dependent on ADR severity and patient group
Patient group	
Elderly	The BNF states that particular vigilance is required to identify adverse reactions in the elderly
Children	All suspected ADRs
Other patient groups	Dependent on ADR severity and patient group
ADR severity	
Fatal	All suspected ADRs
Life threatening	All suspected ADRs
Disabling or incapacitating	All suspected ADRs
Hospitalisation	All suspected ADRs
Prolonging hospital stay	All suspected ADRs
Congenital abnormality	All suspected ADRs
Other ADR	If fits drug type or patient group

ADR, adverse drug reaction; BNF, *British National Formulary*.

Newer drugs and vaccines will be identified with the black triangle symbol. These are newly licenced drugs which require additional monitoring by the European Medicines Agency. Drugs normally retain a black triangle for 5 years, but this can be extended if required.

STOP AND THINK

Would you report an ADR of a rash caused by furosemide in an elderly person? Should you?

DRUG INTERACTIONS

A drug interaction occurs when the effects of one drug are changed by the presence of another drug, food or drink. The changes can be pharmacokinetic or pharmacodynamic.

PHARMACOKINETIC INTERACTIONS

Absorption

Drugs that change the pH of GI fluid can change the rate and amount of absorption of other drugs. If a drug relies on the acidic environment of the stomach to undergo dissolution and absorption, then the action of another drug that raises the pH of the GI fluid will reduce the rate and amount of absorption of the first drug. Examples of drugs which are affected by this type of interaction are proton-pump inhibitors reducing the oral absorption of ketoconazole.

Some drugs tend to react directly with the contents of the stomach, either food or other drugs, to form a chelate or a complex that is not absorbed. Tetracyclines will form a chelate with calcium ions found in milk and also with iron. This results in greatly reduced absorption of tetracycline and reduced action in the body.

PRACTICE APPLICATION

Patients who are being fed with an enteral feed, for example a nasogastric feed, must have their feeds turned off 2 hours before a dose of ciprofloxacin and the feed restarted 2 hours after the dose. The nasogastric line must be flushed well with water before and after the ciprofloxacin dose.

Drugs that have an effect on GI motility, for example metoclopramide, may change the rate and amount of oral absorption of some drugs. The absorption rate may be either increased or decreased, depending on where the drug is absorbed in the GI tract.

Distribution

If two drugs are given which are highly bound to plasma proteins, they will compete for the binding sites on the plasma proteins. The drug that is less successful at binding to plasma proteins will have a higher proportion of free drug available to have a therapeutic action.

Metabolism

Most drug metabolism takes place in the liver, by liver enzymes. The action of these liver enzymes can be inhibited or enhanced (induced) by the presence of other drugs. In the presence of a strong enzyme inducer, other drugs normally metabolised by the same enzyme system will be metabolised to a much greater extent, therefore reducing the plasma concentration of those drugs. Conversely, in the presence of a strong enzyme inhibitor, the plasma concentration of other drugs can be increased.

The cytochrome P450 enzyme system is particularly susceptible to enzyme inhibition or induction by drugs. There are many subtypes of the cytochrome P450 enzyme and drugs that are metabolised by a particular subtype are usually affected by the presence of other drugs metabolised by the same subtype (Chapter 9). An example of this type of interaction is where rifampicin induces liver enzymes, resulting in possible contraception failure where patients are taking oral contraceptives. Warfarin metabolism is also affected by both enzyme inducers and inhibitors; it is usual to monitor the international normalised ratio (INR) more closely when a known interacting drug is added to the regime of a patient taking warfarin. There are also drug–food interactions because of the cytochrome P450 enzyme system. Grapefruit juice is an inhibitor of one of the enzyme cytochrome P450 subtypes, and so patients who are taking drugs that are also metabolised via this subtype should be advised not to drink grapefruit juice. This includes some statins and ciclosporin.

Elimination

Drugs can affect various stages of elimination. Particular interactions to note are listed in Table 13.4.

PHARMACODYNAMIC INTERACTIONS

As you know from Chapter 7, drugs can be either agonists or antagonists at receptors. So logically, we can see that if a patient is given a drug that is an agonist and another drug that is an antagonist at the same receptor, these two drugs will antagonise each other. An example of this is giving an asthmatic patient who uses a β-agonist inhaler, for example salbutamol, a β-blocker. There are many other examples of such interactions, some of which are used therapeutically.

PRACTICE APPLICATION

Naloxone is an opioid antagonist and is used in opioid overdose to compete for the opioid receptors, displace the opioid and prevent it having a further effect.

If two drugs which act in a similar way are given to a patient, their action could be additive or synergistic and result in an excessive therapeutic effect. Examples of these are NSAIDs, warfarin and clopidogrel, which can have an additive effect on increasing bleeding risk if given together. Another example is drugs that can prolong the QT interval on an ECG, for example terfenadine

Table 13.4   Drug interactions caused by alterations in elimination

Drug 1	Drug 2	Mechanism of interaction	Outcome
Salicylates (e.g., aspirin)	Methotrexate	Competition for the same renal tubular secretion pathway	Methotrexate toxicity
NSAIDs (e.g., ibuprofen)	Lithium	Changes in renal blood flow due to reduced prostaglandins	Increased lithium levels
Sodium bicarbonate	Salicylates	Alkalinisation of urine	Increased elimination
Digoxin	Verapamil	Inhibition of drug transporter proteins	Increased digoxin levels

and fluconazole, which when given together can cause a serious cardiac arrhythmia called torsade de pointes. Terfenadine has fallen out of common use because of this serious drug interaction.

Antidepressants are particularly problematic when it comes to drug interactions. Drugs which affect serotonin, for example selective serotonin reuptake inhibitors (SSRIs), can cause serotonin syndrome if they are given concurrently or abruptly stopped. Monoamine oxidase inhibitor (MAOI) antidepressants also affect serotonin, so for this reason they are rarely given in combination with an SSRI. MAOIs are also the subject of interactions with foods containing tyramine, an amino acid. The body requires monoamine oxidase to metabolise tyramine into inactive metabolites and in patients who are taking MAOIs, this metabolism cannot take place. Ecstasy and some drugs that can be bought over the counter in a pharmacy, for example pseudoephedrine, can also cause an interaction with the MAOI, resulting in hypertensive crisis.

MANAGEMENT OF INTERACTIONS

The appendix in the back of the BNF gives a good summary of drug interactions. When prescribing a new drug for a patient, consider the other drugs the patient is on and ensure there will be no serious interaction in the combination you are proposing. If there is an interaction, it is important to consider the possible effect on your specific patient and if there is an alternative drug that can be used, this should be chosen.

If a patient has been maintained on two drugs that are known to interact, it is likely that the doses of both drugs have been adjusted for the interaction. It is not usually necessary to change the therapy of such patients unless they start to exhibit signs or symptoms of an interaction.

SUMMARY

- Adverse drug reactions (ADRs) can be split into two classes: type A and type B.
- Type A ADRs are predictable, dose-dependent and usually reversible when the causative drug is stopped.
- Type B ADRs are unpredictable, can occur at any dose, sometimes occurring after the causative drug has been stopped, and may be irreversible.
- Pharmaceutical causes of ADRs are usually related to dangerous excipients or a poor manufacturing process.
- Pharmacokinetic causes of ADRs usually occur in the metabolism and elimination stages.
- The cytochrome P450 enzyme system is affected by genetic changes, and drugs metabolised by this system can cause ADRs in certain patient groups.
- Pharmacodynamic causes of ADRs usually result in type B ADRs.
- Patients presenting with suspected ADR should have a thorough history of drug use taken to identify the causative drug.
- Management of an ADR involves careful risk/benefit analysis to decide whether the causative drug should be continued or not.
- The MHRA collects data about ADRs through the Yellow Card scheme.
- A drug interaction occurs when the effects of one drug are changed by the presence of another drug, food or drink.
- Pharmacokinetic mechanisms of drug interactions can occur at any stage of the pharmacokinetic process.

- Pharmacodynamic mechanisms of drug interactions include synergistic or additive effects, agonist and antagonist effects, and specific effects on the neurotransmitter systems.

- When adding a new drug into a patient's therapy, it is important to consider potential drug interactions.

- Patients who have been maintained on two interacting drugs will probably be stabilised and do not necessarily need their therapy changing.

ACTIVITY

1. Which of the following statements regarding type A adverse drug reactions are correct?

They are predictable	True/False
They have low incidence	True/False
They have low mortality	True/False
They can be managed by dose reduction	True/False
They have low morbidity	True/False

2. Which of the following statements regarding the pharmacokinetic mechanisms of adverse drug reactions are correct?

Dose reduction may be necessary in renal impairment	True/False
Increases in drug plasma concentrations result in type A ADRs	True/False
The cytochrome P450 enzyme system is important in ADRs	True/False
Pharmacokinetic ADRs result mainly in type B ADRs	True/False
There is genetic variation in the way isoniazid is metabolised	True/False

3. Which of the following statements about how ADRs should be managed are correct?

The patient will know exactly which drug is causing their ADR	True/False
The causative drug must always be stopped	True/False
The causative drug must always be slowly withdrawn	True/False
You must only report definite ADRs to the MHRA	True/False
Anyone can report an ADR to the MHRA	True/False

4. Which of the following statements about drug interaction mechanisms a re correct?

Synergy is where the effects of two drugs cancel each other out	True/False
The formation of chelates in the GI tract aids drug absorption	True/False
Methotrexate and aspirin have an important interaction	True/False
Cytochrome P450 interactions affect the metabolism of various drugs	True/False
Patients taking oral contraceptives must use extra contraceptive methods when they are taking rifampicin	True/False

5. Which of the following statements about the management of drug interactions are correct?

Patients taking MAOIs must not excessively eat foods containing tyramine	True/False
When starting new drugs, prescribers must disregard any other drugs the patient is taking	True/False
The BNF is a useful reference source for identifying drug interactions	True/False
Patients taking simvastatin should drink lots of grapefruit juice	True/False
There are no drug interactions with warfarin	True/False

REFERENCE

Whittlesea, C. and Hodson, K. (2018) *Clinical Pharmacy and Therapeutics*. 6th edn. Elsevier, London.

FURTHER READING

Başaran, N., Pasli, D. and Başaran, A.A. (2022) Unpredictable adverse effects of herbal products. *Food Chem Toxicol* 159:112762.

Baxter, K., Preston, C.L. and Stockley, I.H. (2013) *Stockley's Drug Interactions: A source book of interactions, their mechanisms, clinical importance and management*, 10th edn. Pharmaceutical Press, London.

Hersh, E.V., Pinto, A. and Moore, P.A. (2007) Adverse drug interactions involving common prescription and over-the-counter analgesic agents. *Clin Ther* 29:2477–2497.

Moore, N., Pollack, C. and Butkerait, P. (2015) Adverse drug reactions and drug–drug interactions with over-the-counter NSAIDs. *Ther Clin Risk Manag* 11:1061–1075.

Walker, L.E. and Pirmohamed, M. (2023) Increasing trend in hospitalisation due to adverse drug reactions: Can we stem the tide? *Drug Ther Bull* 61(6):87–91.

USEFUL WEBSITES

British National Formulary (online). BMJ Group and Pharmaceutical Press, London. https://bnf.nice.org.uk/.

Medicines and Healthcare products Regulatory Agency. https://www.gov.uk/government/organisations/medicines-and-healthcare-products-regulatory-agency

CHAPTER 14

Introduction to the Autonomic Nervous System

Joanne Lymn

LEARNING OUTCOMES

By the end of this chapter the reader should be able to:

- describe the role of the autonomic nervous system within the body

- name the two branches of the autonomic nervous system, the neurotransmitters they release and the receptors they bind to

- describe the effects of the autonomic nervous system on the major organs of the body

- understand the mechanism of neurotransmission within the autonomic nervous system and how this may be terminated.

THE NERVOUS SYSTEM

The nervous system of the body can be divided into two branches (Figure 14.1):

- the central nervous system (CNS), which consists of the brain and spinal cord

- the peripheral nervous system, which comprises all the other nerves in the body and connects the CNS and body tissues.

The peripheral nervous system can itself be divided into two components: the somatic nervous system and the autonomic nervous system. The main difference between these two systems is that the somatic system can be described as regulating voluntary movements, those movements which we choose to make. The autonomic nervous system, on the other hand, is involved in regulating involuntary body systems.

In other words, the somatic nervous system acts to relay messages between the CNS and the skin and skeletal muscles, and is involved with regulating responses over which we have conscious control. The autonomic nervous system is responsible for relaying messages between the CNS and the internal organs of the body and as such regulates responses which occur without any conscious control on our part.

THE AUTONOMIC NERVOUS SYSTEM

The main functions of the autonomic nervous system are regulation of:

- the heartbeat

- the contraction and relaxation of smooth muscle

- energy metabolism

- the production of exocrine (and some endocrine) secretions.

The New Prescriber: An Integrated Approach to Medical and Non-medical Prescribing, Second Edition.
Edited by Joanne Lymn, Alison Mostyn, Roger Knaggs, Michael Randall, and Dianne Bowskill.
© 2024 John Wiley & Sons Ltd. Published 2024 by John Wiley & Sons Ltd.

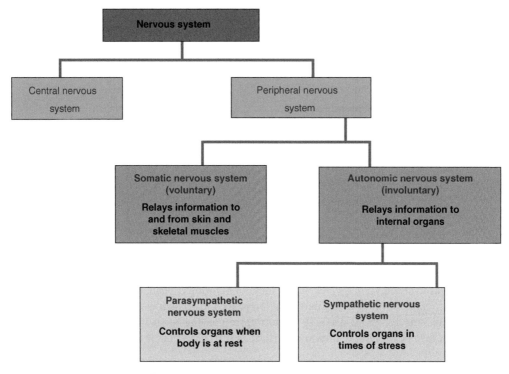

FIGURE 14.1   The divisions of the nervous system.

The autonomic nervous system also plays a role in regulating renin release from the juxtaglomerular cells of the kidney.

STOP AND THINK

- Where in the body do we find smooth muscle?

- What do we mean by exocrine secretions?

- Can you list the exocrine secretions of the body?

The autonomic nervous system can be further divided into two components.

The parasympathetic nervous system
This is most active when the body is relaxed and is often referred to as the 'rest and digest' system: imagine lying on the settee watching the television after lunch on a Sunday.

The sympathetic nervous system
This is referred to as the 'fight/flight/fright' system and is at its most active when the body is under stress: imagine being in a pharmacology exam!
It should be remembered, however, that both of these systems are operating continuously and together to effectively regulate body function.

ACTION OF THE AUTONOMIC NERVOUS SYSTEM ON BODY ORGANS

The parasympathetic and sympathetic nervous systems produce opposing responses on a number of organs of the body (Table 14.1). Perhaps the easiest way of remembering these actions is to think of the systems in terms of 'rest and digest' and 'fight/flight/fright'. If we take the sympathetic

Table 14.1 Opposing actions of the parasympathetic and sympathetic nervous systems on body organs

Organ	Parasympathetic	Sympathetic
Eye	Constriction of pupil	Dilation of pupil
Heart	Decreased heart rate and force of contraction	Increased heart rate and force of contraction
Lungs	Bronchconstriction	Bronchodilation
Gastrointestinal tract	Increased motility of smooth muscle	Decreased motility of smooth muscle
	Relaxation of internal anal sphincter	
	Gastric acid secretion	Constriction of anal sphincters
Bladder	Contraction of detruser	Relaxation of detruser
	Relaxation of internal sphincter	Constriction of internal sphincter

nervous system as an example, this is active in stressful situations of 'fight/flight/fright'. In evolutionary terms this meant exactly what it says: a fight/flight for life. Under these circumstances the heart rate needs to speed up to deliver more blood (containing oxygen and nutrients) to the body so that you can make a run for it. Similarly, the lungs need to dilate to get as much oxygen into the body as possible and the pupil needs to dilate to give you the requisite far vision. Under these circumstances the body has more important priorities than digestion of the last meal and elimination of waste.

It would be a mistake, however, to assume that the parasympathetic and sympathetic systems have opposing effects throughout the body. There are a number of body functions that are regulated by only one of these systems.

SYMPATHETIC NERVOUS SYSTEM

Table 14.2 shows the unopposed action of the sympathetic nervous system on body functions. Again, these responses make sense in terms of the 'fight/flight/fright' model.

- The regulation of blood vessel contractility allows blood to be redistributed away from the visceral beds and into the skeletal muscle beds.

- Glycogenolysis and lipolysis release fuel molecules for ready use by the body in this emergency situation.

Table 14.2 Actions of the sympathetic nervous system on body functions that are not opposed by the parasympathetic nervous system

Component	Action
Blood vessels	Dilation of blood vessels in the skeletal muscle beds
	Contraction of blood vessels of skin and visceral beds
Liver	Stimulation of glycogen breakdown into glucose (glycogenolysis)
Fat	Stimulation of the breakdown of fats into ready fuel molecules (lipolysis)
Kidney	Secretion of renin
Mast cells	Inhibition of histamine release
Sweat glands	Stimulation of sweat production

Table 14.3   Action of the parasympathetic nervous system on body functions

Component	Action
Blood vessels	No direct innervation by the parasympathetic system, but this system stimulates the production of nitric oxide from endothelial cells, rvesulting in generalised vasodilation
Lacrimal gland	Stimulation of tear production
Salivary gland	Stimulation of saliva production
Gastrointestinal tract	Stimulation of gastric acid production

- Inhibition of histamine release from mast cells is important as histamine acts as a bronchocon-strictor and this would impede the bronchodilation required.

- Renin acts ultimately to increase the formation of angiotensin II (Chapter 17), which enhances the constriction of peripheral blood vessels, thus supporting the redistribution of the blood to the skeletal muscle beds.

- Stimulation of sweat production helps to keep the body cool, which is critical in this type of 'fight/flight/fright' response.

STOP AND THINK

Why does the sympathetic nervous system increase blood flow to the skeletal muscle beds?

PARASYMPATHETIC NERVOUS SYSTEM

Table 14.3 shows the action of the parasympathetic nervous system on body function. The parasympathetic nervous system is responsible for stimulating the production of all exocrine secretions of the body, with the exception of sweat.

NEURON STRUCTURE

The autonomic nervous system is made up of nerve cells or neurons. Neurons all have a similar structure, which can be divided into three main parts (Figure 14.2).

- *The cell body*. This is sometimes referred to as the 'soma' and contains the nucleus of the neuron as well as cytoplasmic organelles including mitochondria and ribosomes. It is worth remembering that even though neurons have nuclei and can synthesise proteins, they cannot divide.

- *The dendrites*. These are highly branched projections from the cell body that act as signal receivers and carry messages to the cell body.

- *The axon*. This is a long projection of the cell that carries messages away from the cell body. The axon is usually covered by a myelin sheath that prevents the message dissipating and speeds up the rate of transmission. The axon terminal may be branched to allow connection with the dendrites of a number of other neurons.

NEURON FUNCTION

Neurons are the specialised cells that transmit signals to and from the brain at high speed. The message or signal transmitted by neurons takes the form of electrical impulses that are transmitted down the axon and are known as action potentials. An action potential is generated as a result of

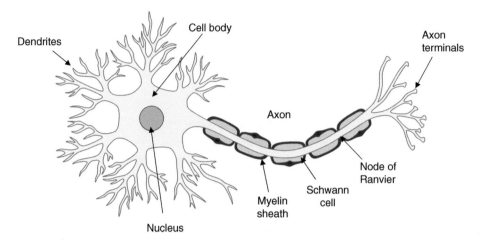

FIGURE 14.2 Typical structure of a neuron, or nerve cell, the fundamental component of the autonomic nervous system. Copyright © motifolio.com.

changes in the ionic composition of both the internal environment of the neuron and the immediate external environment following the movement of sodium and potassium ions across the membrane of the neuron (Chapter 21). Although transmission down an axon is electrical, there is no physical connection between different nerves; they do not actually touch each other and so transmission of the signal from one neuron to another, or from a neuron to a muscle or gland, occurs not by electrical transmission but by chemical transmission. This process of chemical transmission is hugely important in pharmacology. The junction between two neurons or between a neuron and a tissue is called the synapse or chemical synapse (Figure 14.3).

Chemical transmitters, or neurotransmitters, are stored 'prepacked' in lipid packages called vesicles at the axon terminal. As the electrical impulse travels down the axon, it promotes the opening of calcium channels in the membrane and hence calcium enters the axon terminal.

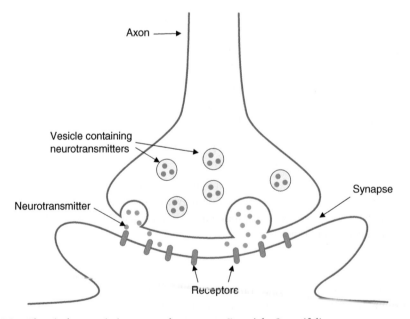

FIGURE 14.3 Chemical transmission across the synapse. Copyright © motifolio.com.

This increase in calcium stimulates the fusion of the lipid vesicles with the plasma membrane and the consequent release of neurotransmitter into the synapse. The released neurotransmitter diffuses across the synapse and binds to specific receptors on the neuron or specialised cell of the tissue, thus transmitting the message to the next cell.

NEURONS IN THE AUTONOMIC NERVOUS SYSTEM

The autonomic nervous system (both the parasympathetic and the sympathetic branches) is made up of two neurons in sequence. The cell body of the first neuron (called the preganglionic neuron) is always in the CNS and it is the region of the CNS in which the cell body of this neuron is located which determines whether it is parasympathetic or sympathetic. Parasympathetic nerves arise in the cranial and sacral regions of the spinal cord and sympathetic nerves arise in the thoracic and lumbar regions.

The second neuron in the sequence is known as the postganglionic neuron. In the parasympathetic nervous system, the preganglionic neuron synapses at a single postganglionic neuron, which is relatively close to the final intended target of the stimulation (muscle or gland), making the axon of the postganglionic neuron relatively short. In the sympathetic nervous system, however, the preganglionic neuron may synapse at several postganglionic neurons, the axons of which are very long as this synapse is some distance from the intended target.

The chemical transmitter released from the preganglionic neuron is always acetylcholine (ACh), which diffuses across the synapse and binds to nicotinic acetylcholine receptors (nAChR) on the postganglionic neuron regardless of whether it is a parasympathetic or sympathetic nerve.

The differences between the two systems occur at the synapse of the postganglionic neuron with the cells of the organ or gland. It is here that the two systems release different neurotransmitters:

- The parasympathetic nervous system continues to use acetylcholine as its neurotransmitter at the neuroeffector junction but the receptors on the muscle/gland are muscarinic (M) receptors.

- The sympathetic nervous system uses noradrenaline (NA) as the neurotransmitter at the neuroeffector junction and the receptors to which this binds on the muscles are known as adrenergic receptors or adrenoceptors.

There are two exceptions to this rule in the sympathetic nervous system.

- *The adrenal medulla.* Following acetylcholine binding to nicotinic receptors on the adrenal medulla, adrenaline is released into the bloodstream. This adrenaline can then act on adrenergic receptors in the lungs. This is extremely important as there is no direct innervation of the lungs by the sympathetic nervous system; what we mean by this is that there are no sympathetic nerves which go directly to the lungs. Hence the reaction of the lungs to sympathetic nervous system stimulation is entirely as a result of the release of adrenaline into the bloodstream.

- *The sweat glands.* These are similar to the lacrimal and salivary glands stimulated by the parasympathetic nervous system in that they continue to utilise acetylcholine as a neurotransmitter and this binds to muscarinic receptors on the cells of the sweat glands (Figure 14.4).

PRACTICE APPLICATION

Drugs which mimic the effects of the autonomic nervous system are used clinically for the treatment of many different conditions, including respiratory disease, myasthenia gravis, Alzheimer's disease and cardiovascular disease.

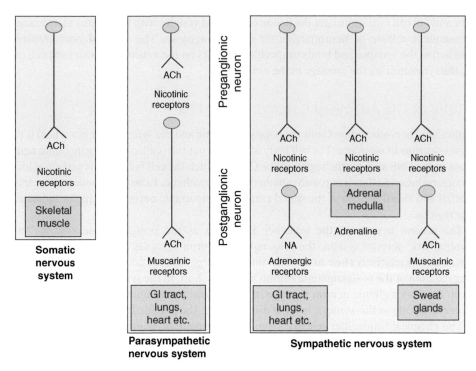

FIGURE 14.4   Receptor types and neurotransmitters of the autonomic nervous system (adapted from *Rang and Dale's Pharmacology*, 10th edn). ACh, acetylcholine; GI, gastrointestinal; NA, noradrenaline.

CHOLINERGIC TRANSMISSION

This term refers to neurotransmission that utilises acetylcholine as the neurotransmitter. From what we have learned so far we know that cholinergic transmission is important for:

- transmission from the preganglionic to the postganglionic neuron (in both the parasympathetic and sympathetic nervous systems)

- transmission from the postganglionic neuron to the effector muscle/gland in the parasympathetic nervous system

- transmission to the sweat glands in the sympathetic nervous system

- transmission to the skeletal muscles (somatic nervous system).

Acetylcholine is stored in vesicles in the axon terminals. As the electrical signal passes down the axon, calcium channels in the terminal membranes open and calcium enters the axon terminals. This increase in calcium promotes the fusion of lipid vesicles with the plasma membrane and acetylcholine is released. Acetylcholine then diffuses across the gap and binds to either nicotinic (on neuron) or muscarinic (on muscles or glands) receptors to stimulate a response.

The body has to have a mechanism by which this response is turned off otherwise acetylcholine would be continually binding and stimulating a response and this is clearly not the case. Acetylcholine is broken down at both the synapse and the neuroeffector junctions by the enzyme acetylcholinesterase, which converts it into acetate and choline. If you remember back to the beginning of the pharmacology section (Chapter 7), we talked about the 'lock and key' hypothesis and that molecules have to be the right shape to fit the receptor and signal a response.

Neither acetate nor choline individually are the right shape to fit properly into either the nicotinic or muscarinic receptors and hence these molecules cannot generate a response, they are not the right 'key' (Figure 14.5).

In terms of pharmacology, we can use a number of different types of drugs to either increase or decrease cholinergic transmission in the body (Table 14.4).

Thinking about the use of muscarinic agonists and antagonists clinically to induce responses in the body, it is important to note that muscarinic receptors can be separated into five different receptor subtypes, known as M_1, M_2, M_3, M_4 and M_5. Whilst all receptor subtypes can be found within the CNS they are differentially located in the peripheral nervous system, raising the possibility that receptor subtype selective drugs could modulate response in specific tissues. This remains an emerging area of pharmacology, but an example of this would be the use of M_3 receptor antagonists in the treatment of an overactive bladder.

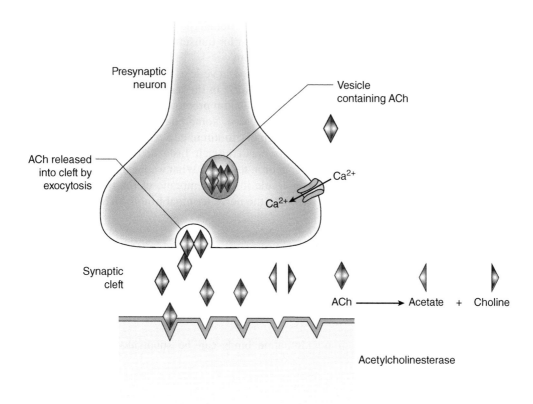

FIGURE 14.5 Acetylcholine transmission is turned off by the action of the enzyme acetylcholinesterase. ACh, acetylcholine.

Table 14.4   Drug groups that can be used clinically to modulate cholinergic transmission in the body

Muscarinic agonists	Mimic the action of acetylcholine at muscarinic receptors in the body and hence act to enhance the normal response at these receptors
Muscarinic antagonists	Similar in shape to acetylcholine and so compete with acetylcholine for muscarinic receptors, but will not stimulate a response and hence result in a reduced response at these receptors
Nicotinic agonists (depolarising muscle relaxants)	Mimic the action of acetylcholine at nicotinic receptors of the neuromuscular junction, but remain bound at these receptors for much longer than acetylcholine, which results in prolonged depolarisation and muscle block
Nicotinic antagonists (non-depolarising muscle relaxants).	Compete with acetylcholine for binding at nicotinic receptors
Anticholineserase drugs	Inhibit the acetylcholinesterase enzyme in the cleft or at the neuroeffector junction, which prevents acetylcholine from being broken down, increasing the amount of acetylcholine and prolonging the action of acetylcholine

NORADRENERGIC TRANSMISSION

This term refers to neurotransmission that utilises noradrenaline as the neurotransmitter. Consequently, noradrenergic transmission is important for transmission from the postganglionic neuron to the muscle in the sympathetic nervous system.

Just as with acetylcholine, noradrenaline is stored in vesicles in the axon terminals. As the electrical signal passes down the axon, calcium channels in the terminal membranes open and calcium enters the axon terminals. This increase in calcium promotes the fusion of lipid vesicles with the plasma membrane and noradrenaline is released. Noradrenaline then diffuses across the gap and binds to adrenergic receptors, or adrenoceptors, to stimulate a response. Unlike acetylcholine, noradrenaline is not broken down by an enzyme in the cleft. Instead, this signalling is 'turned off' by the reuptake of noradrenaline into the neuron terminal. What we mean by this is that noradrenaline in the cleft binds to a carrier molecule in the membrane of the pre-synaptic axon terminal and this carries noradrenaline back into the nerve terminal from which it was released (Figure 14.6).

STOP AND THINK

Given the mechanisms of inactivation in the autonomic nervous system, how do you think drugs might act to increase this neurotransmission clinically?

The adrenoceptors to which noradrenaline binds can be subdivided into alpha- and beta-receptor subtypes.

Alpha-adrenoceptors

There are two types of alpha-adrenoceptor, known as alpha-1 (α_1) and alpha-2 (α_2). The α_1-receptors are located on blood vessels, in the gastrointestinal tract and bladder and in the eye. Stimulation of these receptors results in smooth muscle contraction. The α_2-receptors are located on nerve terminals (autoreceptors), in the brain and on platelets. Stimulation of these receptors results in termination of neurotransmitter release from the nerve terminals, inhibition of sympathetic outflow from the central nervous system and platelet aggregation.

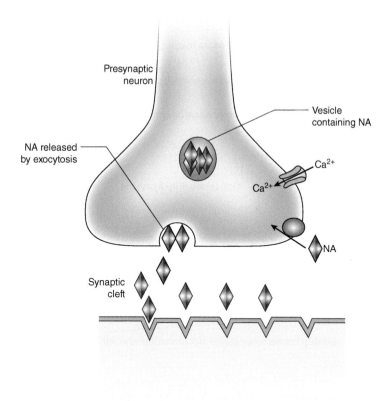

FIGURE 14.6   Noradrenergic transmission is turned off by the reuptake of noradrenaline into the neuron. NA, noradrenaline.

Beta-receptors

There are three different types of beta-receptor known as beta-1 (β_1), beta-2 (β_2) and beta-3 (β_3). β_1-receptors are located mainly in the heart, with some located in the kidney. Stimulation of these receptors increases heart rate directly and peripheral vascular resistance indirectly through renin release from the juxtaglomerular cells of the kidney. β_3-receptors are located mainly in fat, with stimulation of these receptors resulting in lipolysis or breakdown of fat. These receptors are the subject of much drug research. β_2-receptors, on the other hand, are located throughout the rest of the body. Stimulation of these receptors results in relaxation of smooth muscle (blood vessels, bronchi, gastrointestinal tract, detrusor muscle), glycogenolysis (liver), inhibition of histamine release (mast cells), tremor (skeletal muscle) and increased neurotransmitter release (nerve terminals).

The division of adrenoceptors into different subtypes is pharmacologically and clinically of enormous importance, with drugs being designed to act at selective receptor subtypes.

PRACTICE APPLICATION

The division of adrenoceptors into subtypes is important clinically.

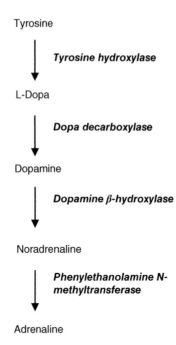

FIGURE 14.7 The relationship between dopamine, noradrenaline and adrenaline.

Table 14.5 Drug groups that can be used clinically to modulate noradrenergic transmission in the body

Adrenoceptor agonists	Mimic the action of noradrenaline and adrenaline at adrenoceptors in the body and hence act to enhance the normal response at these receptors
Adrenoceptor antagonists	Similar in shape to noradrenaline and adrenaline and so will compete with these ligands for adrenoceptors. They will not, however, stimulate a response and hence result in a reduced response at these receptors
Drugs that increase noradrenaline synthesis	Increase the synthesis of noradrenaline in the nerve terminal. Following electrical stimulation more noradrenaline will be released at the neuroeffector junction, thus enhancing the response at adrenoceptors
Drugs that increase noradrenaline release	Stimulate noradrenaline release from the nerve terminal, thus acting to stimulate the response at adrenoceptors
Reuptake inhibitors *(this mechanism is particularly important in the central nervous system)*	Inhibit the carrier protein that moves noradrenaline back into the nerve terminal, resulting in an increase in noradrenaline at the neuroeffector junction and enhancing the stimulation of adrenoceptors

The other aspect of noradrenergic transmission that needs to be considered here is the synthesis of noradrenaline (Figure 14.7). A number of drugs used clinically act by inhibiting enzymes in this pathway.

In terms of pharmacology, we can use a number of different types of drugs to either increase or decrease noradrenergic transmission in the body (Table 14.5).

SUMMARY

- The autonomic nervous system is divided into two branches – the parasympathetic and the sympathetic – and these exert different effects on the organs of the body.

- Anatomically, the autonomic nervous system consists of two neurons: the preganglionic neuron (with its cell body in the central nervous system) and the postganglionic neuron.

- Neurotransmitters are released from the neuron by a process called exocytosis, which requires high levels of calcium.

- The activity of acetylcholine is terminated by the action of the enzyme acetylcholinesterase in the synapse.

- Acetylcholinesterase breaks acetylcholine down into acetate and choline.

- The activity of noradrenaline is terminated by reuptake into the nerve terminal by a carrier molecule.

- Acetylcholine is released from all preganglionic nerves and binds to nicotinic receptors.

- Acetylcholine is released from the postganglionic nerves of the parasympathetic nervous system (and the sympathetic nerves innervating the sweat glands) and binds to muscarinic receptors.

- Noradrenaline is released from the postganglionic nerves of the sympathetic nervous system and binds to adrenoceptors.

- Adrenaline is not a neurotransmitter but a hormone whose release into the bloodstream is stimulated by the action of the sympathetic nervous system on the adrenal glands.

- Classification of adrenoceptors into different subtypes is clinically important.

ACTIVITY

Are the following statements true or false?

1. The two main neurotransmitters that operate in the autonomic nervous system are acetylcholine and adrenaline. True/False

2. The sympathetic and parasympathetic nervous systems have opposing effects on gastrointestinal smooth muscle motility. True/False

3. The sympathetic and parasympathetic nervous systems both act to stimulate sweat production. True/False

4. Neurotransmitters in the autonomic nervous system are released into the synapse by exocytosis. True/False

5. Acetylcholine is inactivated by enzymes within the synaptic cleft. True/False

6. Side effects of muscarinic agonists include constipation and urinary retention. True/False

7. Drugs that act as agonists at adrenoceptors activate the 'fight/flight/fright' response. True/False

8. Drugs acting at nicotinic receptors affect both the sympathetic and parasympathetic nervous systems. True/False

9. Drugs that act as antagonists at β-adrenoceptors induce bronchodilation.   True/False

10. The action of noradrenaline is curtailed by reuptake into the nerve terminal.   True/False

11. Oympathetic nervous system stimulation to the bladder relaxes the detrusor muscle and constricts the sphincter.   True/False

12. The parasympathetic nervous system stimulates glycogenolysis in the liver.   True/False

13. There is direct sympathetic innervation of the lungs.   True/False

14. Drugs which bind to β-1-receptors modulate heart rate.   True/False

15. Muscarinic receptors are located on the postganglionic neuron of the parasympathetic nervous system.   True/False

FURTHER READING

Abrams, P., Andersson, K.E., Buccafusco, J.J., et al. (2006) Muscarinic receptors: their distribution and function in body systems, and the implications for treating overactive bladder. *Br J Pharmacol* 148:565–578.

Booij, L.H.D.J. (1996) *Neuromuscular Transmission*. BMJ Books, London.

Eglen, R.M. (2006) Muscarinic receptor subtypes in neuronal and non-neuronal cholinergic function. *Auton Autocoid Pharmacol* 26:219–233.

Foster, R.W. (2003) *Basic Pharmacology*, 4th edn. Arnold, London.

Kruk, Z.L. and Pycock, C.J. (1991) *Neurotransmitters and Drugs*, 3rd edn. Chapman and Hall, London.

McGavock, H. (2017) *How Drugs Work. Basic Pharmacology for Healthcare Professionals*, 4th edn. CRC Press, Taylor & Francis Group, Boca Raton.

Page, C.P., Curtis, M.J., Sutter, M.C., et al. (2006) *Integrated Pharmacology*, 3rd edn. Mosby, London.

Ritter, J.M., Flower, R., Henderson, G., et al. (2023) *Rang and Dale's Pharmacology*, 10th edn. Elsevier, Amsterdam.

Ross, J., Horton-Szar, D. and Smith, C. (2015) *Crash Course: Nervous System*, 4th edn. Mosby, London.

Webster, R.A. and Jordan, C.C. (1989) *Neurotransmitters, Drugs and Disease*. Wiley-Blackwell, London.

Zimmerman, H. (1994) *Synaptic Transmission: Cellular and Molecular Basis*. Oxford University Press, New York.

Clinical Application of the Principles of the Autonomic Nervous Systems

CHAPTER 15

Joanne Lymn

LEARNING OUTCOMES

By the end of this chapter the reader should understand:

- how drugs that target receptors within the parasympathetic nervous system can be used clinically

- why drugs that target receptors within the parasympathetic nervous system have certain cautions and contra-indications

- how the hydrolysis of acetylcholine may be regulated for clinical effect

- how drugs that target receptors within the sympathetic nervous system can be used clinically

- why drugs that target receptors within the sympathetic nervous system have certain cautions and contraindications

- how the synthesis, release and reuptake of noradrenaline may be regulated for clinical effect.

This chapter describes how the autonomic nervous system can be manipulated for clinical effect. The autonomic nervous system is an ideal starting point for developing an understanding of why drugs have certain side effects and why specific cautions and contraindications are listed. The drug groups we are going to cover in this chapter are those that act through the modulation of both the parasympathetic and the sympathetic nervous systems (Table 15.1).

DRUGS WHICH TARGET THE PARASYMPATHETIC NERVOUS SYSTEM AND CHOLINERGIC TRANSMISSION

MUSCARINIC AGONISTS

These drugs mimic the action of acetylcholine at muscarinic receptors in the body and are sometimes referred to as parasympathomimetic. There are only two examples of this type of drug in clinical use these days: bethanechol and pilocarpine. Bethanechol is listed in the *British National Formulary* (BNF) for the treatment of urinary retention (although it is considered less suitable for prescribing, having been superseded by catheterisation). Pilocarpine is listed for the oral treatment of xerostomia (dry mouth) following irradiation for head and neck cancer, dry mouth and dry eyes in Sjögren's syndrome and as eye drops for the production of miosis (pupil constriction) in primary angle-closure glaucoma.

The New Prescriber: An Integrated Approach to Medical and Non-medical Prescribing, Second Edition.
Edited by Joanne Lymn, Alison Mostyn, Roger Knaggs, Michael Randall, and Dianne Bowskill.
© 2024 John Wiley & Sons Ltd. Published 2024 by John Wiley & Sons Ltd.

Table 15.1 Groups of drugs used clinically that target the action of the parasympathetic and sympathetic nervous systems

Parasympathetic nervous system	Sympathetic nervous system
Muscarinic agonists	Noradrenergic agonists
Muscarinic antagonists	Noradrenergic antagonists
Anticholinesterase drugs	Drugs affecting noradrenaline synthesis
	Drugs affecting noradrenaline release
	Drugs affecting noradrenaline uptake

If we recap on the effect of muscarinic agonists in the body (Table 15.2), we know that that the parasympathetic nervous system acts to:

- promote micturation by contracting the detrusor muscle of the bladder and relaxing the bladder sphincter
- stimulate saliva production
- constrict the pupil.

Muscarinic agonists are non-selective, however, and so bind to and stimulate the activity of muscarinic receptors throughout the body. These drugs mimic the effects of acetylcholine, which is the endogenous agonist, at these receptors. This explains why the same class of drugs can be used clinically to produce very different effects.

Similarly, it also explains why diarrhoea, abdominal pain and increased lacrimation are amongst the side effects listed in the BNF for bethanechol and oral pilocarpine. Stimulation of the muscarinic receptors in the gastrointestinal (GI) tract will increase the motility of the GI tract and relax the sphincters, which may lead to diarrhoea and colicky pain, while stimulation of the receptors on the lacrimal glands will result in increased tear production.

The BNF lists asthma and chronic obstructive pulmonary disease (COPD) under cautions for oral pilpocarpine treatment. This is because stimulation of the muscarinic receptors in the lungs results in bronchoconstriction. While the level of bronchoconstriction produced may not affect healthy adults, it may be significant in patients with asthma and COPD who already have impaired lung function.

Table 15.2 Effect of the parasympathetic nervous system on body organs

Organ	Effect of the parasympathetic nervous system
Heart	Decreased heart rate and force of contraction
Lungs	Bronchoconstriction
Gastrointestinal tract	Increased motility of smooth muscle, relaxation of sphincters
Bladder	Contraction of detruser muscle, relaxation of sphincters
Eye	Constriction of pupil
Salivary glands	Stimulate secretion
Lacrimal glands	Stimulate secretion

STOP AND THINK

Why do you think these side effects are only rare when using pilocarpine eye drops?

MUSCARINIC ANTAGONISTS

These drugs compete with acetylcholine for binding to the muscarinic receptors on body organs but when bound to the receptor, they do not stimulate a response. These drugs are competitive antagonists (Chapter 7). They exhibit similar affinity for the muscarinic receptors but have reduced efficacy and consequently reduce or inhibit the response of the parasympathetic nervous system, effectively exhibiting the opposite effect of muscarinic agonists (Table 15.3). Whilst most muscarinic antagonists are considered non-selective, binding to all muscarinic receptor subtypes, progress has been made in producing muscarinic antagonists that have some receptor selectivity (M_3-receptor antagonists) and these are starting to be used more commonly clinically.

There are a number of muscarinic antagonists in clinical use today, including solifenacin, tropicamide and tiotropium.

PRACTICE APPLICATION

Tropicamide hydrochloride is listed as part of the *Optometrists' Formulary*.

Solifenacin

Solifenacin succinate, given orally, is indicated by the BNF for use in the treatment of urinary frequency, urgency and incontinence. As a muscarinic antagonist with selectivity for the M_3-receptor subtype, solifenacin decreases the contraction of the detrusor and inhibits the relaxation of the urethral sphincter normally seen following parasympathetic stimulation, thus relaxing the bladder and allowing more urine to be stored and reducing the urge to micturate.

STOP AND THINK

Why might GI discomfort be a side effect of solifenacin treatment?

Table 15.3   Effect of muscarinic antagonists on body organs and associated potential clinical effects

Body organ	Effect of muscarinic antagonist	Potential side effect
Heart	Increased heart rate and force of contraction	Tachycardia
Gastrointestinal tract	Decreased motility of the gastrointestinal tract	Constipation
	Contraction of the sphincters	
Bladder	Relaxation of the detruser muscle	Urinary retention
	Constriction of the sphincter	
Salivary gland	Decreased saliva production	Dry mouth
Lacrimal gland	Decreased tear production	Dry eyes

Table 15.4 Clinical effect of overstimulation of muscarinic receptors by anticholinesterase drugs

Organ	Possible clinical effect of overstimulation of receptors
Heart	Bradycardia
Lungs	Shortness of breath
Gastrointestinal tract	Diarrhoea
Bladder	Urinary frequency
Eye	Loss of far vision
Salivary glands	Excessive saliva production
Lacrimal glands	Watery eyes

Tiotropium bromide

Tiotropium bromide is an example of a muscarinic antagonist, used clinically in the management of COPD and severe asthma, acute bronchospasm and severe or life-threatening asthma. Tiotropium binds to the muscarinic receptors in the lungs and prevents the bronchoconstriction induced by acetylcholine.

Table 15.3 demonstrates that dry mouth, urinary retention and constipation are typical anti-muscarinic side effects resulting from the fact that tiotropium can bind to muscarinic receptors in all these areas and prevent the action of acetylcholine. These side effects are only rarely experienced with tiotropium as it is given by inhalation and therefore is delivered directly to its site of action (a topical response). In addition, the chemical structure of tiotropium is such that it has a quaternary amine, which makes it large and charged; it is not therefore absorbed very well across membranes and so rarely enters the systemic circulation.

ANTICHOLINESTERASE DRUGS

These drugs inhibit the action of cholinesterase enzymes in the cleft. They reduce the breakdown of acetylcholine and increase cholinergic transmission (at both nicotinic and muscarinic receptors). Examples of these drugs are neostigmine, pyridostigmine and donepezil, and they are used clinically to:

- reverse the effects of non-depolarising neuromuscular blockers (nicotinic antagonists)
- treat myasthenia gravis
- treat mild-moderate dementia in Alzheimer's disease.

Because these drugs inhibit the breakdown of acetylcholine peripherally as well as at the neuromuscular junction, they increase muscarinic effects throughout the body (Table 15.4), resulting in side effects such as increased salivation, diarrhoea and abdominal cramps.

Asthma is listed as a caution for the use of anticholinesterase drugs in the treatment of both myasthenia gravis and Alzheimer's disease because the reduced breakdown of acetylcholine in the lungs will result in prolonged bronchoconstriction.

DRUGS WHICH TARGET THE SYMPATHETIC NERVOUS SYSTEM AND NORADRENERGIC TRANSMISSION

ADRENERGIC AGONISTS

These drugs mimic the action of adrenaline and noradrenaline in the body and produce effects that are similar to stimulation of the sympathetic nervous system. These drugs are often called directly acting sympathomimetics. They are often selective for a specific receptor subgroup (either α_1 or β_2) and hence the effects of these drugs relate to the receptor subtype they bind to (Table 15.5).

Table 15.5 Effect of the sympathetic nervous system on the body and the specific receptor subtype that is responsible for the effect

Organ	Effect of sympathetic nervous system	Receptor subtype
Heart	Increased heart rate and force of contraction	β_1
Lungs	Bronchodilation in response to adrenaline released from the adrenal gland	β_2
Gastrointestinal tract	Decreased motility of smooth muscle	β_2
	Contraction of sphincter	α_1
Bladder	Relaxation of detruser muscle	β_2
	Contraction of sphincter	α_1
Eye	Dilation of pupil (contraction of ciliary muscle)	α_1
Blood vessels	Contraction of skin and visceral beds	α_1
	Dilation of skeletal muscle beds	β_2
Liver	Glycogenolysis	β_2
Fat	Lipolysis	β_3
Kidney	Renin secretion	β_1/β_2
Sweat	Secretion	Muscarinic
Mast cells	Inhibition of histamine release	β_2
Skeletal muscle	Tremor	β_2

Phenylephrine

This is an α_1-specific adrenoceptor agonist currently used for eye examination because it causes mydriasis (dilates the pupil). Phenylephrine is also used in topical nasal decongestants, which can be bought over the counter. Its use in this context is due to its ability to constrict the blood vessels of the nasal mucosa, resulting in reduced oedema and easing the blockage of nasal passages. While side effects are limited because of the topical nature of phenylephrine use, systemic side effects can occur following repeated and excessive use.

Salbutamol

Salbutamol is a selective β_2-agonist that is used clinically to treat both asthma and COPD. Its action in the respiratory system is to produce bronchodilation by mimicking the action of the sympathetic nervous system. It should be remembered, however, that selectivity is not the same as specificity so whilst salbutamol is more likely to bind to (has a greater affinity for) β_2-receptors, it is still able to bind to and stimulate the β_1-receptors in the heart, resulting in arrhythmias being listed as a side effect.

STOP AND THINK

Salbutamol is generally delivered by inhalation. Can you think of two reasons why this route of administration might be preferred to the oral route?

Diabetes is also listed as a caution for salbutamol use. Table 15.5 shows that stimulation of β_2-receptors in the liver results in glycogenolysis or the breakdown of glycogen into glucose. This may lead to changes in the patient's insulin requirement and hyperglycaemia. Because this glucose cannot be taken up and used by the tissues, it can lead to fatty acids within the tissues being broken down, with the production of ketone bodies leading to ketoacidosis.

ADRENERGIC ANTAGONISTS

These drugs act by blocking adrenaline and noradrenaline binding to adrenoceptors in the body and thus inhibit or reduce the effects of the sympathetic nervous system. These drugs either bind to α-receptors (α-blockers), or β-receptors (β-blockers) and can be used clinically in the management of cardiovascular disease and other conditions. The side effects related to the use of these drugs vary, to a certain extent, depending on the type of adrenergic antagonist used (Table 15.6) and the characteristics of the individual drugs.

Prazosin, doxazosin, tamsulosin

These drugs are all antagonists at α_1-receptors. Prazosin and doxazocin are indicated for the treatment of hypertension and all three drugs are indicated for the treatment of benign prostatic hyperplasia.

In terms of their cardiovascular action, blocking α_1-receptors prevents noradrenaline from binding to these receptors and causing vasoconstriction. This results in vasodilation of peripheral arteries, thus reducing peripheral vascular resistance and reducing blood pressure (Chapter 17). In benign prostatic hyperplasia α-blockers are used to relax the prostate muscle and bladder sphincter, making it easier to pass urine.

Celiprolol, pindolol, acebutolol

These drugs are partial agonists and so are able to act as both agonists and antagonists at β-adrenergic receptors, they are said to possess intrinsic sympathomimetic activity. As a result, these drugs tend to cause less bradycardia than other β-blockers, and whilst rarely used these drugs are still indicated for the treatment of hypertension and angina.

Labetalol, carvedilol

These drugs are non-specific adrenergic receptor antagonists and thus have affinity for both α- and β-adrenoceptors. They will therefore bind to α- and β-receptors in the body, blocking the action of noradrenaline and adrenaline at both these receptor subtypes. These drugs are used clinically to treat hypertension and angina. Carvedilol is used to treat chronic heart failure (Chapter 17). They reduce both cardiac output, by blocking the action of nordarenaline at the β_1-receptors in the heart and thus reducing heart rate, and peripheral vascular resistance, by blocking the action of noradrenaline on the β_1-receptors in the peripheral vasculature, thus promoting vasodilatation.

Table 15.6 Some side effects of the different forms of adrenoceptor antagonists linked to the receptor subtypes they bind to

Side effect	Non-specific adrenergic antagonists	β-receptor antagonists	Cardioselective β-blockers
Bronchoconstriction	+++	+++	+
Gastrointestinal disturbances	++	++	+
Disturbances of micturation	+++	++	+
Visual disturbances	++	–	–
Nasal stuffiness	++	–	–

STOP AND THINK

Why might the inhibition of renin production by the kidney be important in the clinical action of these drugs in treating hypertension?

Propranolol, timolol

These drugs are β-receptor antagonists, which are indicated for use in the treatment of hypertension and angina, although are more commonly used to treat the physical symptoms of anxiety. The difference between these drugs and labetalol and carvedilol is that propranolol and timolol are solely β-adrenoceptor antagonists and so do not have effects on the α-receptors. Consequently, they do not have the extra vasodilating effect of the mixed receptor antagonists.

Atenolol, bisoprolol, metoprolol, nebivolol

These drugs are cardioselective β-receptor antagonists, which means that they have a greater affinity for the β_1-receptors in the heart than for the β_2-receptors elsewhere in the body. Bisoprolol is widely used in both ischaemic heart disease and chronic heart failure (Chapter 17).

Asthma is listed in the BNF as a contraindication for the use of β-adrenoceptors because these drugs may block the β_2-receptors in the lungs, thus preventing the natural bronchodilation that occurs through adrenaline. While this does not present a problem in normal individuals, it can be dangerous in asthmatics. The use of β-adrenoceptor antagonists in asthmatics would also lessen the effectiveness of treating bronchoconstriction by β_2-agonists.

STOP AND THINK

Why do you think uncontrolled heart failure is listed as a contraindication for the use of β-adrenoceptor antagonists?

Some β-adrenoceptor blocking drugs are associated with sleep disturbances and nightmares, while others are not. This is likely explained by the lipid solubility of the drugs. Propranolol and metoprolol are relatively lipid soluble and hence can cross the blood–brain barrier (BBB), resulting in sleep disturbance and nightmares. Atenolol, on the other hand, is much more water-soluble (polar) and does not easily cross the BBB so it is associated with fewer central nervous system-type side effects.

PRACTICE APPLICATION

The difference in lipid solubility of β-adrenoceptor antagonists might impact drug handling in the elderly. The more water-soluble drugs such as atenolol, celiprolol, nadolol and solatol may require dose reduction in the elderly.

DRUGS AFFECTING NORADRENALINE SYNTHESIS

An example of a drug that affects noradrenaline synthesis and can be used clinically is co-careldopa, which is a mixture of carbidopa, a DOPA decarboxylase inhibitor, and levodopa. DOPA decarboxylase inhibitors prevent levodopa (L-Dopa) from being converted into dopamine (Figure 15.1).

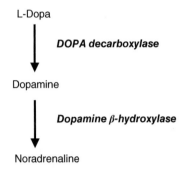

FIGURE 15.1   Production of noradrenaline from L-Dopa.

Co-careldopa can be used in the treatment of Parkinson's disease, which results from an imbalance between the neurotransmitters dopamine and acetylcholine and is often treated by increasing dopamine levels (Chapter 22). Carbidopa prevents levodopa from being converted into dopamine in the periphery. Carbidopa does not cross the BBB while levodopa does and therefore results in higher concentrations of dopamine in the brain, with lower concentrations of levodopa. It also reduces the peripheral side effects of levodopa treatment, which might include sympatho-mimetic effects.

DRUGS AFFECTING NORADRENALINE RELEASE

These drugs stimulate noradrenaline release from nerve terminals in the absence of nerve stimulation and are known as indirectly acting sympathomimetics. They are similar in shape to noradrenaline and can therefore be taken up into the nerve terminal by the reuptake carrier protein. Once in the nerve terminal, they displace noradrenaline from the vesicles in which it is stored. The increase in free noradrenaline content of the neuron results in its release into the neuroeffector junction by a carrier protein, where it can bind to and stimulate adrenocep-tors. Ephedrine is an example of such a sympathomimetic drug and is used in the treatment of nasal congestion.

DRUGS AFFECTING NORADRENALINE UPTAKE

These drugs decrease the reuptake of noradrenaline into the nerve terminal by inhibiting the action of the carrier protein. This increases the action of noradrenaline at the receptor. Imipramine is an example of a drug that affects noradrenaline uptake that is still listed clinically for the treatment of nocturnal enuresis in children. In this case, the action of imipramine relaxes the detrusor muscle and constricts the sphincter, thereby increasing the capacity of the bladder. Imip-ramine does not solely inhibit the carrier protein responsible for noradrenaline reuptake but also acts as an antagonist at a number of other types of receptors and it is this action that is responsible for most of the side effects of the drug.

SUMMARY

- Drug groups that act by mimicking the action of acetylcholine on body organs are musca-rinic agonists.

- Muscarinic agonists are non-selective and competitive.

- Drug groups that act by reducing the action of acetylcholine on body organs are muscarinic antagonists.

- Muscarinic antagonists are used to treat urinary frequency, asthma and chronic obstructive pulmonary disease.

- Typical side effects of muscarinic antagonists include dry mouth, constipation and urinary retention.

- Anticholinesterase drugs inhibit the action of acteylcholinesterase, thereby increasing the level of acetylcholine.

- Anticholinesterase drugs can be used to reverse non-depolarising neuromuscular blockade and to treat both myasthenia gravis and Alzheimer's disease.

- Drug groups that act by mimicking the action of adrenaline and noradrenaline on body organs are adrenergic agonists. Drug groups that act by reducing the action of adrenaline and noradrenaline on body organs are adrenergic antagonists.

- Division of adrenergic receptors into specific subgroups is clinically very important.

- Adrenergic antagonists can be divided into non-selective adrenergic antagonists, β-receptor antagonists and cardioselective β-receptor antagonists. Side effects differ between these types of antagonists.

- DOPA decarboxylase inhibitors prevent the formation of dopamine, noradrenaline and adrenaline from levodopa, and are used in the treatment of Parkinson's disease.

- Drugs that stimulate the release of nordarenaline in the absence of nerve stimulation, such as ephedrine, are commonly used to treat nasal congestion.

- Inhibition of the carrier protein in the nerve terminal prevents the reuptake of noradrenaline, thus prolonging its effects. Noradrenaline reuptake inhibitors are used clinically to treat nocturnal enuresis in children.

ACTIVITY

1. Tropicamide, a muscarinic antagonist, is used as eye drops to facilitate the examination of the fundus of the eye. Why do you think tropicamide is useful in these circumstances?

2. Why is bradycardia listed as a caution for the use of anticholinesterase drugs?

3. Salbutamol mimics the action of which of the following chemicals?

    (a) Noradrenaline

    (b) Acetylcholine

    (c) Adrenaline

4. One of the most common side effects of salbutamol use is fine tremor. Can you explain why this might be the case?

5. Why would the use of β-adrenoceptor antagonists lessen the effect of salbutamol in the lungs?

6. Why would ephedrine be useful for the treatment of nasal congestion?

FURTHER READING

Abrams, P. and Andersson, K.E. (2007) Muscarinic receptor antagonists for overactive bladder. *BJU Int* 100:987–1006.

Ågesen, F.N., Weeke, P.E., Tfelt-Hansen, P. and Tfelt-Hansen, J. (2019) Pharmacokinetic variability of beta-adrenergic blocking agents used in cardiology. *Pharmacol Res Perspect* 7(4):e00496.

Andrus, M.R. and Loyed, J.V. (2008) Use of beta-adrenoceptor antagonists in older patients with chronic obstructive pulmonary disease and cardiovascular co-morbidity: safety issues. *Drugs Aging* 25:131–144.

Anzueto, A. and Miravitlles, M. (2020) Tiotropium in chronic obstructive pulmonary disease: a review of clinical development. *Respir Res* 29(1):199.

Armstrong, M.J. and Okun, M.S. (2020) Diagnosis and treatment of Parkinson disease: A review. *JAMA* 323(6):548–560.

Barker, R.A. (1993) *Neuroscience: An Illustrated Guide.* Ellis Horwood, New York.

Barnes, P.J. (2004) Distribution of receptor targets in the lung. *Proc Am Thorac Soc* 1:345–351.

British National Formulary. London, BMJ Group and Pharmaceutical Press. https://bnf.nice.org.uk/.

Davies, A.N. and Thompson, J. (2015) Parasympathomimetic drugs for the treatment of salivary gland dysfunction due to radiotherapy. *Cochrane Database Syst Rev.* https://doi.org/10.1002/14651858.CD003782.pub3.

Dusser, D. and Ducharme, F.D. (2019) Safety of tiotropium in patients with asthma. *Ther Adv Respir Dis* 13:1753466618824010.

Kruk, Z.L. and Pycock, C.J. (1991) *Neurotransmitters and Drugs*, 3rd edn. Chapman and Hall, London.

Li, H., Xu, T.-Y., Li, Y., et al. (2022) Role of α1-blockers in the current management of hypertension. *J Clin Hypertens (Greenwich)* 24(9):1180–1186.

Luo, D., Liu, L., Han, P., Wei, Q and Shen, H. (2012) Solifenacin for overactive bladder: a systematic review and meta-analysis. *Int Urogynecol J* 23(8):983–991.

Marques, L. and Vale, N. (2022) Salbutamol in the management of asthma: A review. *Int Mol Sci* 23(22):14207.

Page, C.P., Curtis, M.J., Sutter, M.C., et al. (2006) *Integrated Pharmacology*, 3rd edn. Mosby, London.

Ritter, J.M., Flower, R., Henderson, G., et al. (2023) *Rang and Dale's Pharmacology*, 10th edn. Elsevier, Amsterdam.

Romi, F., Gilhus, N.E. and Aarli, J.A. (2005) Myasthenia gravis: clinical, immunological, and therapeutic advances. *Acta Neurol Scand* 111:134–141.

Samir, M., Mahmoud, M.A. and Elawady, H. (2021) Can the combined treatment of solfenacin and imipramine have a role in desmopressin refractory monosymptomatic nocturnal enuresis? A prospective double-blond randomized placebo-controlled study. *Urologia* 88(4):369–373.

Seeberger, L.C. and Hauser, R.A. (2007) Optimizing bioavailability in the treatment of Parkinson's disease. *Neuropharmacology* 53:791–800.

Sharma, K. (2019) Cholinesterase inhibitors as Alzheimer's therapeutics (Review). *Mol Med Rep* 20(2):1479–1487.

Webster, R.A. and Jordan, C.C. (1989) *Neurotransmitters, Drugs and Disease.* Blackwell Scientific, Oxford.

The Gastrointestinal System

CHAPTER 16

Michael Randall

LEARNING OUTCOMES

By the end of this chapter the reader should be able to:

- explain the physiological control of gastric acid secretion
- describe the mechanism of action, pharmacokinetics, unwanted effects and clinical uses of:
  - antacids
  - histamine (H_2) receptor antagonists
  - proton pump inhibitors
  - misoprostol
  - triple therapy
- describe the role of *Helicobacter pylori* and non-steroidal anti-inflammatory drugs in peptic ulceration
- understand in broad terms the control of the vomiting reflex

- identify the four main receptor types involved in the vomiting process and their location
- describe the mechanism of action, pharmacokinetics, unwanted effects and clinical uses of:
  - histamine H_1 receptor antagonists
  - muscarinic receptor antagonists
  - $5HT_3$ receptor antagonists
  - D_2 receptor antagonists
- describe the mechanism of action, pharmacokinetics, unwanted effects and clinical uses of laxative agents
- understand the mechanism of action, pharmacokinetics, unwanted effects and clinical uses of antimotility agents.

Gastrointestinal pharmacology encompasses the management of diseases of the stomach, nausea and vomiting, constipation and diarrhoea.

DYSPEPSIA

Dyspepsia describes upper gastrointestinal symptoms, such as heartburn, nausea, discomfort and wind, and may be referred to as 'indigestion'. Gastro-oesophageal reflux disease (GORD) involves reflux of the gastric contents into the oesophagus, which leads symptoms of a burning pain or 'heartburn' due to acidic damage to the oesophagus. It tends to be worsened by eating, certain foods, and by both obesity and pregnancy (due to increased intra-abdominal pressure).

Peptic ulcer disease is more serious and involves erosion of the stomach or duodenal lining. The leading cause of peptic ulceration is infection with the Gram-negative bacterium *Helicobacter pylori*, which is the cause of ~95% of cases in duodenal ulceration and 70–80% of cases in of gastric ulceration. The infection leads to chronic inflammation (gastritis) and gastric damage, leading to ulceration. The second leading cause is the ulcerogenic effects of non-steroidal anti-inflammatory drugs (NSAIDs).

The New Prescriber: An Integrated Approach to Medical and Non-medical Prescribing, Second Edition.
Edited by Joanne Lymn, Alison Mostyn, Roger Knaggs, Michael Randall, and Dianne Bowskill.
© 2024 John Wiley & Sons Ltd. Published 2024 by John Wiley & Sons Ltd.

CONTROL OF GASTRIC ACID SECRETION

Gastric acid secretion is under tight parasympathetic, hormonal and local control, which leads to the activation of proton pumps (H^+/K^+ adenosine triphosphatases [ATPases]) and the efflux of protons from the parietal cells into the gastric lumen, leading to a pH around 1.5 (Figure 16.1). Control of gastric acid secretion is required to ensure that acid is released in relation to food. There are four control mechanisms:

- Parasympathetic: Acetylcholine from the vagus nerve acts at muscarinic M_3 receptors on parietal cells to stimulate the proton pump and cause acid secretion.

- Hormonal: Gastrin is a polypeptide hormone released by the G cells of the stomach, duodenum and pancreas to stimulate cholecystokinin B (CCK_2) receptors on parietal cells to stimulate gastric acid secretion.

- Autocrine: Histamine is released by enterochromaffin-like cells to stimulate histamine H_2 receptors on parietal cells to stimulate gastric acid secretion.

- Cytoprotection: This protects the stomach against the gastric acid. It involves the local release of prostaglandins, which modulate the proton pump (Figure 16.1). The prostanoids are also cytoprotective via the release of mucus to protect and bicarbonate release to oppose the acid.

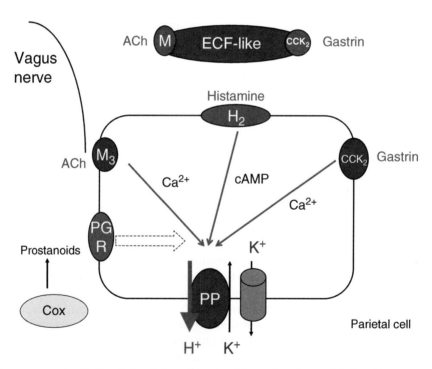

FIGURE 16.1 A parietal cell and stimulation of gastric acid secretion via acetylcholine (via muscarinic receptors, coupled to an increase in intracellular calcium), histamine (via histamine H_2 receptors, coupled to an increase in cAMP) and gastrin (via CCK_2 receptors, coupled to an increases in intracellular calcium) and modulation via prostanoids. ACh, acetylcholine; cAMP, cyclic adenosine monophosphate; CCK_2, cholecystokinin B; Cox, cyclooxygenase; ECF, enterochromaffin-like cell; M, muscarinic; M_3, muscarinic M_3; PGR, prostaglandin receptor; PP, proton pump.

PHARMACOLOGICAL BASIS OF MANAGEMENT

ANTACIDS

Antacids are alkalis that provide rapid relief of dyspepsia by neutralising the acid by a simple acid–base reaction and so remove the symptoms, but they do not lead to a cure. Examples of antacids include sodium bicarbonate and magnesium hydroxide.

ALGINATES

These are mucopolysaccharides and are usually combined with antacids, for example Gaviscon and Peptac. The alginic acid forms a viscous raft that floats on the gastric contents, protecting the oesophagus during reflux. Accordingly, alginates are used in GORD to reduce the impact of reflux.

H$_2$-RECEPTOR ANTAGONISTS

These are competitive histamine H$_2$-receptor antagonists that inhibit histamine-induced gastric acid secretion (Figure 16.2). The suppression of acid release provides symptomatic relief in dyspepsia. Famotidine is the most commonly used agent as it has fewer drug interactions than the prototypical agent cimetidine, which is rarely used. The once commonly used ranitidine is no longer widely available.

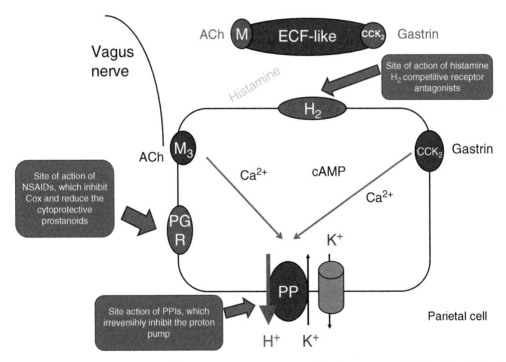

FIGURE 16.2   The sites of action of histamine H$_2$-receptor antagonists (to compete with histamine-induced activation of the proton pump), proton pump inhibitors (PPIs) to irreversibly inhibit the proton pump (PP) and the ulcerogenic effects of non-steroidal anti-inflammatory drugs via inhibition of cyclooxygenase (Cox), which produces cytoprotective prostanoids, which modulate the PP. ACh, acetylcholine; cAMP, cyclic adenosine monophosphate; CCK$_2$, cholecystokinin B; ECF, enterochromaffin-like cell; M, muscarinic; M$_3$, muscarinic M$_3$; PGR, prostaglandin receptor.

PROTON PUMP INHIBITORS

Proton pump inhibitors (PPIs; e.g., lansoprazole, omeprazole [esomeprazole as its *S*-isomer], pantoprazole) are the most effective acid suppressors as they inhibit the final common pathway (Figure 16.2). PPIs irreversibly inhibit the proton pump (H^+/K^+ ATPase), which leads to long-lasting suppression of proton secretion. The chemical properties of PPIs, defined by their pKa values, means that they are only converted to active drugs at acidic pH, which means that their actions are largely confined to the gastric mucosa. This results in a high level of selectivity and limited side effects. However, PPIs are unstable in gastric acid and so are administered as gastro-resistant capsules to avoid being degraded as the drug enters the stomach, and the pH-dependent formulation leads to selective release in the duodenum. Following absorption, PPIs act systemically and are activated in the region of the parietal cells as described above. Given this formulation, the PPI capsule must be swallowed whole to ensure delivery to the duodenum.

PPIs are very safe and effective drugs, and a number of them (e.g., omeprazole and pantoprazole) are available in pharmacies for a maximum of 4 weeks' usage. Esomeprazole, which is the active enantiomer of omeprazole (although clinically they are equally effective), is widely available in the UK in many retail outlets.

PPIs are generally well tolerated, but side effects can include diarrhoea. PPIs have some significant drug interactions, some of which occur via inhibition of cytochrome P450. In addition, bioactivation of the antiplatelet drug clopidogrel (Chapter 18) is thought to be reduced by both omeprazole and esomeprazole, and alternatives such as pantoprazole or lansoprazole should be used instead with clopidogrel.

There has been concern around the long-term use of PPIs and bone mineralisation, increasing fracture risk (Lespessailles and Toumi 2022). Given this concern, PPIs should not be used long term, especially in patients at risk of osteoporosis and fractures.

PROSTAGLANDIN ANALOGUES

Misoprostol is a stable prostaglandin analogue E_1 that mimics the action of the cytoprotective prostanoids, stimulates the production of bicarbonate and reduces the activity of the proton pump by reducing cAMP levels. Misoprostol is contraindicated in women of childbearing age as it can stimulate uterine contractions.

NON-ULCER DYSPEPSIA

In the absence of ulceration, dyspepsia is managed by using the optimum acid suppressor, which gives control of symptoms. Given the safety profile and effectiveness of PPIs, they are often used.

PRACTICE APPLICATION

Triple therapy of *H. pylori* infection

The treatment of patients with peptic ulceration who are infected with *H. pylori*, is called triple therapy and leads to eradication of the infection and cure. Triple therapy usually involves a PPI plus two antibacterial agents from clarithromycin, amoxicillin or metronidazole for 1–2 weeks. Triple therapy is associated with 90% eradication rates.

STOP AND THINK

What factors determine the choice of which antibiotics to use in triple therapy?

PRACTICE APPLICATION

Prevention of NSAID-induced ulceration

NSAID use is the second leading cause of peptic ulceration (Chapter 26). The production of the cytoprotective protanoids via cyclooxygenase is inhibited by NSAIDs, protection is decreased and this can lead to ulceration (Figure 16.2). Concurrent *H. pylori* infection also predisposes towards NSAID-induced damage and so this should be investigated. For NSAID-induced damage, the initial approach is to stop the NSAID and switch to paracetamol for pain relief if this is required. If the patient must continue with the NSAID or low-dose aspirin, or is initially identified as being at a high risk (>65 years, past ulcer, concomitant oral steroids, selective serotonin reuptake inhibitors or venlafaxine), then prophylaxis which PPIs (or sometimes misoprostol) are commonly used.

NAUSEA AND VOMITING

Nausea and vomiting are common occurrences and may reflect simple disease (e.g., after exposure to bacterial toxins), be associated with motion (travel sickness) or reflect more serious underlying pathology. Causes of nausea and vomiting include alcohol intoxication, viral and bacterial gastrointestinal infections, motion sickness, peptic ulceration, pregnancy, migraine, vestibular disorders including Ménière's disease, and head trauma. One key area in therapeutics is the association of nausea and vomiting as a side effect of a range of drug therapies, including:

- anticancer drugs
- digoxin
- erythromycin
- levodopa
- opioids
- selective serotonin reuptake inhibitors.

The vomiting pathway is under common, central control, leading to a highly coordinated physiological response, involving respiratory, salivary and gastric control, and resulting in the expulsion of gastric contents. Given the range of causative factors, there are several mechanisms of nausea, including:

- local irritation of the stomach involving visceral afferent fibres
- the central effects of toxins on the chemoreceptor trigger zone (CTZ)
- the conflict between visual and balance information, which is thought to occur in motion sickness.

Vomiting is under the control of the vomiting centre, which receives a direct input from visceral afferent nerves and is also regulated by the CTZ. The CTZ is, in turn, sensitive to circulating drugs and toxins, and receives input from the vestibular nuclei, which is linked to the labyrinth of the inner ear.

PHARMACOLOGICAL BASIS OF MANAGEMENT

Antiemetic drugs encompass a range of different drug classes, with different sites of action within the vomiting pathway. The site of action determines the circumstances in which an agent is effective (Figure 16.3).

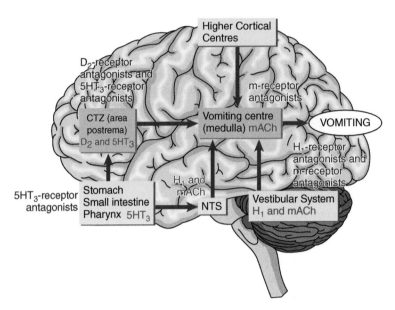

FIGURE 16.3   The sites of action of the four main classes of antiemetic drugs. 5-HT$_3$, 5-hydroxytryptamine 5-HT$_3$ receptor; CTZ, chemoreceptor trigger zone; D$_2$, dopamine D$_2$ receptor; mACh, muscarinic acetylcholine receptor; m-receptor, muscarinic receptor; NTS, nucleus of tractus solitarius.

HISTAMINE H$_1$-RECEPTOR ANTAGONISTS

These agents (e.g., cinnarizine, cyclizine, promethazine) are older sedative antihistamines that also have appreciable antimuscarinic activity, which contributes towards their use as antiemetics. They act on the vestibular nuclei and are effective in motion sickness. Cyclizine is often used in severe vomiting during pregnancy.

ANTIMUSCARINIC AGENTS

Antimuscarinic agents (e.g., hyoscine) act in both the vomiting centre and the vestibular apparatus, making them highly effective in motion sickness.

STOP AND THINK

What side effects would you expect from antimuscarinic drugs?

DOPAMINE RECEPTOR ANTAGONISTS

These agents (e.g., domperidone, metoclopramide, prochlorperazine) block dopamine receptors in the CTZ. However, the blockade of central dopamine receptors is associated with extrapyramidal effects and drug-induced Parkinsonism. This is less of an issue with domperidone, which has limited access to the central nervous system (CNS). The potential for neurological side effects of metoclopramide mean that its use is restricted and limited to short-term usage. Dopamine receptor antagonists are effective against anticancer drug-induced emesis.

5-HYDROXYTRYPTAMINE RECEPTOR ANTAGONISTS

These agents (e.g., ondansetron) block 5-hydroxytryptamine (5-HT), acting at 5-HT$_3$ receptors in the gut and CNS, and are particularly effective against anticancer drugs, which may cause the release of 5-HT in the gastrointestinal tract, and also in postoperative nausea and vomiting.

DIARRHOEA

Diarrhoea involves the frequent passing of watery stools. This, especially in vulnerable patients, can lead to dehydration, which can be life-threatening. Indeed, the key to management is rehydration.

Acute diarrhoea is often infectious, for example rotaviruses damage villi in the small-bowel and adhesive enterotoxigenic bacteria (such as cholera and *Escherichia coli*) adhere to the brush border, and lead to ion and water secretion from the lower gastrointestinal tract.

Other causes of diarrhoea include the following:

- Antibiotic-associated diarrhoea is a common side effect of antibiotics and is usually mild. Antibiotics alter the balance of gut flora, which can lead to pathogenic bacteria thriving, leading to infection. A serious event here involves the growth of *Clostridium difficile*, which may present as severe and bloody diarrhoea in pseudomembranous colitis. All patients receiving antibiotics should be counselled that mild diarrhoea is a common side effect but should be alert to serious bloody diarrhoea.

- PPIs are also associated with causing diarrhoea, especially in older or more vulnerable patients. As PPIs raise gastric pH, they reduce the bactericidal effects of stomach acid, which can lead to infection.

- Orlistat, an anti-obesity drug, inhibits pancreatic lipases to prevent the breakdown of fat and this may lead to steatorrhoea (fatty diarrhoea), which may be part of its therapeutic action by ensuring that the patient avoids fatty food.

- The gastroprotective agent misoprostol activates prostanoid receptors in the intestines, increasing cAMP, which may lead to secretory diarrhoea.

PHARMACOLOGICAL BASIS OF THE MANAGEMENT OF DIARRHOEA

The first step in the management of acute diarrhoea, where a simple cause such as an adverse drug reaction can be identified, is to remove the cause and the condition may resolve. The cornerstone of therapy is oral rehydration therapy (ORT).

ORAL REHYDRATION THERAPY

ORT involves a specific mixture of electrolytes and glucose, which must be made up to a specific osmolality. The presence of glucose in ORT is to allow sodium to be co-transported with glucose by the epithelial sodium-glucose linked transporter-1 and this is followed by water, leading to rehydration.

ANTIBIOTICS

Many simple gastrointestinal infections are viral, and antibiotics are of no value. As noted above, antibiotics themselves can lead to diarrhoea. If, however, a bacterial causative organism is identified by stool cultures, this can guide the appropriate use of antibiotics.

ANTIMOTILITY AGENTS

Antimotility agents, including the opioid loperamide, are widely used to provide symptomatic relief. This is achieved by slowing down gastrointestinal motility and allowing the absorption of fluid. The symptomatic relief allows bowel control and prevents diarrhoea from interfering with daily activities. Despite the widespread use of loperamide, it does not alter the time course of infective diarrhoea and could potentially prolong the infection, as there is reduced flushing of the bowels.

Opioids reduce gastrointestinal motility via the activation of presynaptic μ-opioid receptor inhibition of parasympathetic nerves, leading to reduced release of acetylcholine. Although loperamide is an opioid, it does not have central effects as it does not penetrate the blood–brain barrier and is largely retained in the gastrointestinal tract by enterohepatic cycling.

CONSTIPATION

Constipation is defined as altered bowel habits with reduced frequency (e.g., fewer than three motions per week) and the passing of hardened faeces. In the simplest case, constipation may reflect an inadequate intake of roughage in the diet. Other causes may be psychological (resulting from painful defecation associated with haemorrhoids or anal fissure), irritable bowel syndrome (IBS), pregnancy, postoperative (secondary to immobility, dehydration or constipating drugs), associated with ageing, caused by serious bowel pathology such as carcinoma of the bowel, secondary fluid restriction in renal failure or induced by drug treatment. Drugs that may cause constipation include:

- opioids, commonly associated with constipation by reducing gastrointestinal motility as described above, therefore patients taking opioids are commonly co-prescribed laxatives

- antimuscarinic drugs, including tricyclic antidepressants and older antihistamines, which reduce gastrointestinal motility by blocking the muscarinic receptors, stimulated by the parasympathetic nervous system

- diuretics, which have a dehydrating effect

- calcium channel blockers, which relax the smooth muscle of the lower gastrointestinal tract.

MANAGEMENT

The best approach to constipation is a balanced diet with non-starch polysaccharides and fluid or adding bulking agents (e.g., methylcellulose) to the diet. Exercise might also help. Otherwise, laxatives may be indicated.

OSMOTIC LAXATIVES

Lactulose is a disaccharide and when it enters the colon it is converted by bacteria to lactic and acetic acids, which osmotically raise the fluid volume. This increase in fluid volume leads to larger and softer stools. The effects of lactulose are delayed by a day or two.

Macrogols include polyethylene glycol polymers, which absorb and retain fluid in the gastrointestinal tract and so increase the volume of the stools.

STIMULANT LAXATIVES: SENNA EXTRACTS AND SODIUM PICOSULPHATE

These provide rapid relief of symptoms. Senna extracts enter the colon and are metabolized to anthracene derivatives, which stimulate gastrointestinal activity by irritation. Sodium picosulphate is also an irritant that stimulates lower gastrointestinal activity.

SUMMARY

- Proton pump inhibitors are very safe and effective drugs, widely used in dyspepsia.

- Peptic ulcer disease is largely associated with *H. pylori* infection and can be successfully treated with triple therapy of a proton pump inhibitor plus two antibiotics.

- NSAID-induced ulceration is one of the most significant adverse drug reactions therefore NSAID use should be carefully managed and prophylaxis should be used in at-risk patients.

- Antiemetics have a significant role in limiting drug-induced emesis.

- The mainstay of therapy for diarrhoea is oral rehydration therapy. Antimotility agents are used but only provide symptomatic relief.

- Constipation can often be managed by lifestyle changes but for certain drug-induced cases, co-prescribing laxatives should be considered.

ACTIVITY

1. A patient is prescribed a proton pump inhibitor, which ONE of the following is a relevant counselling point:

   (a) A dry cough is a common side effect.

   (b) Avoid alcohol as the medicine interacts with alcohol.

   (c) Do not take with aspirin-containing products.

   (d) Swallow the capsule whole.

   (e) You should expect rapid relief within a few minutes.

2. In choosing triple therapy, which ONE the following would influence the choice of antibacterials?

   (a) Concurrent asthma

   (b) Penicillin allergy

   (c) The co-prescribed proton pump inhibitor

   (d) The microbiome

   (e) The presence of MRSA in the gastric mucosa

3. For which ONE of the following classes of drugs would you counsel a patient that constipation is a common side effect?

   (a) Metformin

   (b) Opioids

   (c) Paracetamol

   (d) Prostaglandin analogues

   (e) Proton pump inhibitors

REFERENCE

Lespessailles, E. and Toumi, H. (2022) Proton pump inhibitors and bone health: an update narrative review. *Int J Mol Sci* 23:10733.

FURTHER READING

Brunton, L. and Knollmann, B. (2022) *Goodman and Gilman's The Pharmacological Basis of Therapeutics*, 14th edn. McGraw Hill, New York.

Ritter, J.M., Flower, R., Henderson, G., et al. (2023) *Rang and Dale's Pharmacology*, 10th edn. Elsevier, Amsterdam.

GUIDANCE

NICE (2014) Gastro-oesophageal reflux disease and dyspepsia in adults: investigation and management. NICE Guideline 184. https://www.nice.org.uk/guidance/cg184.

Cardiovascular Drugs and Diseases

CHAPTER 17

Richard Roberts

LEARNING OUTCOMES

By the end of this chapter the reader should be able to:

- describe the homeostatic factors involved in the regulation of blood pressure

- describe the pathophysiology of chronic heart failure

- discuss the clinical use of drugs for the treatment of hypertension, hypercholesterolaemia, ischaemic heart disease and chronic heart failure

- understand the mechanism of action and major adverse effects of:

  o calcium channel inhibitors

  o angiotensin-converting enzyme inhibitors/angiotensin receptor antagonists

  o β-adrenoceptor antagonists

  o diuretics (loop diuretics, thiazide and potassium-sparing agents)

  o digoxin

  o nitrates

  o statins

  o cholesterol uptake inhibitors

  o sodium glucose 2 transporter inhibitors

  o neutral endopeptidase inhibitors such as sacubitril

- critically apply current clinical guidelines for cardiovascular conditions.

Cardiovascular disease is a leading cause of morbidity and mortality. Cardiovascular disease ranges from hypertension to ischaemic heart disease, stroke and chronic heart failure. Indeed, hypertension alongside dyslipidaemia is a risk factor for myocardial infarction, stroke and heart failure. Cardiovascular disease is associated with lifestyle and ageing, and risk is also related to sex, genetics and ethnicity. This chapter considers how therapy can reduce cardiovascular risk and manage cardiovascular disease.

REGULATION OF BLOOD PRESSURE

To understand hypertension and its treatment, we first consider the physiology of blood pressure regulation. Blood pressure is determined by both cardiac output and total peripheral resistance (TPR):

$$\text{blood pressure} = \text{cardiac output} \times \text{total peripheral resistance}$$

The New Prescriber: An Integrated Approach to Medical and Non-medical Prescribing, Second Edition.
Edited by Joanne Lymn, Alison Mostyn, Roger Knaggs, Michael Randall, and Dianne Bowskill.
© 2024 John Wiley & Sons Ltd. Published 2024 by John Wiley & Sons Ltd.

peripheral resistance is determined by both the level of 'tone' or constriction in the vasculature, and the volume of circulating blood. Vasoconstriction leads to increased TPR, and reduced excretion of fluid by the kidneys leads to increased blood volume.

Cardiac output is determined by both the force of contraction of the ventricles and heart rate, therefore reducing both of these factors will lead to a reduction in blood pressure.

RENIN-ANGIOTENSIN-ALDOSTERONE SYSTEM

The renin-angiotensin-aldosterone system (RAAS) plays an important role in the regulation of fluid retention, electrolyte balance and blood pressure. Renin is released from the kidney in response to a reduction in blood pressure, a decrease in renal perfusion or a decrease in sodium levels (Figure 17.1). It is a proteolytic enzyme that cleaves angiotensinogen to produce angiotensin I. Angiotensin I is in turn cleaved by angiotensin-converting enzyme (ACE) to produce angiotensin II. Angiotensin II acts

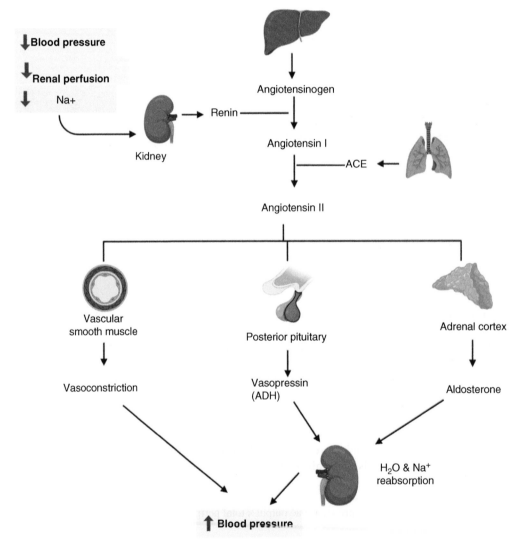

FIGURE 17.1 Outline of the role of the renin-angiotensin-aldosterone system in the control of blood pressure. Created in Biorender. ACE, angiotensin-converting enzyme, ADH, antidiuretic hormone.

at AT1 receptors and has numerous functions, including vasoconstriction, stimulation of the release of aldosterone from the adrenal cortex (Figure 17.1) and release of vasopressin from the posterior pituitary, all of which contribute to an increase in blood pressure. Aldosterone acts on the distal convoluted tubule in the kidney to promote sodium reabsorption and, as a result, water reabsorption. Vasopressin also contributes to retention of water in the kidneys, reducing urine output.

CARDIAC OUTPUT AND REGULATION BY THE AUTONOMIC NERVOUS SYSTEM

Sympathetic innervation of the heart leads to an increase in heart rate and force of contraction of the ventricles (Chapter 14). β_1-adenoceptors in the sino-atrial node are activated by noradrenaline and adrenaline, and increase the rate of closure of K^+ channels, which reduces the duration between action potentials, thus increasing heart rate. There is also increased conduction through the atrio-ventricular node, thus reducing the time between atrial contraction and ventricular contraction. β_1-adenoceptors on ventricular cardiac muscle increase the force of contraction of the ventricles. Overall, there is an increase in cardiac output. Parasympathetic innervation releases acetylcholine, which acts on muscarinic M_1 receptors in the sino-atrial node to reduce the rate of closing of K^+ channels, thus increasing the duration between action potentials and reducing heart rate. The funny current (If) is a pacemaker current in the sino-atrial node that regulates the level of Na^+ and K^+ across the cardiac muscle membrane, therefore inhibiting this channel can lead to a reduction in heart rate.

HYPERTENSION

Hypertension is defined as a blood pressure which is associated with significant cardiovascular risk. The increased pressure in the vasculature leads to increased growth of the smooth muscle in blood vessels (remodelling), increased size of the left ventricle in the heart (ventricular hypertrophy) and increased pressure in the renal vascular bed. This leads to enhanced contraction of blood vessels, increased risk of heart failure and renal damage, respectively. There is also increased risk of stroke and myocardial infarction. The aim of treatment of a patient with high blood pressure is therefore to reduce the risk of the development of these changes. Hypertension can be either essential (primary) or secondary. Secondary hypertension is secondary to another condition or drug treatment (e.g., with corticosteroids and non-steroidal anti-inflammatory drugs) and therefore has a known cause, for example renal disease, Cushing's syndrome or hyperthyroidism. The cause of essential (primary) hypertension is not known but may be multifactorial, such as lifestyle (exercise, diet, smoking, weight).

Patients with a sustained blood pressure of 140/90 mmHg (or average ambulatory/home blood pressure measurement of 135/85 mmHg) are classed as hypertensive. Initial treatment for patients with stage 1 hypertension (>140/90 and <160/100 mmHg should be lifestyle changes (e.g., quitting smoking, dietary changes, weight loss). Patients with stage 2 hypertension >160/100 mmHg (or average ambulatory blood pressure measurement of 150/95 mmHg) or with a blood pressure of >140/90 and <160/100 mmHg with end organ damage should be started on pharmacological therapy (NICE 2019).

PRACTICE APPLICATION

NICE guidelines follow the AC(D) rules, depending on the age or ethnicity of the patient (Figure 17.2). At Step 1, patients aged less than 55 years should be started on an ACE inhibitor/AT_1 receptor antagonist (A), whereas patients over the age of 55 should be started on a calcium channel inhibitor. Patients of Afro-Caribbean heritage should be started on a calcium channel inhibitor (C), regardless of their age, as hypertension in this ethnic group tends to be associated with low renin levels. Most patients do not reach

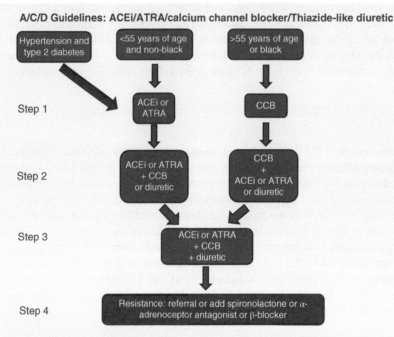

FIGURE 17.2 Summary of the NICE guidelines (2019) for the treatment of hypertension. ACEi, angiotensin converting enzyme inhibitor; ATRA, angiotensin receptor antagonist; CCB, calcium channel blocker.

their target after initial treatment and so move to Step 2, which involves adding the other drug class or a thiazide-like diuretic (D). Step 3 involves A + C + D and Step 4 may involve additional therapies, including α- or β-adrenoceptor antagonists, or the mineralocorticoid receptor antagonist, spironolactone or referral to secondary care. Patients with diabetes are initially treated with an ACE inhibitor/AT_1 receptor antagonist, as these agents are renoprotective against diabetic nephropathy.

CALCIUM CHANNEL INHIBITORS

Calcium channel inhibitors (also known as blockers and antagonists) are widely used in hypertension and ischaemic heart disease. They can be broadly divided into rate-limiting calcium channel inhibitors (so-called because of their cardiac slowing effects) and dihydropyridines (Table 17.1).

Table 17.1 Examples of drugs in the main subclassification of calcium channel inhibitors

Dihydropyridines	Amlodipine
	Felodipine
	Nifedipine
Rate-limiting calcium channel inhibitors	Verapamil
	Diltiazem

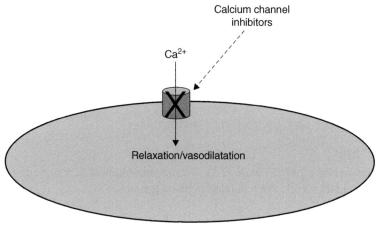

FIGURE 17.3 The action of calcium channel inhibitors to inhibit entry of calcium via voltage-operated calcium channels into vascular smooth muscle, leading to vasodilatation.

Mechanism of action

Smooth muscle contraction is caused by an increase in intracellular calcium through release from intracellular stores and via influx through calcium channels. Voltage-gated calcium channels are a major mechanism for influx of extracellular calcium into smooth muscle cells, therefore inhibiting these calcium channels will lead to a reduction in the influx of calcium and, hence, an inhibition of contraction (Figure 17.3). Inhibition of vascular smooth muscle contraction in blood vessels will mean that there is greater relaxation of blood vessels and thus less pressure within the vasculature. Dihydropyridine-type calcium channel inhibitors act at the dihydropyridine binding site on L-type voltage gated calcium channels. By reducing calcium influx and thus reducing vascular smooth muscle contraction, they reduce total peripheral resistance, thereby reducing blood pressure.

Inhibition of calcium influx in the coronary circulation leads to relaxation of the coronary arteries, thereby increasing blood flow. This is beneficial in angina, in which there is impaired blood flow. Verapamil has some selectivity for calcium channels in the heart, leading to a reduction in heart rate. As blood flows through the coronary circulation during diastole, reducing the heart rate increases the diastolic time period, giving more time for blood to flow through the coronary arteries. Diltiazem, on the other hand, has equal effects on both heart and vascular calcium channels.

Side effects

Most of the side effects of calcium channel inhibitors relate to the inhibition of smooth muscle contraction. Peripheral oedema, with ankle swelling, is common due to precapillary vasodilatation raising capillary pressure and reducing fluid reabsorption. Inhibition of gastrointestinal smooth muscle leads to a reduction in movement of faecal content, which leads to constipation. Verapamil is contraindicated in heart failure because of its negative inotropic effects, which could reduce cardiac output further in this condition.

Amlodipine, verapamil and diltiazem inhibit CYP3A4 (Chapter 9), which leads to an increase in plasma levels of simvastatin and therefore an increased risk of myopathy. The maximum dose of simvastatin should be reduced to 20 mg daily to compensate for the reduced metabolism.

DRUGS THAT AFFECT THE RAAS

The RAAS is targeted by both ACE inhibitors (e.g., ramipril) and angiotensin (AT1) receptor antagonists (e.g., candesartan). ACE inhibitors were introduced in the 1980s and AT1 receptor antagonists in the 1990s. They are broadly equivalent in terms of effectiveness but have different side-effect profiles.

ANGIOTENSIN-CONVERTING ENZYME INHIBITORS

Mechanism of action

ACE is a component of the RAAS (Figure 17.1), therefore inhibition of ACE prevents the formation of angiotensin II and thus leads to a reduction in blood pressure.

Side effects

ACE also metabolises bradykinin and therefore inhibition of ACE leads to an increase in levels of this peptide. Bradykinin is a potent vasodilator and so increasing the levels of bradykinin contributes to the blood pressure-reducing effects of ACE inhibitors. However, bradykinin also induces cough, which can be problematic for around 10% of patients. In these patients, angiotensin receptor antagonists would be an alternative treatment. These drugs inhibit the effects of angiotensin II at the AT1 receptor, without altering bradykinin levels, and therefore without inducing cough.

ACE inhibitors can cause a large drop in blood pressure on first exposure to the drug (first-dose hypotension) in a small number of patients, therefore patients are often advised to take the first dose at night so that they are lying down if hypotension occurs. This first-dose hypotension is worse if the patient is taking a diuretic concurrently. In this case, patients would be advised to stop taking the diuretic until they are stabilised on the ACE inhibitor.

ACE inhibitors can also increase vascular permeability through the effects of bradykinin, leading to angioedema. This can result in swelling of the lips and tongue. This is a rare, serious adverse event that is more prevalent in patients of African or Caribbean heritage.

There is a risk of hyperkalaemia with ACE inhibitors (and angiotensin receptor antagonists, see below), particularly if taken with potassium supplements or in combination with potassium-sparing diuretics, or in patients with impaired renal function. ACE inhibitors may also lead to an impairment of renal function, although they may be beneficial in diabetic nephropathy. Side effects may be more severe in patients with impaired renal function, therefore electrolytes and renal function should be measured before initiation of treatment and before dose adjustment, and should be monitored during treatment.

ACE inhibitors and angiotensin receptor antagonists should not be used in patients with bilateral renal stenosis due to risks of severe hypotension and reduction in glomerular filtration, which could exacerbate the condition.

ANGIOTENSIN RECEPTOR ANTAGONISTS (SARTANS)

Mechanism of action

Angiotensin receptor antagonists (also known as ARBs or sartans, e.g., candesartan, losartan and valsartan) antagonise the AT1 receptor, thereby preventing the effects of angiotensin II on the production of aldosterone and vasopressin, and preventing the vasocontractile effects of angiotensin II. As indicated above, they are far less likely to produce the cough or angioedema side effects seen with ACE inhibitors.

DIURETICS (SEE CHAPTER 19)

THIAZIDES AND THIAZIDE-LIKE

Thiazide diuretics (notably bendroflumethiazide) have been used for many years in the treatment of hypertension, but due to their association with worsening or uncovering diabetes they are now used as second-line agents, with thiazide-like agents (e.g., chlortalidone and indapamide) now being preferred.

Mechanism of action

These drugs act on the distal convoluted tubule in the kidney, where they inhibit the sodium/ chloride symporter, reducing the reabsorption of these ions from the urine (Figure 17.4). This alters the osmotic gradient such that less water is reabsorbed from the urine, increasing diuresis. This leads to a reduction in blood volume and therefore a reduction in blood pressure. These diuretics also lead to vasodilatation, which contributes to the blood pressure-reducing effect. The mechanism of this vasodilatation is unknown, but it lasts after drug treatment has been stopped, suggesting an adaptive mechanism.

    The retention of sodium in the urine leads to a reuptake of sodium in exchange for potassium in the collecting duct, leading to reduced plasma potassium levels. The reduction in plasma volume

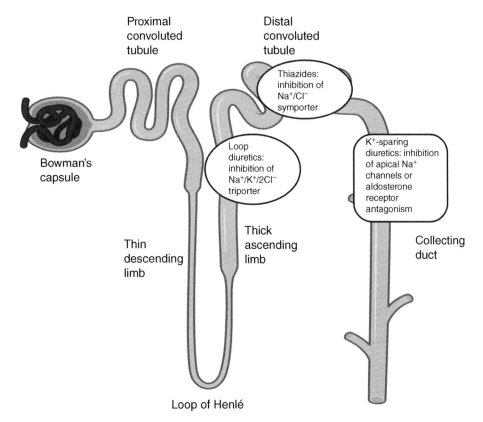

FIGURE 17.4   The renal nephron showing the main sites of diuretic action in the management of cardiovascular diseases. Loop diuretics are commonly used in chronic heart failure associated with pulmonary oedema, thiazides and thiazide-like diuretics are second-line antihypertensives, potassium (K)-sparing agents are sometimes used with loop diuretics or thiazides to prevent potassium loss and aldosterone receptor antagonists are also used to oppose the actions of aldosterone in chronic heart failure. Created in Biorender.

caused by diuretics leads to a compensatory increase in renin and therefore activation of the RAAS. This increase in RAAS is likely to contribute to the reabsorption of sodium and loss of potassium.

Thiazides and thiazide-like diuretics require a certain level of renal function for them to be effective, as they require excretion in the proximal tubules to reach their site of action. They should therefore be avoided in patients with eGFR <30 mL/min/1.72 m^2.

Side effects

Owing to the increased loss of potassium from the kidneys, patients are at risk of hypokalaemia, therefore electrolytes should be monitored regularly.

All diuretics will increase urination and therefore patients should be advised to take them at a time of day which will lead to least impact. For example, they should be taken first thing in the morning so that the increased urination does not impact on sleep at night.

Thiazides and thiazide-like diuretics can worsen diabetes and gout. Elderly patients are more likely to develop side effects and therefore patients should be started at a lower dose.

POTASSIUM-SPARING DIURETICS

Mechanism of action

Potassium-sparing diuretics (e.g., amiloride) block the epithelial sodium channel in the collecting duct in the kidney to prevent reabsorption of sodium, therefore preventing reabsorption of water (Figure 17.4). As sodium is not being exchanged for potassium in the collecting duct, these drugs prevent loss of potassium.

Other potassium-sparing diuretics include mineralocorticoid receptor antagonists (such as spironolactone), which block the actions of aldosterone, which is a sodium-retaining/potassium-losing steroid hormone (see below).

Side effects

Potassium-sparing diuretics have increased risk of hyperkalaemia, particularly when used alongside ACE inhibitors or potassium supplements, therefore electrolytes should be monitored. The risk of hyperkalaemia is increased with decreased renal function and so should be avoided in severe renal impairment.

β-ADRENOCEPTOR ANTAGONISTS (β-BLOCKERS)

β-adrenoceptor antagonists (e.g., atenolol or bisoprolol) have been used for many years in cardiovascular disease. They were originally the agents of choice in hypertension, but are now only used in hypertension with concurrent ischaemic heart disease or failure, and in refractory hypertension (uncontrolled hypertension despite the use of five or more antihypertensive drugs). Labetalol is also used in pregnancy-associated hypertension.

Mechanism of action

β_1-adrenoceptors in the heart increase heart rate and force of contractions, leading to increased cardiac output and hence increased blood pressure (Chapter 14). β-adrenoceptor antagonists prevent the effects of adrenaline and noradrenaline on the heart, reducing cardiac output. Non-selective antagonists such as propranolol also antagonise β_2-adrenoceptors in the lungs and can lead to breathlessness. β_1-adrenoceptor antagonists have some degree of selectivity for the β_1-adrenoceptors in the heart over the β_2-adrenoceptors in the lungs, but they are contraindicated in patients with asthma. Part of their antihypertensive effects are via inhibition of renin release and reduced activity of the RAAS. They are less effective at reducing blood pressure compared to ACE inhibitors and calcium channel inhibitors, and are no longer recommended as first-line antihypertensives.

Side effects

β-adrenoceptor antagonists can also lead to fatigue due to effects on β-adrenoceptors in skeletal muscle, cold extremities due to antagonism of β-adrenoceptors in the vasculature and sleep disturbances, including nightmares.

β-adrenoceptor antagonists can lead to alteration of glucose metabolism. Furthermore, as hypoglycaemia leads to stimulation of the sympathetic nervous system, antagonism of β-adrenoceptors can lead to a masking of the symptoms of hypoglycaemia such that patients with diabetes may be unaware that they are becoming hypoglycaemic, therefore they should be used with caution in patients with diabetes.

STOP AND THINK

β-blockers can worsen respiratory diseases. In which conditions should β-blockers be avoided or used with caution?

α-ADRENOCEPTOR ANTAGONISTS

α-adrenoceptors (α_1- and α_2-adrenoceptors) stimulate vasoconstriction and therefore contribute to an increase in blood pressure. Selective α_1-adrenoceptor antagonists such as prazosin can be used for patients with difficult to treat hypertension. However, they are associated with several side effects, including blurred vision, drowsiness and dizziness, gastrointestinal disturbances and heart palpitations.

Dyslipidaemia

High plasma cholesterol is associated with an increased risk of cardiovascular disease, in particular an increase in low-density lipoprotein (LDL)-cholesterol (LDL-C) and a decrease in high-density lipoprotein (HDL)-C. Hypercholesterolaemia increases the risk of developing atherosclerosis, which leads to an increased risk of ischaemic heart disease.

Lipid transport and atherosclerosis

Lipids, including cholesterol, are transported around the body as a mixture of lipid and protein known as lipoproteins. LDLs transport cholesterol from the liver to peripheral tissues whereas HDLs transport cholesterol from the peripheries back to the liver. Very low-density lipoproteins are involved in the transport of triglycerides around the body. As LDLs transport cholesterol to the peripheries, an increase in LDL-C is associated with an increased risk of cholesterol accumulating in the walls of blood vessels. In contrast, as HDLs transport cholesterol from the peripheries back to the liver for metabolism, an increase in HDL-C is associated with reduced risk of atherosclerosis.

Damage to the endothelial layer of blood vessels caused by high blood pressure, turbulent flow of blood or oxidative stress caused by, for example, smoking or diabetes leads to an inflammatory response. Reactive oxygen species produced by inflammatory cells oxidise LDL-C, which then gets engulfed by phagocytic macrophages. The cholesterol droplets in these macrophages give rise to the name 'foam cells'. These foam cells are deposited in the wall of the blood vessel, which is the start of the formation of an atherosclerotic plaque.

Cardiovascular risk can be assessed by the QRISK-3 tool (https://qrisk.org/) and takes account of the ratio of total cholesterol (TC) to HDL-C, systolic blood pressure and other parameters to determine the risk of developing cardiovascular disease over the next 10 years.

The following are risk factors for atherosclerosis:

• genetics

• dyslipidaemia (raised LDL or reduced levels of HDL)

• hypertension

• smoking

• obesity

• hyperglycaemia

• reduced physical activity.

TREATMENT OF HYPERCHOLESTEROLAEMIA

Cholesterol is synthesised in the liver from 3-hydroxy-3-methyl-glutaryl CoA (HMG-CoA). The initial step in the synthesis utilises HMG-CoA reductase to convert HMG-CoA into mevalonate (Figure 17.5). Cholesterol is ultimately synthesised from mevalonate through a series of enzymes.

HMG-COA REDUCTASE INHIBITORS (STATINS)

Mechanism of action

Statins (e.g., simvastatin, atorvastatin and pravastatin) inhibit HMG-CoA reductase, which, as outlined above, is the first step in the synthesis of cholesterol. The reduction in cholesterol synthesis due to inhibition of this enzyme leads to an upregulation of LDL-C receptors on the hepatocytes in the liver, resulting in an increased uptake of LDL-C from the plasma into the liver.

Numerous clinical trials have demonstrated the effects of statins on reducing mortality from cardiovascular disease in patients with raised cholesterol levels. The Heart Protection Study (Heart Protection Study Collaborative Group 2002) also demonstrated a reduction in mortality in patients who are at risk of myocardial infarction due to high blood pressure, type 2

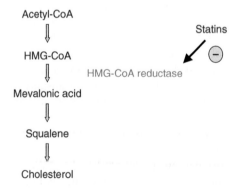

FIGURE 17.5 Statins inhibit 3-hydroxy-3-methyl-glutaryl CoA (HMG-CoA) as the first committed step in cholesterol synthesis.

diabetes or coronary heart disease, but with cholesterol levels classed as being in the normal range. This trial indicates that statins have beneficial effects even in patients who do not have hypercholesterolaemia.

Cholesterol synthesis in the body is highest at night, therefore most statins should be taken in the evening before going to bed. Atorvastatin is an exception because it has a longer plasma half-life.

Side effects and monitoring

Although muscle pain is common with statins, a rare side effect of statin use is an increased breakdown of skeletal muscle, resulting in rhabdomyolysis. Breakdown products released from the skeletal muscle can lead to kidney damage and renal failure. Patients taking statins should report any unexpected muscle pain. To reduce the risk of rhabdomyolysis, the lowest effective dose of statin should be used, and dose adjustment might be necessary with concomitant treatment with drugs known to inhibit the metabolism of statins (e.g., calcium channel inhibitors, see previous section). Creatine kinase levels should be measured in patients who are at risk of myopathy or who have persistent, unexplained muscle pain before initiation of treatment on statins.

Grapefruit juice inhibits simvastatin metabolism and therefore produces a transient increase in plasma levels of the drug (Chapter 9), therefore patients should be advised not to consume grapefruit or grapefruit juice whilst taking simvastatin.

Liver function tests should be carried out before and after initiation of treatment with statins (after 3 and 12 months).

CHOLESTEROL UPTAKE INHIBITORS

Mechanism of action

Cholesterol uptake inhibitors (e.g., ezetimibe) inhibit the Niemann–Pick C1-like 1 sterol transporter in the gastrointestinal tract to reduce the uptake of cholesterol from the diet. In general, an increase in dietary cholesterol does not contribute to an increase in plasma cholesterol levels as the body adapts to the increased intake by reducing the reuptake of bile. As bile salts are synthesised from cholesterol, a reduced reuptake of bile requires the liver to synthesise new bile salts from cholesterol, thereby reducing plasma cholesterol levels. However, a cholesterol uptake inhibitor can help to reduce plasma cholesterol levels further in patients already being treated with a statin due to the combination of reducing uptake from the diet and reducing cholesterol synthesis in the liver. To this end, combination drugs containing simvastatin and ezetimibe are available.

Side effects

Risk of rhabdomyolysis is greater if ezetimibe is taken alongside a statin, therefore patients should report any unexplained muscle pain, as with statin therapy alone.

Reduced absorption of cholesterol from the gastrointestinal tract can lead to gastrointestinal disturbances.

PROPROTEIN CONVERTASE SUBTILISIN/KEXIN TYPE 9 INHIBITORS

Proprotein convertase subtilisin/kexin type 9 (PCSK9) is an enzyme that contributes to the breakdown of LDL receptors in hepatocytes. Inhibition of this enzyme, by drugs such as the monoclonal antibodies alirocumab and evolocumab, and the siRNA inhibitor inclisiran, will lead to an increase in the number of LDL receptors. This in turn will lead to an increased uptake of LDL-C into the liver. PCSK9 inhibitors are used by specialists as add-on therapies for patients with difficult to treat hypercholesterolaemia.

Mechanism of action

Alirocumab and evolocumab are monoclonal antibodies targeting PCSK9, reducing its activity. They are given by subcutaneous injection every 2–4 weeks.

Inclisiran is a small interfering RNA (siRNA) that inhibits the synthesis of PCSK9. It is given by subcutaneous injection. The second dose is given after 3 months and then every 6 months for subsequent doses.

PRACTICE APPLICATION:

Who to treat?
The QRISK3 (https://qrisk.org/) calculator should be used to determine whether or not a patient requires pharmacological treatment. This takes into account the patient's biological sex, ethnicity, age, smoking status, concurrent diseases (e.g., diabetes or renal disease), weight, systolic blood pressure and TC:HDL-C ratio.

Initial advice for patients with hypercholesterolaemia should be lifestyle changes, including weight loss, exercise, quitting smoking and reducing alcohol intake. NICE guidelines recommend low-intensity atorvastatin treatment (20 mg) to patients with >10% risk of developing cardiovascular disease in the next 10 years. All patients with cardiovascular disease should receive high-intensity therapy with atorvastatin 80 mg.

Congestive (chronic) heart failure

Congestive (chronic) heart failure can occur because of remodelling of the heart due to chronic hypertension or as a result of ischaemic heart disease or cardiomyopathy. Chronic hypertension can lead to enlargement of the cardiac muscle in the left ventricle (ventricular hypertrophy) in response to the increased workload of the heart required to pump against the higher pressure in the vasculature. Ventricular hypertrophy ultimately leads to an impairment of cardiac muscle contraction, resulting in a reduction in cardiac output.

Heart failure can be due to left or right ventricular failure, or a combination of both. Left ventricular failure leads to reduced blood pressure and reduced renal perfusion, leading to activation of the RAAS. Activation of the RAAS leads to vasoconstriction (through angiotensin II acting on AT1 receptors on vascular smooth muscle) and retention of water through the effects of aldosterone on the kidneys. Both of these lead to an increase in both pre-load and after-load on the heart, and therefore an increase in workload of the heart. However, as the heart is in failure, it is unable to cope with this increase in workload, which results in a further reduction in cardiac output. The sympathetic nervous system is also activated to stimulate the heart in an attempt to increase cardiac output. The reduction in peripheral blood pressure and retention of fluid in the kidneys contributes to peripheral oedema. Right ventricular failure can be the result of pulmonary hypertension. Reduced output from the right ventricle leads to a reduction in pulmonary blood pressure, contributing to pulmonary oedema.

The aim of treatment in heart failure is to reduce the workload on the heart, thus preserving heart function and reducing the symptoms.

LOOP DIURETICS (CHAPTER 19)

Mechanism of action

Loop diuretics (e.g., furosemide) inhibit the sodium/potassium/chloride co-transporter in the thick, ascending limb of the loop of Henlé in the kidney, preventing the reabsorption of these ions from the urine and so also reducing reabsorption of water (Figure 17.4). This leads to increased diuresis and a reduction in blood volume. Loop diuretics are used in heart failure to counteract the water retention and oedema caused by activation of the RAAS. A reduction in blood volume leads to a reduction in both pre- and after load in the heart, thereby reducing the workload of the heart. This helps to preserve cardiac function, as well as reducing the symptoms of fluid retention, such as oedema.

As with other diuretics, patients should be aware of the impact of increased urination on lifestyle and sleep.

Side effects

Postural hypotension is a key adverse event and is associated with dizziness and falls, especially in older patients. Patients should be advised to get up slowly from sitting to standing.

DRUGS TARGETING THE RAAS

ACE INHIBITORS

ACE inhibitors are useful in heart failure to counter the activation of the RAAS in response to reduced blood pressure and renal perfusion. Inhibition of angiotensin II production leads to a reduction in both pre- and after-load on the heart, thereby reducing workload. AT1 receptor antagonists are used as an alternative to ACE inhibitors. In the longer term, ACE inhibitors and AT1 receptor antagonists oppose the adverse effects of angiotensin II on myocytes associated with neurohormonal adaptation.

β-ADRENOCEPTOR ANTAGONISTS (β-BLOCKERS)

The β-adrenoceptor antagonists bisoprolol, carvedilol and nebivolol are licensed for first-line therapy in heart failure and are initiated at very low doses.

Mechanism of action

The mechanism by which these antagonists work to improve heart failure is unclear, but the mechanism may be due to counteracting the increased in sympathetic activity, which is associated with increased cardiac workload and myocyte toxicity. β_1-adrenoceptors increase the heart rate and force of contraction of the ventricles, thus increasing cardiac output, therefore β-adrenoceptor antagonists decrease cardiac output. As cardiac output is already decreased in heart failure, β-adrenoceptor antagonists licenced for heart failure should be used with care, with a low dose used initially and the dose slowly titrated upwards until the maximum tolerated dose is achieved ('start low and go slow'). The symptoms of heart failure may worsen with initial treatment, but chronic treatment leads to an overall improvement in cardiac function. However, patients should be monitored carefully during the initial treatment and dose titration to ensure that cardiac function does not worsen.

STOP AND THINK

β-blockers used to be contraindicated in heart failure. How are they now used safely and effectively in heart failure?

MINERALOCORTICOID RECEPTOR ANTAGONISTS

Mineralocorticoid receptor antagonists such as eplerenone and spironolactone are antagonists of the aldosterone receptor, preventing the effects of aldosterone on fluid retention in the kidneys, and counteracting the activation of the RAAS in heart failure (Figure 17.4). Aldosterone receptor antagonists are also beneficial in reducing fibrosis of cardiac muscle, which leads to stiffening of the heart muscle in heart failure.

Side effects

As with other drugs that target the RAAS, mineralocorticoid receptor antagonists can lead to hyperkalaemia, therefore electrolytes should be monitored before and 1 week after initiation of treatment. Electrolytes should then be monitored monthly for the first 3 months and then every 3 months for the first year. Thereafter, monitoring can be done every 6 months.

Mineralocorticoid receptor antagonists can cause acute renal failure, therefore creatinine levels should also be monitored before and during treatment, alongside electrolytes.

NEUTRAL ENDOPEPTIDASE INHIBITORS

Sacubitril is a neprilysin inhibitor that inhibits the breakdown of beneficial natriuretic peptides and bradykinin. Sacubitril is often used in combination with the AT1 receptor antagonist valsartan.

IVABRADINE

Ivabradine inhibits If or pacemaker current in the sino-atrial node. This results in a bradycardic effect. Slowing the heart rate allows more time for the ventricles to fill with blood.

SODIUM-GLUCOSE CO-TRANSPORTER 2 INHIBITORS

This class of drugs was initially used in type 2 diabetes as they inhibit the sodium-glucose co-transporter 2 in the proximal tubule, preventing the reabsorption of glucose and reducing hypoglycaemia. There is good evidence that the sodium-glucose co-transporter 2 inhibitor dapagliflozin improves outcomes in heart failure. The beneficial mechanism is uncertain but proposed mechanisms have included diuresis, a direct effect on the heart, a decrease in afterload and improved myocardial energetics.

DIGOXIN

The cardiac glycosides are derived from the foxglove plant and have been used for centuries for the management of heart failure, but their role is now in the management of atrial fibrillation in refractory heart failure.

Mechanism of action

Digoxin is a cardiac glycoside that inhibits the Na^+-K^+ ATPase pump in cardiac muscle. This leads to an increase in the influx of calcium into cardiac muscle, increasing the force of contraction. Digoxin improves symptoms of heart failure but does not affect mortality. It has a low therapeutic index and so is reserved for patients with severe heart failure with concurrent atrial fibrillation.

Digoxin also reduces the heart rate by reducing the conduction of the action potential through the atrio-ventricular node. This can be beneficial in atrial fibrillation as it allows more time for blood to move from the atria into the ventricles before the ventricles contract. However, the reduction in heart rate can be problematic, particularly in patients with heart failure, and so the dose needs to be adjusted.

Side effects

The reduction in the heart rate is the most common manifestation of digoxin toxicity. Dose adjustment should be carried out to ensure the heart rate does not drop below 60 bpm.

Increases in plasma calcium (hypercalcaemia) and decreases in plasma potassium levels (hypokalaemia) or magnesium levels (hypomagnesaema) can enhance the effects of digoxin, leading to toxicity.

Alteration of the action potential through the heart can lead to arrhythmias. Central nervous system disorders, including dizziness, nausea and vomiting, are common. Dosing is normally once a day, but the dose can be divided to reduce nausea.

PRACTICE APPLICATION

The management of heart failure is an evolving area. ACE inhibitors/AT1 receptor antagonists and licenced β-blockers (typically bisoprolol) have established first-line roles, with diuretics being added for relief of symptomatic oedema (NICE 2018). More recently, NICE has also approved both sodium-glucose co-transporter 2 inhibitors (NICE 2021) and sacubitril with valsartan (Entresto) (NICE 2016), and these agents are increasingly used. Add-on therapies include mineralocorticoid receptor antagonists, digoxin (for patients with atrial fibrillation) and ivabradine (for patients in sinus rhythm).

ISCHAEMIC HEART DISEASE

Angina pectoris is defined as a chest pain or discomfort that is made worse by exertion and/or stress and is relieved by rest or nitrates. Stable angina is caused by reduced blood flow through the coronary circulation due to an atheroma, leading to a transient ischaemia when blood flow does not meet demand during an increase in cardiac workload. Unstable angina is caused by the rupture of an atherosclerotic plaque, leading to the formation of a platelet plug that blocks the coronary circulation. This produces a rapid reduction in blood flow, but the platelet plug can also dislodge to restore blood flow. Variant angina, or Prinzmetal's angina, is caused by spasm of the coronary artery, leading to reduced blood flow. This is often not associated with exercise or stress and can occur when the patient is at rest.

NITRATES (E.G., GLYCERYL TRINITRATE OR ISOSORBIDE MONONITRATE)

Mechanism of action

These drugs lead to an increase in nitric oxide (NO) in the blood vessels, which stimulates vasodilatation (Figure 17.6). Vasodilatation in the coronary circulation improves coronary blood flow to the area of ischaemia, producing a rapid reduction in symptoms. Vasodilatation in the venous system also reduces the workload on the heart, reducing the requirements for oxygen. Glyceryl trinitrate (GTN) can be administered as a tablet or a spray under the tongue. Sublingual absorption is rapid and by-passes first-pass metabolism in the liver (Chapter 9), and so produces a rapid relief of symptoms during an attack of angina. However, the effects are short-lived so GTN is only used for symptomatic relief. Sustained release patches of GTN are also available, which can be used for prophylaxis.

Isosobide mononitrate produces a slower, but more sustained increase in NO, and can be used for prophylactic treatment of angina. Longer-acting nitrates can lead to nitrate tolerance whereby the effects of nitrates are lost. Development of tolerance is rapid, but reversible. Patients are advised to have a nitrate-free period lasting 8 hours to prevent tolerance. Ideally this would be at night when the patient is at rest and therefore less likely to have an angina attack.

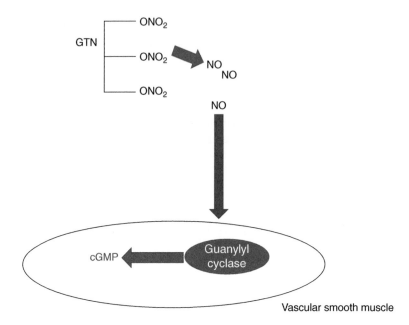

FIGURE 17.6 Mode action of glyceryl trinitrate (GTN) via the release of nitric oxide (NO) to cause relaxation of vascular smooth muscle via activation of guanylyl cyclase and increasing cyclic guanosine monophosphate (cGMP).

Side effects

As nitrates can cause rapid vasodilatation, patients can suffer from dizziness and postural hypotension, therefore they should be advised to sit down after taking nitrate. Dilation of the blood vessels in the brain can lead to a throbbing headache.

β-ADRENOCEPTOR ANTAGONISTS (β-BLOCKERS)

β-adrenoceptor antagonists can be used to prevent an attack of angina and are drugs of first choice for prevention. Antagonism of the β_1-adrenoceptors in the heart leads to a reduction in heart rate and force of contraction, and therefore reduces the workload of the heart. This reduces the requirements for oxygen such that the delivery of oxygen through the coronary circulation is more able to meet the demand. Furthermore, as coronary blood flow occurs during diastole, reducing the heart rate increases the duration of diastole, thereby allowing more time for the blood to flow through the coronary circulation.

Side effects

The side effects of β-adrenoceptor antagonists are covered in the section on hypertension. As discussed before, β-adrenoceptor antagonists, including β_1-adrenoceptor selective antagonists, are contraindicated in patients with asthma due to the increased risk of bronchoconstriction. In this case, a rate-limiting calcium channel inhibitor would be preferable.

CALCIUM CHANNEL INHIBITORS

Mechanism of action

Calcium channel inhibitors prevent contraction of the coronary arteries, thereby promoting vasodilatation and therefore improving coronary blood flow. Furthermore, the reduction in blood pressure in the peripheral circulation will reduce the workload of the heart, thus reducing oxygen requirements so that delivery is more able to meet demand.

Rate-limiting calcium channel inhibitors such as verapamil also reduce the heart rate, reducing the demand for oxygen from the cardiac muscle and increasing diastole. This is an alternative for a β-adrenoceptor antagonist in a patient with asthma.

Calcium channel inhibitors also reduce coronary artery spasm and therefore can be used in the treatment of variant angina.

In refractory angina, β-blockers and calcium channel inhibitors are used in combination. However, in using the combination, rate-limiting calcium channel inhibitors are avoided because their negative inotropic effects when combined with those of β-blockers can lead to fatal asystole. As dihydropyridines are devoid of cardiac effects, they can used in combination with β-blockers.

POTASSIUM CHANNEL ACTIVATORS

Nicorandil is a combined K_{ATP} channel activator and nitric oxide donor. Activation of the K_{ATP} channel leads to efflux of potassium ions from vascular smooth muscle. The resultant hyperpolarisation leads to inhibition of the voltage-gated calcium channels, which are normally opened in response to depolarisation. Closing these channels leads to inhibition of vasoconstriction and promotion of vasodilatation in the peripheral circulation and coronary circulation. Combined with the release of nitric oxide, this leads to a reduction in the workload of the heart and increased coronary blood flow.

Side effects

Peripheral vasodilatation can lead to increased blood flow to the skin, causing flushing. Similarly, vasodilatation in the brain can lead to headache and dizziness. Nausea and vomiting are also common.

IF CHANNEL INHIBITORS

Ivabradine is an inhibitor of the If or funny current channels in the cardiac pacemaker cells. The If channel is a hyperpolarization-activated cyclic nucleotide-gated channel. Inhibition of these channels leads to a reduction in heart rate and therefore a reduction in cardiac workload and increased diastole.

Side effects

As ivabradine reduces the heart rate, it should not be given to patients with a heart rate below 75 bpm. Bradycardia is common, therefore heart rate should be monitored at rest and should not be allowed to drop below 50 bpm. Dose adjustment may be required.

Ivabradine can lead to the development of atrial fibrillation and can cause blurred vision and dizziness.

SUMMARY

- The treatment of hypertension follows the A/C(D) algorithm (which takes account of age and ethnicity) in otherwise healthy patients. ACE inhibitors/ AT1 receptor antagonists are recommended for patients with concurrent diabetes.

- ACE inhibitors/AT1 receptor antagonists have a central role in the management of hypertension and chronic heart failure.

- Calcium channel inhibitors are effective antihypertensives and beneficial in ischaemic heart disease.

- Statins are recommended for patients who are at >10% risk of a cardiovascular event, irrespective of their cholesterol level.

- β-blockers are beneficial in ischaemic heart disease.

- Patients with chronic heart failure are routinely treated with ACE inhibitors/AT1 receptor antagonists, certain licenced β-blockers and diuretics. Mineralocorticoid receptor antagonists, neutral endopeptidase inhibitors and sodium-glucose co-transporter-2 inhibitors are widely used.

ACTIVITY

1. Which ONE of the following classes of drugs is associated with causing hyperkalaemia?

   (a) AT1 receptor antagonists (e.g., losartan)

   (b) Calcium channel inhibitors (e.g., amlodipine)

   (c) Loop diuretics (e.g., furosemide)

   (d) Potassium channel activators (e.g., nicorandil)

   (e) Thiazide-like diuretics (e.g., indapamide)

2. Which ONE of the following is a common side effect of ACE inhibitors (e.g., ramipril)?

   (a) Ankle swelling

   (b) Constipation

   (c) Cough

   (d) Hyperglycaemia

   (e) Negative inotropy

3. Which ONE of the following classes of drug is now being used in the management of chronic heart failure?

   (a) Endocannabinoids (e.g., anandamide)

   (b) Peroxisome proliferator-activated receptor γ agonists (e.g., pioglitazone)

   (c) Potassium channel activators (e.g., nicorandil)

   (d) Rate-limiting calcium channel inhibitors (e.g., verapamil)

   (e) Sodium-glucose co-transporter 2 inhibitors (e.g., dapagliflozin)

4. Which ONE of the following is a key counselling point for statin therapy?

   (a) Ankle swelling is a key side effect

   (b) Dizziness on standing is a common side effect

   (c) Headaches are a common side effect

   (d) Report unexplained muscle pain

   (e) Statins should be taken first thing in the morning

REFERENCES

Heart Protection Study Collaborative Group (2002) MRC/ BHF Heart Protection Study of cholesterol lowering with simvastatin in 20 536 high-risk individuals: a randomised placebo controlled trial. *Lancet* 360:7–22.

NICE Guidance (2018). Chronic heart failure in adults: diagnosis and management. NICE guideline 106. https://www.nice.org.uk/guidance/ng106.

NICE guidance (2019). Hypertension in adults: assessment and management. NICE guideline 136. https://www.nice.org.uk/guidance/ng136.

NICE Technology appraisal (2016). Sacubitril valsartan for treating symptomatic chronic heart failure with reduced ejection fraction. Technology appraisal guidance 388. https://www.nice.org.uk/guidance/ta388.

NICE Technology appraisal (2021). Dapagliflozin for treating chronic heart failure with reduced ejection fraction. Technology appraisal guidance 679. https://www.nice.org.uk/guidance/ta679

FURTHER READING

Brunton, L. and Knollmann, B. (2022) *Goodman and Gilman's The Pharmacological Basis of Therapeutics*, 14th edn. McGraw Hill.

Ritter, J.M., Flower, R., Henderson, G., et al. (2023) *Rang and Dale's Pharmacology*, 10th edn. Elsevier, Amsterdam.

USEFUL WEBSITE

Calculation of a patient's 10-year risk of a cardiovascular event: https://qrisk.org/.

| CHAPTER 18 | # Haemostasis and Thrombosis |

Michael Randall

LEARNING OUTCOMES

By the end of this chapter the reader should be able to:

- understand the terms haemostasis and thrombosis, and differentiate between them
- understand the coagulation cascade and the action of specific anticoagulant drugs within this cascade
- understand the process of platelet activation and the action of specific antiplatelet drugs
- understand the process of fibrinolysis and the action of specific fibrinolytic drugs.

HAEMOSTASIS

Haemostasis is a normal physiological response to arrest blood loss in response to vascular damage. The process of haemostasis consists of three separate stages (vasoconstriction, platelet adhesion and aggregation, and coagulation leading to fibrin formation) which occur in a logical manner.

VASOCONSTRICTION

This makes perfect sense physiologically. Haemostasis is the arrest of blood loss so the most obvious and logical step is the reduction of blood flow through the damaged vessel(s), which can be readily achieved by vasoconstriction.

ADHESION AND ACTIVATION OF PLATELETS

Platelets do not normally adhere to the endothelial surface of blood vessels, but once endothelial damage has occurred, a number of chemicals are released which attract platelets to the damaged area. These platelets adhere to the damaged endothelial surface and in doing so become 'activated'. These activated platelets attract more platelets to the area (platelet aggregation) and a 'platelet plug' is formed which 'plugs' the damaged area of the vessel, thus further reducing blood loss.

COAGULATION

Fibrin formation is the end-product of the coagulation cascade and is important in solidifying and stabilizing the platelet plug.

THROMBOSIS

Thrombosis, on the other hand, is defined as the pathological formation of a clot in the absence of bleeding. There are three key factors that predispose to thrombosis formation and were originally described by the German physician Rudolf Virchow. These are known today as Virchow's triad:

- injury to vessel wall, such as following the rupture of an atherosclerotic plaque
- altered blood flow, such as in leg veins on long-haul flights
- abnormal coagulability of blood, such as in the latter stages of pregnancy or following the use of oral contraceptives.

Thrombi can be classified as either arterial or venous, depending on which type of blood vessel they occur in. These different thrombi cause different clinical problems and are slightly different in their cellular make-up.

ARTERIAL THROMBI

These consist mainly of platelets and white blood cells, and are generally the result of endothelial injury, which itself is usually the result of underlying atherosclerotic disease. Arterial thrombi result in:

- myocardial infarction
- stroke
- peripheral ischaemia.

Therapy is largely via antiplatelet drugs.

VENOUS THROMBI

These consist of platelets and both white and red blood cells, and are the result of blood stasis. Venous thrombi result in:

- deep vein thrombosis
- pulmonary embolism.

Therapy is largely via anticoagulants.

CARDIOEMBOLIC THROMBI

This is the formation of blood clots within the heart and is often associated with atrial fibrillation (AF). Clot formation in the left atria of the heart may lead to clots breaking off and passing into the cerebral circulation, which is a risk factor for transient ischaemic attacks and strokes. Indeed, in AF the annual risk of a stroke is around 4%. Clots formed in the right atria may pass into the pulmonary circulation, leading to a pulmonary embolism. Based on the risk of stroke due to thrombosis (calculated by the congestive heart failure, hypertension, age ≥ 75 [doubled], diabetes, stroke [doubled], vascular disease, age 65 to 74 and sex category [female] [CHA_2DS_2-VASc] score), patients with atrial fibrillation are usually prescribed anticoagulants.

ROLE OF THE COAGULATION CASCADE IN THROMBOSIS AND HAEMOSTASIS

While it is relatively uncommon to use drugs that promote haemostasis, drugs that prevent thrombosis are commonly used clinically. Antithrombotic therapy can be divided into three separate classes that act on different aspects of thrombosis formation:

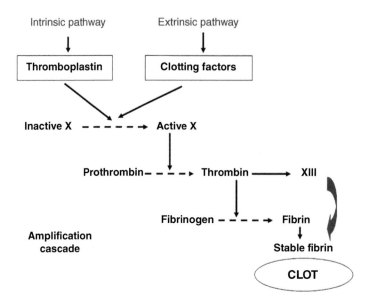

FIGURE 18.1 A simplified diagram showing the extrinsic and intrinsic pathways feeding into coagulation. Each step represents an amplification, for example thromboplastin activates many inactive Factor X coagulation factors to form active Factor X, which then activates prothrombin to thrombin. Factor XIII leads to the stabilization of fibrin, which forms the scaffold of the clot.

- to reduce blood coagulation (anticoagulants)
- to alter platelet function (antiplatelet drugs)
- to break down the fibrin meshwork (fibrinolytics).

Before discussing exactly how these different classes of drugs act, it is important to understand the function of the coagulation cascade. There are actually two pathways of blood coagulation (Figure 18.1). The intrinsic pathway is important in the clotting of shed blood, while the extrinsic pathway is the most important coagulation pathway in vivo. The two pathways then converge to form a common pathway.

There are two important factors to remember in relation to the coagulation cascade.

1. The blood already contains all the necessary components for coagulation, albeit in inactive forms. These inactive precursors are activated by proteolysis, or cleavage, of the inactive form into a shorter active protein. Each active factor then cleaves the next inactive factor in the cascade.

2. Each step involves a substantial amplification and many of the steps involve serine protease activity.

3. In terms of the extrinsic pathway of coagulation, it is the binding of tissue factor to factor VII in the presence of calcium that converts factor VII to VIIa, which can then act on factor X to produce factor Xa, and so on.

4. Vitamin K is an important co-factor in the synthesis of functional coagulation factors. Vitamin K is a fat soluble vitamin, the name of which is derived from the German word 'Koagulation', and the action of this vitamin on coagulation factors is crucial for their calcium-binding properties. Activation of coagulation factors is a calcium-dependent process.

ANTICOAGULANT DRUGS

These drugs prevent the production of fibrin by inhibiting the action of the clotting cascade. If fibrin is not produced, then the platelet plug does not solidify and can be relatively easily disrupted by the normal flow of blood through the vessel. There are three main types of anticoagulant drugs: those which can be administered orally (direct oral anticoagulants [DOACs], e.g., rivaroxaban, and coumarins, e.g., warfarin), and those which can only be administered parenterally (e.g., heparin). These drugs prevent the formation of venous thrombi and are therefore used to treat and prevent deep vein thrombosis and pulmonary embolism. They are also widely used in atrial fibrillation.

DIRECT ORAL ANTICOAGULANTS

DOACs (e.g., rivaroxaban) have largely replaced warfarin as the oral anticoagulant of choice. DO-ACs directly inhibit the coagulation cascade, with rivaroxaban inhibiting activated Factor X and dabigatran inhibiting thrombin (Figure 18.2). DOACs appear to be equally effective as warfarin at preventing thrombosis. Unlike warfarin, DOACs have a rapid onset of action, as opposed to the 2–3-day delay with warfarin. The only real barrier to the use of DOACs has been the challenges around reversing their effects but expensive antidotes to DOACs are now available.

PHARMACOKINETICS

As noted above, DOACs are given orally and at fixed doses. Dabigatran has relatively low bioavailability therefore capsules should be swallowed whole to optimise this. It is given twice daily for treatment and prevention of deep vein thrombosis and pulmonary embolisms, and is largely cleared via the renal route. Both rivaroxaban and apixaban have much greater bioavailability and are largely cleared via the hepatic route (CYP3A4).

DOACs have far fewer drug interactions and they do not require extensive monitoring, with their actions being much more predictable between patients. However, there are some interactions via either P-glycoprotein (dabigatran, rivaroxaban and apixaban) and CYP3A4 (rivaroxaban and apixaban) and these should be checked for. For example, the activity of rivaroxaban and apixaban can be increased by inhibitors (e.g., erythromycin) or reduced by inducing agents (e.g., phenytoin, carbamazepine).

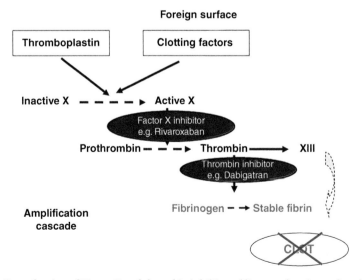

FIGURE 18.2   Sites of action of Factor X and thrombin inhibitors (direct oral anticoagulants) to interrupt the coagulation case and inhibit the formation of a clot.

WARFARIN

Pharmacodynamics

Warfarin has been used for many decades. It is often referred to as a vitamin K antagonist, but it is not an antagonist in the traditional sense in that it does not act on a receptor. Vitamin K needs to be activated by a reductase enzyme (vitamin K epoxide reductase [VKOR] complex) to act as a co-factor in the formation of coagulation factors. In terms of the extrinsic pathway of coagulation, vitamin K is important for the production of all the components of this pathway. Warfarin competes with vitamin K for the reductase enzyme (VKOR complex), thus reducing the level of activity of vitamin K and reducing the production of functional forms of all the relevant coagulation factors.

The therapeutic effects of warfarin take 48–72 hours to occur because it inhibits the formation of new coagulation factors. Warfarin does not have any effect on coagulation factors that have already been made, hence its therapeutic action is delayed until all preformed coagulation factors have been degraded. The delayed onset of action is also important in relation to the reversal of the effects of warfarin following over-anticoagulation.

Vitamin K can be given to reverse the effects of warfarin but this will take several hours because it will allow the formation of new functional coagulation factors but will not affect the activity of preformed factors. Indeed, in an emergency it may be necessary to replace the coagulation factors themselves. The major side effect associated with warfarin use is, perhaps unsurprisingly, haemorrhage. Warfarin has also been shown to be teratogenic.

STOP AND THINK

Why is the use of warfarin contraindicated in women in the first trimester of pregnancy?

Pharmacokinetics

Warfarin is heavily plasma protein bound, being about 99% bound to plasma albumin with a small volume of distribution.

There are two enantiomers of warfarin, the S and R forms, and these forms not only have different potencies but are metabolised by different cytochrome P450 isoenzymes. The S form is three times more potent than the R form and is metabolised by CYP2C9. The less potent R form is metabolised by CYP1A2 and CYP3A4 (Kaminsky and Zhang 1997). This complexity in terms of activity and the number of CYP isoforms involved in metabolism makes warfarin susceptible to a substantial number of drug–drug interactions (Table 18.1). Genetic variations in both inhibition of VKOR complex and cytochrome P450 lead to substantial interindividual variation and so the dose of warfarin is individual to each patient.

Drugs that inhibit the action of CYP isoforms will inhibit the metabolism of warfarin, resulting in an enhanced anticoagulant effect and increasing the risk of bleeding. On the other hand, drugs which induce the activity of CYP isoforms will enhance the metabolism of warfarin, reducing its anticoagulant effect and increasing the risk of clotting. Cranberry juice is thought to inhibit the metabolism of warfarin and should not be consumed by patients taking warfarin. Similarly, there are a number of dietary and herbal products, including St John's wort, ginseng, and gingko, that can induce CYP isoform activity and thus reduce the activity of warfarin. Leafy green vegetables are rich in vitamin K and can oppose the actions of warfarin.

Monitoring warfarin's activity

Warfarin has a narrow therapeutic window, and its activity is monitored by the prothrombin time, expressed as the international normalized ratio (INR), with the patient's prothrombin

Table 18.1   Drug interactions with warfarin which occur through modulation of CYP450 enzyme activity

Interaction with	CYP isoform affected	Effect on warfarin activity
Cimetidine	CYP1A2 and CYP3A4 inhibition	Increased warfarin activity
Macrolides (e.g., clarithromycin)	CYP3A4 inhibition	Increased risk of bleeding
Fluconazole	CYP2C9 inhibition	
Carbamazepine	CYP3A4 induction	Reduced activity of warfarin
Phenytoin	CYP2C9 and CYP3A4 induction	Increased risk of clotting
Rifampicin	CYP2C9 and CYP3A4 induction	

time divided by the normal prothrombin time of 12–14 seconds. As a patient is anticoagulated with warfarin the INR will rise from 1 to a desired target. For example, in the case of atrial fibrillation, the target INR is typically 2.5 and the dose is adjusted to achieve this target via regular monitoring. An interaction due to inhibition of metabolism is likely to increase the INR (requiring a dose reduction or stopping warfarin) and an inducer of metabolism is likely to decrease the INR (requiring an increase in the dose of warfarin). A classic example of an interaction with a cytochrome P450 inhibitor is between macrolides (such as clarithromycin) and warfarin. This interaction is not inevitable but can occur in some patients and so the patient's INR should be monitored 2–3 days after starting the macrolide and the dose of warfarin reduced if there is an increase in the INR. Alternatively, a non-interacting antibacterial might be preferred at the outset.

HEPARINS

Pharmacodynamics

Unlike warfarin, heparins (unfractionated heparin and low molecular weight heparin [LMWH], e.g., enoxaparin) have an immediate anticoagulant effect. This is because they increase the activity of antithrombin III. Antithrombin III is a naturally occurring inhibitor present in the blood as part of the normal physiological mechanisms which regulate blood coagulation. It inhibits serine proteases associated with thrombin and other factors in the clotting cascade, and prevents them from activating the next factor in the cascade. Heparins bind to antithrombin III, changing its three-dimensional shape and making it more likely to bind to thrombin and other coagulation factors, thus increasing its activity. While both unfractionated heparin and LMWH binding to antithrombin II inhibit the action of factor Xa, only unfractionated heparin has a significant effect on thrombin. The immediate onset of the action of heparin is reflected in the processes used to reverse its effects, which essentially involve stopping the administration of heparin. This then reduces the binding to, and activity of, antithrombin II. In an emergency it may be necessary to administer protamine, which acts by binding to the heparin, thus preventing it from binding to antithrombin III.

Unfractionated heparins are monitored by the activated partial thromboplastin time but have largely been replaced by LMWHs, whose action is far more predictable and which do not require routine monitoring.

Pharmacokinetics

Unfractionated heparin is very large in size, relatively polar in nature and is given either intravenously or by subcutaneous injection. It has a short half-life and can exhibit saturation kinetics such that its half-life appears to increase with increasing dose of the drug; consequently, its activity requires monitoring. LMWH, on the other hand, as the name suggests, is smaller in size and has a longer half-life than unfractionated heparin. LMWH is primarily cleared via the kidneys and as such do not exhibit the same saturation kinetics as unfractionated heparin, making activity more consistent and eliminating the need for close monitoring.

STOP AND THINK

Why do you think that neither unfractionated heparin nor LMWH can be given orally?

ROLE OF PLATELETS IN THROMBOSIS AND HAEMOSTASIS

Under normal healthy conditions, platelets do not adhere to the vascular endothelium but following vascular injury, platelets begin to stick to the damaged endothelium. This occurs through the binding of the glycoprotein Ia/IIb receptors on the surface of the platelets to molecules such as von Willebrand factor which are not normally exposed but become so following damage to the endothelium. Once they have started to adhere, platelets become activated and start to secrete chemicals such as adenosine diphosphate (ADP) and thromboxane A_2 (TXA_2), which are pro-aggregatory and promote platelet aggregation. They also upregulate, or increase, the expression of glycoprotein IIb/IIIa receptors on the surface of the platelets and it is to these receptors which fibrinogen binds, causing cross-linking of the platelets and stabilizing the platelet plug (Figure 18.3).

ANTIPLATELET DRUGS

ASPIRIN

Low-dose aspirin, typical dose 75 mg (or a quarter of a standard aspirin tablet), is a widely used antiplatelet drug in secondary prevention of cardiovascular events. Aspirin irreversibly inhibits cyclooxygenase (COX), which in platelets is responsible for the production of the pro-aggregatory molecule thromboxane, TXA_2 (Figure 18.4). Inhibition of COX also inhibits the endothelial production of anti-aggregatory prostacyclin. As platelets do not have a nucleus, they do not have the machinery to make new proteins and hence cannot make new COX to replace those which have been irreversibly inhibited. Thus, the activity of this enzyme is lost for the lifetime of the platelet (around 7–10 days). By contrast, endothelial cells have nuclei and so can regenerate COX within a matter of hours and so result in the production of the protective prostacyclin. Consequently, regular low-dose aspirin permanently inhibits platelet production of TXA_2 and reduces the aggregation of platelets.

ADVERSE EFFECTS

Peptic ulceration

The inhibition of cyclooxygenase by aspirin prevents the formation of prostaglandins in the body. Prostaglandins reduce stomach acid secretion and promote mucus secretion, thus protecting the stomach lining from the effects of acid (Chapter 16). A reduction in prostaglandin production in the stomach can therefore leave patients susceptible to gastrointestinal bleeding. Accordingly, patients at risk of gastric damage who require low-dose aspirin should be considered for gastroprotection via proton pump inhibitors (Chapter 16). The risk of gastric bleeding is so significant that aspirin is only recommended for secondary prevention.

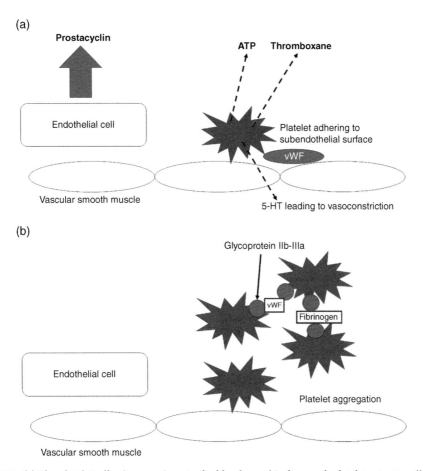

FIGURE 18.3   (a) The platelet adhesion reaction. As the blood vessel is damaged, platelets start to adhere (promoted by von Willebrand's factor [vWF]), then the platelets release adenosine diphosphate (ADP) and thromboxane to recruit other platelets and 5-hydroxytryptamine (5-HT) to promote blood vessel contraction. In health, endothelial cells release prostacyclin to oppose platelet adhesion. (b) The aggregation reaction. The released ADP leads to the expression of glycoprotein IIb-IIIa, which leads to cross-linking of platelets via fibrinogen and vWF.

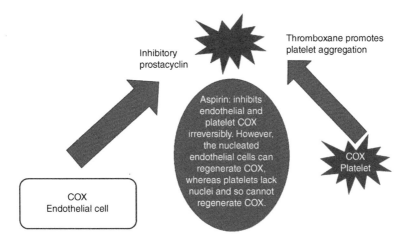

FIGURE 18.4   Action of aspirin to inhibit both endothelial and platelet cyclooxygenase (COX) irreversibly. The endothelial cells can soon regenerate COX and produce prostacyclin, whereas platelets can no longer make COX or thromboxane.

Bronchospasm

The use of aspirin can also result in bronchospasm. This is because the inhibition of the enzyme cyclooxygenase by aspirin can result in a build-up of arachidonic acid in the cell membrane, which may be converted to leukotrienes by the enzyme lipoxygenase. Leukotrienes are bronchoconstrictors (Chapter 20). The bronchoconstriction is often referred to as aspirin allergy and while present in only about 1% of the general population, it can affect around 10% of patients with asthma. Hence the use of aspirin is cautioned in asthmatics and contraindicated in patients with a previous history of hypersensitivity to aspirin or other non-steroidal anti-inflammatory drugs.

Clopidogrel

Clopidogrel acts as an antiplatelet drug by inhibiting the ADP-induced aggregation of platelets. Clopidogrel binds irreversibly to ADP (purinoreceptor $2Y_{12}$) receptors on platelets, preventing the binding of ADP itself. Clopidogrel is a pro-drug and requires metabolism by cytochrome P450 enzymes, particularly CYP3A4, in the liver to be activated. One key interaction here occurs with the proton pump inhibitor omeprazole (Chapter 16) and the combination should be avoided. It is therefore important to consider possible interactions with other drugs. CYP3A4 inducers will speed up the activation of clopidogrel and possibly increase its therapeutic effects while CYP3A4 inhibitors will reduce the activation of clopidogrel, reducing its therapeutic effect (Mullangi and Srinivas 2009).

STOP AND THINK

How might rifampicin and clarithromycin alter the activity of clopidogrel?

PRACTICE APPLICATION

Clopidogrel is widely used as an antiplatelet drug and is often used in conjunction with aspirin for additive effects (dual antiplatelet therapy). Dual antiplatelet therapy is often post-myocardial infarction, to prevent platelet aggregation following the insertion of a stent and following ischaemic stroke. While dual antiplatelet therapy with aspirin is associated with a lower risk of thromboembolic events, it has a higher risk of major bleeding.

Prasugrel

Prasugrel is also an antiplatelet drug with a similar mode of action to clopidogrel via irreversible antagonism of platelet $P2Y_{12}$ receptors. However, prasugrel has fewer drug interactions, less pharmacogenetic variation and a more rapid onset of action. Accordingly, prasugrel is increasingly used in preference to clopidogrel.

Abciximab

This is a monoclonal antibody (signified by the ending 'mab', which stands for monoclonal antibody) to the glycoprotein IIb/IIIa receptors. Abciximab binds to these receptors, preventing cross-linking of platelets and hence the stabilization of the platelet plug. Abciximab is used in angioplasty to prevent platelet aggregation.

FIBRINOLYTIC CASCADE

Activation of the coagulation cascade automatically leads to activation of the fibrinolytic cascade. This cascade leads to the activation of plasminogen and the formation of plasmin, which digests fibrin (and the inactivation of coagulation factors). Thus, activation of the fibrinolytic cascade acts to break down thrombi.

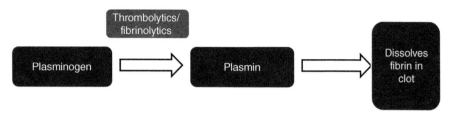

FIGURE 18.5   Mechanism of action of thrombolytic drugs.

Fibrinolytic (thrombolytic) drugs

These drugs have a dynamic action resulting in the breakdown of thrombi. The key example of these drugs is alteplase, which act as a plasminogen activator converting plasminogen to plasmin (Figure 18.5), which then acts to break down fibrin. Alteplase is primarily used in the treatment of acute ischaemic stroke when administered within the first 4.5 hours of the event. This leads to the restoration of blood flow and reduces neuronal loss and the associated neurological deficits. About 85% of strokes are ischaemic strokes, whereas the remainder are haemorrhagic. As alteplase breaks down clots and causes bleeding, it is essential that haemorrhagic stroke is excluded by brain imaging prior to thrombolysis. Thrombolytic drugs have been used for many years in the management of myocardial infarction, but the primary treatment is now percutaneous transluminal coronary angioplasty.

Adverse effects of fibrinolytic drugs

The main adverse effect of fibrinolytic drugs is bleeding. Fibrinolytic drugs act by breaking down blood clots and cannot differentiate between pathological thrombi and normal haemostatic clots. Consequently, the use of fibrinolytic drugs is contraindicated in patients with active bleeding ulcers and those who have undergone recent surgery or trauma.

SUMMARY

- Haemostasis is the body's normal physiological response to vascular damage.
- Thrombosis is the pathological formation of a blood clot in the absence of bleeding.
- The extrinsic pathway of coagulation is the most important pathway in vivo.
- All components of the coagulation cascade are present in the blood in an inactive form and are activated by proteolysis.
- Vitamin K is an important co-factor in the synthesis of functional coagulation factors.
- Anticoagulants act to prevent the formation of fibrin.
- Direct oral anticoagulants have largely replaced warfarin.
- Warfarin competes with vitamin K and reduces the formation of new functional coagulation factors.
- Heparin binds to antithrombin III to have an immediate anticoagulant effect.
- Platelets bind to damaged endothelium and become activated. These activated platelets aggregate to form a platelet plug.
- Aspirin inhibits the activity of cyclooxygenase for the lifetime of the platelet.

- Clopidogrel binds irreversibly to purinoreceptor $2Y_{12}$ receptors to prevent adenosine diphosphate-induced platelet aggregation.
- The fibrinolytic cascade produces plasmin, which acts to break down fibrin.

ACTIVITY

1. Atrial fibrillation is a key risk factor for which one of the following?

   (a) Deep vein thrombosis

   (b) Fibrinolysis

   (c) Ischaemic stroke

   (d) Haemorrhage

   (e) Hypertension

2. Which one of the following is an integral part of the coagulation cascade?

   (a) Adhesion of platelets

   (b) Factor X activates fibrinogen

   (c) Thrombin activates fibrinogen

   (d) Thrombin is converted to fibrinogen

   (e) Thrombin is the final product

3. Which one of the following is a clear advantage of direct oral anticoagulants (DOACs) compared to warfarin?

   (a) DOACs have fewer drug interactions

   (b) DOACs are selective for the vitamin K epoxide reductase complex

   (c) DOACs are cheaper

   (d) DOACs are more easily reversed

   (e) DOACs are not associated with causing bleeding

4. Which one of the following is an important issue in the use of warfarin?

   (a) It acts almost immediately

   (b) It is given by injection

   (c) It is unaffected by inhibitors of cytochrome P450

   (d) It opposes the actions of vitamin K

   (e) It requires monitoring via the activated partial thromboplastin time

5. Which one of the following promotes platelet aggregation?

   (a) Adenosine triphosphate

   (b) Endothelial cyclooxygenase

   (c) Nitric oxide

   (d) Prostacyclin

   (e) Thromboxane

6. Which one of the following is thought to contribute towards the antiplatelet activity of low-dose aspirin?

   (a) Aspirin inhibits the expression of glycoprotein IIb-IIIa

   (b) Aspirin is a thromboxane receptor antagonist

   (c) Aspirin is selective for endothelial cyclooxygenase

   (d) Endothelial cells are resistant to aspirin

   (e) Platelets lack a nucleus

7. Which one of the following is the principal use of the thrombolytic drug alteplase?

   (a) Atrial fibrillation

   (b) Haemorrhagic stroke

   (c) Hypertension

   (d) Ischaemic stroke

   (e) Secondary prevention of myocardial infarction

REFERENCES

Kaminsky, L.S. and Zhang, Z.Y. (1997) Human P450 metabolism of warfarin. *Pharmacol Ther* 73:67–74.

Mullangi, R. and Srinivas, N.R. (2009) Clopidogrel: review of bioanalytical methods, pharmacokinetics/pharmacodynamics, and update on recent trends in drug-drug interaction studies. *Biomed Cromatogr* 23:26–i41.

FURTHER READING

Ageno, W., Crotti, S. and Turpie, A.G. (2004) The safety of antithrombotic therapy during pregnancy. *Expert Opin Drug Saf* 3:113–118.

Baxter, K., Preston, C.L. and Stockley, I.H. (2013) *Stockley's Drug Interactions: a source book of interactions, their mechanisms, clinical importance and management*, 10th edn. Pharmaceutical Press, London.

Brunton, L. and Knollmann, B. (2022) *Goodman and Gilman's The Pharmacological Basis of Therapeutics*, 14th edn. McGraw Hill, New York.

Ritter, J.M., Flower, R., Henderson, G., Loke, Y.K., MacEwan, D., Robinson, E. and Fullerton, J. (2023) *Rang and Dale's Pharmacology*, 10th edn. Elsevier, Amsterdam.

GUIDANCE

British Haematological Society. Clinical guidelines. https://b-s-h.org.uk/guidelines/about-our-guidelines.

CHAPTER 19

The Renal System

Michael Randall

LEARNING OUTCOMES

By the end of this chapter the reader should be able to:

- describe the basic structure and list the functions of the kidneys

- describe the basic principles of glomerular filtration

- assess an individual's renal function using common biochemical measures and grade the severity of renal failure

- describe the effects of renal failure on drug kinetics

- safely adjust drug doses for a patient with renal failure, utilising standard reference materials

- give examples of drugs that require careful dose adjustment in renal failure

- explain the classification of nephrotoxicity into predictable and idiosyncratic reactions.

STRUCTURE AND FUNCTION OF THE KIDNEYS

STRUCTURE OF THE KIDNEYS

The kidneys are situated at the back of the abdomen behind the peritoneum, one on either side of the aorta. Each kidney is 10–12 cm in length and is surrounded by a fibrous capsule. Each capsule is surrounded further by fat (perinephric fat) and by another layer of fibrous tissue (perinephric fascia). An adrenal gland sits on top of each kidney, enclosed by the perinephric fascia. The outer zone of the kidney is called the renal cortex and the inner zone is called the renal medulla. Figure 19.1 shows the kidney in cross-section.

The basic functional unit of the kidney is the nephron (Figure 19.2). Each kidney has between 400,000 and 800,000 nephrons. This number declines with increasing age. Each nephron is composed of a glomerulus, which is a ball of highly porous capillaries, and an associated tubule that leads to the collecting duct. Blood is filtered by the glomerulus to form urine in the Bowman's capsule, which is the start of the tubule. The composition of the urine is continually modified along the length of the tubule by the reabsorption and secretion of substances. A large amount of blood passes through the glomeruli every minute (~25% of the total cardiac output), and approximately 180 litres of glomerular filtrate are produced over a 24-hour period (more than 30 times the average circulating total blood volume!). All but 1–2 litres of this filtrate are reabsorbed by the tubules of the nephrons back into the bloodstream. The whole process allows the plasma to be adequately filtered, but the very efficient reabsorptive processes prevent volume and electrolyte depletion.

A ureter drains the urine from each kidney into the bladder. The ureter arises from the renal pelvis. Each renal pelvis divides into two or three major calyces, which in turn subdivide into two or three minor calyces. The collecting duct of each nephron flows into a papillary duct that opens out on a renal papilla into a minor calyx.

The New Prescriber: An Integrated Approach to Medical and Non-medical Prescribing, Second Edition.
Edited by Joanne Lymn, Alison Mostyn, Roger Knaggs, Michael Randall, and Dianne Bowskill.
© 2024 John Wiley & Sons Ltd. Published 2024 by John Wiley & Sons Ltd.

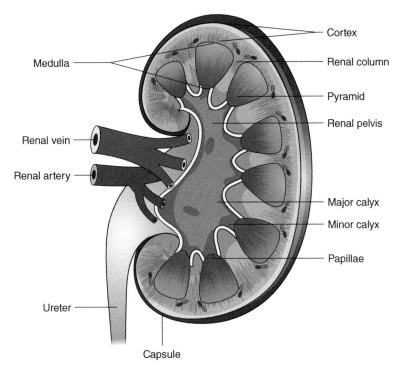

FIGURE 19.1   Frontal cross-section of the human kidney.

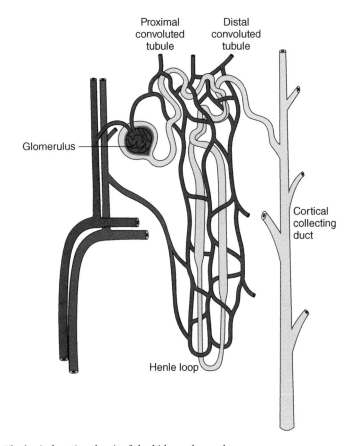

FIGURE 19.2   The basic functional unit of the kidney, the nephron.

Table 19.1 Functions of the kidneys

Function type	Description of function
Regulatory	Control of body fluid volume and composition
	Regulation of water, sodium, potassium, hloride, magnesium and phosphate excretion
	Regulation of acid-base balance through the reabsorption of bicarbonate and the excretion of hydrogen ions
Excretory	Excretion of waste products and drugs
Endocrine	Production of hormones, e.g., erythropoietin (stimulates red blood cell production), renin (converts angiotensinogen to angiotensin I) and prostaglandins (powerful vasodilatory agents in the kidney)
Metabolic	Metabolism of vitamin D to the potent active form and of small molecular weight proteins

FUNCTIONS OF THE KIDNEYS

The kidneys have a number of very important functions (Table 19.1). Their principal role is the regulation of the volume and composition of body fluid to maintain a stable extracellular environment and the elimination of waste material.

RISK FACTORS FOR KIDNEY DISEASE

There are a number of factors that make the chances of a person developing kidney disease more likely. If you are considering prescribing medication for a patient in one of these groups, it would be sensible to check their renal function first.

- Increasing age: kidney function declines with increasing age.
- Ethnic group: kidney disease is more common amongst the Asian population.
- Diabetes (type 1 and type 2, especially if longstanding).
- Hypertension.
- Vascular disease, for example heart disease and stroke.

STOP AND THINK

Think about the patients you see in your day-to-day work. Are they at risk of kidney disease? How are you going to determine those individuals for whom you need to take kidney function into account when prescribing?

THE PRINCIPLES OF GLOMERULAR FILTRATION

Blood enters the glomerulus via an afferent arteriole and leaves via an efferent arteriole. The high hydrostatic pressure in the glomerular capillaries exceeds the opposing pressures within them and the Bowman's capsule, resulting in water, ions and small molecules being driven across the filtration barrier into the Bowman's capsule. Pressure changes within the afferent and efferent arterioles affect glomerular filtration. Pressure in the glomerular capillaries is reduced by afferent arteriolar constriction and increased by efferent arteriolar constriction.

Table 19.2   Examples of substances filtered and not filtered by the kidneys

Filtered	Not filtered
Water	Plasma proteins
Electrolytes	Red blood cells
Urea	While blood cells
Creatinine	

The molecular size of a substance and its electrical charge, protein binding, configuration and rigidity determine whether it crosses the filtration barrier and enters the filtrate or remains in the blood (Table 19.2). The filtration barrier has a net negative electrical charge, meaning that the movement of negatively charged molecules is restricted relative to those molecules with a positive or neutral charge.

The glomerular filtration rate (GFR) is a measure of the rate at which the blood is filtered by the kidneys. The GFR is therefore an important indicator of kidney function. The normal GFR depends on age, sex and body size, but is approximately 120 ml/min. There are a number of ways of estimating the GFR, each of which has its own limitations, and these are discussed in more detail below.

ASSESSING KIDNEY FUNCTION

Serum Urea and Creatinine

Serum urea and creatinine have commonly been used to estimate kidney function. Both are substances produced by the body and excreted by the kidney, and can be measured easily in the laboratory. Urea (measured in mmol/l) is a small molecule produced by the liver that is the waste product of protein metabolism. Creatinine (measured in µmol/l) is derived from creatine, which is a component of muscle cells. The blood levels of both can be affected by a number of factors. Urea levels are raised, for example, in dehydration and in gastrointestinal bleeding, and tend to be low if someone is malnourished or in liver disease. Creatinine levels are affected by muscle mass and values tend to be higher in people with a large muscle bulk.

When kidney function is impaired, urea and creatinine accumulate in the blood. However, due to the physiological reserve of the kidneys, the level of neither substance rises substantially until the level of renal function has deteriorated significantly, that is, when the GFR has fallen to around 30 ml/min. This limits their usefulness in assessing kidney function.

Clearance Methods

Clearance (CL) is defined as the volume of plasma from which a substance is completely removed or cleared by the kidneys per unit time. The ideal marker for measuring clearance is freely filtered by the glomerulus and is not reabsorbed, secreted, synthesised or metabolised by the tubules. For such substances, the amount filtered by the glomerulus is equal to the amount excreted in the urine.

There is no naturally occurring ideal marker to measure clearance, so creatinine has traditionally been used to estimate the GFR. Creatinine is used because its rate of production is typically very constant and serum levels and urinary output therefore vary very little throughout a 24-hour period. However, because a small amount of creatinine is secreted by the tubules, GFR measured by creatinine clearance can be overestimated. This is more pronounced when the GFR is low as tubular secretion of creatinine increases. Urine is collected over a 24-hour period and the urinary creatinine level is measured. A 24-hour urinary collection also indicates urine flow in millilitres per minute. A plasma creatinine level is measured at some point in the 24-hour period. Using the formula below, the creatinine clearance can be calculated:

$$\text{creatinine clearance} = \frac{U \times V}{P}$$

where V is the rate of urine flow, U is the urine concentration of creatinine and P is the plasma concentration of creatinine. The normal range of values for men is 90–140 ml/min and for women is 80–125 ml/min.

Estimation Equations

GFR and creatinine clearance can also be predicted from estimation equations using the plasma creatinine. These are the methods commonly used in everyday practice.

The Cockcroft–Gault equation allows rapid estimation of the creatinine clearance from the plasma creatinine in a patient with a stable creatinine level. This formula incorporates the patient's weight:

$$C_{cr}\left(\text{ml/m in}\right) = \frac{\left(140 - \text{age}\right) \times \text{weight}\left(\text{kg}\right) \times f}{\text{plasma creatinine}\left(\mu\text{mol/l}\right)}$$

where C_{cr} is the estimated creatinine clearance. The normal average f for men is 1.23 and for women is 1.04.

The Cockcroft–Gault equation takes into account the increasing creatinine production with increasing weight, and the decline in creatinine production with age. However, the equation does not adjust for body surface area.

More recently, an equation to predict the GFR from the plasma creatinine concentration has been developed from data obtained in the Modification of Diet in Renal Disease (MDRD) study. The formula, which takes into account body surface area, calculates the estimated GFR (eGFR) using the patient's age, sex and creatinine levels, and also makes an adjustment if the patient is Afro-Caribbean. The *British National Formulary* usually uses either eGFR or creatinine clearance to account for renal function.

There are limitations to both of these estimation equations. They are less accurate in certain populations, including individuals with a normal GFR, children, pregnant women, elderly patients, specific ethnic groups and those with an unusual body shape and/or weight, for example morbid obesity and amputees. Neither of the equations is validated in acute kidney injury (acute renal failure). In these situations, alternative methods for calculating the GFR should be considered, for example clearance methods.

DRUG USE IN PATIENTS WITH RENAL IMPAIRMENT

Drug prescribing for patients with renal impairment is problematic for a number of reasons. People with impaired renal function usually have other medical problems, for example diabetes, are often elderly and take many different types of medication. This in itself predisposes them to increased adverse effects from medicines. However, in renal impairment, the body often handles drugs differently, leading to further increased risk of drug toxicity. These combined effects mean that patients with impaired kidney function are a high-risk group for drug management. Many of the adverse effects, however, are predictable and can be avoided or minimised by careful medicine prescribing and use.

STOP AND THINK

Think about drugs that you might prescribe in practice. Which drugs may require dose reduction in renal impairment? Where are you going to find the necessary information to recommend altered doses for these drugs?

Renal impairment can affect all four pharmacokinetic parameters: absorption, distribution, metabolism and excretion.

ABSORPTION

Generally of little clinical significance, with notable exceptions, for example the intestinal absorption of both dietary and supplemental iron is significantly reduced in CKD.

DISTRIBUTION

Volumes of distribution may be altered due to fluid overload, reduced albumin and altered protein binding. This can impact significantly on drug distribution. For example, phenytoin is ordinarily 90% protein bound with the unbound 10% being the active drug. In renal impairment, low albumin levels and high levels of urea (molecules of which may bind to albumin) leave fewer binding sites for drugs, thus a much smaller proportion of the drug is protein bound. Care needs to be taken when interpreting phenytoin levels (low levels may not necessarily be subtherapeutic). Ideally, a free-fraction serum level should be taken but, as this is often not available, a total serum level can be interpreted, bearing in mind albumin and urea levels.

METABOLISM

The kidney is a site of drug metabolism but in most cases this is minimal compared to the liver. However, there are examples where the loss of renal metabolism can be seen clinically. For example, patients with renal impairment may need smaller doses of insulin as insulin is partially metabolised by the kidney.

EXCRETION

The kidney is the major organ involved in drug elimination from the body. Drugs and/or their metabolites that are excreted by the renal route are excreted more slowly in patients with kidney disease and if this is not taken into account, it can lead to accumulation in the body (Figure 19.3).

It is therefore necessary to adjust the dosing of drugs cleared by the kidneys, which can be done either by increasing the dosage interval (Figure 19.4) or by reducing the dose (Figure 19.5).

DRUG DOSING IN RENAL IMPAIRMENT

Now that you are aware of the effect that renal failure may have on the kinetics of a drug, it is important to be able to apply this in practice. The extent to which the kinetics is altered depends on:

- the properties of the drug
- the severity of the patient's renal impairment.

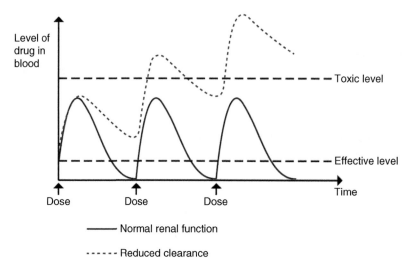

FIGURE 19.3   Accumulation of drug in renal failure.

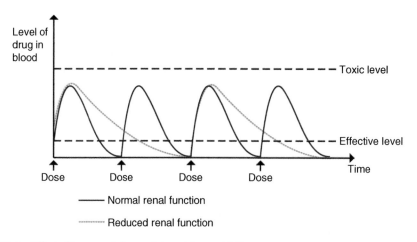

FIGURE 19.4   Effect of increased dosage interval in renal failure.

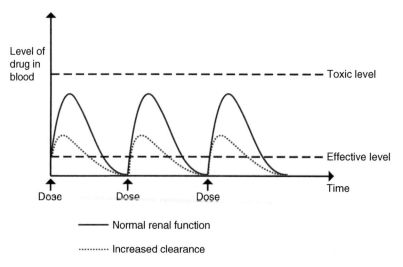

FIGURE 19.5   Effect of decreased dose in renal failure.

eGFR has a valuable role to play in highlighting patients with CKD who may require dose adjustment. However, the MDRD formula differs from the Cockcroft–Gault equation because it gives a GFR estimate normalised for a body surface area of 1.73 m², whereas Cockcroft–Gault estimates individual creatinine clearances. In patients of an average height and build, there is good correlation between the two equations and for the majority of drugs in patients of average weight, either calculation can be used to determine drug dosing. However, eGFR should not be used for calculating drug doses in patients at extremes of weight nor for potentially toxic drugs of a narrow therapeutic index. In these circumstances the difference between the two equations may be clinically significant and Cockcroft–Gault estimates should be used to avoid potential drug over/under doses.

PRACTICE APPLICATION

It is important to remember the limitations of both the eGFR and Cockcroft–Gault estimation equations. When using either equation, creatinine levels should be stable and the clinical picture should always be taken into account.

Once you have an estimate of the patient's renal function, there are a number of reference sources that can guide you on whether or not you need to adjust the dose of the drug you wish to prescribe. The most readily available source for most will be the *British National Formulary* in which guidance on the use and dosing of drugs in renal failure is provided. Where possible, values for eGFR, creatinine clearance or other measures of renal function are included.

One key example of dosing in renal impairment is metformin. Metformin is the drug of first choice in type 2 diabetes but is potentially inappropriate in patients with eGFR <30 ml/min/1.73m² due to the risk of lactic acidosis. Whilst managing strategies involve dose reductions for largely renally excreted drugs, in the case of aminoglycloside antibiotics such as gentamicin, the usual strategy is to increase the dose interval.

Manufacturers often provide information on dosing in renal impairment in their Summary of Product Characteristics. These are available free online at emc.medicines.org.uk, which is a very useful website when further information is required.

Further specialist reference sources may be available from specialist renal units or medicines information centres.

Drug Dosing in Dialysis

Prescribing for patients on dialysis is further complicated as many drugs are cleared from the body by dialysis. When prescribing drugs for patients in this situation, it is important to consult specialist literature or seek advice from your local renal unit.

EXAMPLES OF DRUGS THAT MAY NEED DOSE ADJUSTING IN RENAL IMPAIRMENT

Not all drugs will need dose adjusting for patients with chronic kidney disease. Whether or not dose reduction is required depends on what proportion of the drug is excreted by the kidney in an active form and how toxic the drug is if it accumulates. For example, a drug that is largely metabolised in the liver, with minimal dose-related side effects, is likely to need no dose reduction and careful monitoring of side effects is sufficient. Conversely, drugs that are cleared by the kidneys with a narrow therapeutic index may need very precise dose adjustment and monitoring of both efficacy and side effects (Table 19.3).

Table 19.3 Examples of drugs that need careful dose adjustment in renal failure

Antibiotics, e.g. gentamicin, vancomycin, levofloxacin,
Gabapentin
Low molecular weight heparins
Digoxin
Opioids

MONITORING

Sensitivity to some drugs is increased in renal impairment even if accumulation does not occur and patients with CKD can be extremely sensitive to the side effects of drugs. Therefore, even when guidance on dosing is followed, it is imperative that the patient is monitored for signs of drug toxicity and doses adjusted/alternative drugs used as appropriate.

NEPHROTOXICITY

There are a number of drugs which should be avoided completely or used with great caution in people with impaired kidney function. This is because they may themselves cause a further deterioration in kidney function or can be directly harmful to the kidneys if they accumulate should their excretion be impaired. This is called nephrotoxicity, which can be either predictable or idiosyncratic.

PRACTICE APPLICATION

Patients with impaired renal function excrete drugs more slowly and are highly susceptible to the effects of nephrotoxic drugs.

Predictable

The harmful effect of the drug on the kidneys can be predicted (often this is dose or level related). Examples of drugs causing predictable nephrotoxicity and which therefore which should be avoided or used with caution are shown in Table 19.4.

Table 19.4 Drugs that cause predictable nephrotoxicity

Drug group	Mechanism
Non-steroidal anti-inflammatory drugs, e.g. ibuprofen and diclofenac	Can cause a critical reduction in glomerular perfusion by inhibiting prostaglandin production
ACE inhibitors and angiotensin II receptor blockers, e.g. ramipril, lisinopril, candesartan, losartan	Can cause acute kidney injury by altering renal blood flow in patients with renovascular disease
Aminoglycoside antibiotics, e.g gentamicin	Directly toxic to the kidneys if the serum levels are high because of reduced clearance
Ciclosporin	Causes chronic glomerular damage and scarring in the kidney

Idiosyncratic

The harmful effect of the drug on the kidney is unexpected. These are rare events which occur in susceptible individuals. Examples of drugs causing idiosyncratic nephrotoxicity include:

- antibiotics, for example penicillins
- non-steroidal anti-inflammatory drugs
- diuretics
- proton pump inhibitors, for example lansoprazole.

STOP AND THINK

Are any of the drugs that you might prescribe in practice nephrotoxic? What factors will you need to consider before prescribing these drugs and what parameters might you need to monitor?

USE OF DIURETICS IN RENAL FAILURE

Diuretics are drugs that cause a net loss of sodium and water from the body by an action on the kidney. They are commonly used in chronic kidney disease to treat hypertension, increase urine output and prevent fluid accumulation.

Diuretics can be split into three families: loop diuretics, thiazide-like diuretics and potassium sparing diuretics (Table 19.5). All three classes of diuretic (with the exception of spironolactone and eplerenone) act from within the tubular lumen and therefore must reach their site of action by being secreted into the proximal tubule. This secretion is lessened in the failing kidney and so the response to diuretics is reduced in CKD.

In practice, this means that thiazide-like diuretics are generally ineffective if the creatinine clearance is less than 30 ml/min unless used in combination with a loop diuretic, so the former are rarely used in patients with moderate to severe renal impairment. Use of loop diuretics is widespread, but the doses required are often much higher than those used in the general population (e.g., furosemide doses of up to 500 mg daily).

Table 19.5 Actions of the three classes of diuretic drugs

	Loop	Thiazide-like	Potassium sparing
Examples	Furosemide	Indapamide	Spironolactone
	Bumetanide		Eplerenone
			Amiloride
Site of action	Thick segment of the loop of Henle	Distal convoluted tubule	Collecting duct
Mechanism of action	Inhibits sodium reabsorption	Inhibits sodium reabsorption	Spironolactone/eplerenone are aldosterone (mineralocorticoid receptor) antagonists
			Amiloride blocks sodium channels
Effect on plasma potassium levels	Decreased	Decreased	Increased

The use of potassium-sparing diuretics is limited in kidney disease as patients often cannot tolerate the increased potassium levels they cause and so potassium should be monitored extremely closely if these diuretics are required.

Renal patients on diuretic therapy must not be allowed to become dehydrated as this may worsen existing renal failure.

SUMMARY

- The nephron is the basic functional unit of the kidney and consists of a glomerulus and an associated tubule that leads to the collecting duct.

- The main role of the kidney is regulating body fluid volume and composition.

- Glomerular filtration rate (GFR) is an important indicator of kidney function.

- Creatinine clearance can be predicted from the Cockcroft–Gault equation.

- Kidney disease can be divided into five stages according to the eGFR.

- Renal impairment does not generally affect drug absorption or metabolism.

- Drug distribution can be altered in renal impairment due to fluid overload and reduced plasma albumin concentration.

- Many drugs are excreted more slowly in renal impairment and drug dosages may need to be adjusted accordingly.

- Drugs that need careful dose adjustment in renal impairment include some antibiotics, gabapentin, digoxin, opioids and low molecular weight heparins.

- Drugs that cause nephrotoxicity should be avoided or used with great caution in people with impaired kidney function.

- Diuretics exert their pharmacological action from within the lumen of the tubule.

- Doses of diuretics may need to be higher in patients with renal impairment.

- It is important to identify patients at risk of kidney disease before you start prescribing.

- Check whether careful dose adjustment or caution is required for the drug you wish to prescribe. If you find that dose adjustment is necessary, use eGFR or Cockcroft–Gault where appropriate to estimate the degree of renal function and follow dosage guidance in the available reference sources.

ACTIVITY

1. In addition to its regulatory and excretory roles, the kidney is also a synthetic and metabolic organ. True/False

2. Kidney disease is more common amongst Caucasian populations. True/False

3. The molecular weight and electronic charge of a molecule partly determine if it is filtered by the kidney. True/False

4. Creatinine is a substance produced by the body that is both filtered and actively secreted by the kidneys. True/False

5. The Cockcroft–Gault equation gives an estimation of creatinine clearance normalised for body surface area. True/False

6. Renal impairment can affect all four ADME- Absorption, distribution, metabolism and excretion pharmacokinetic parameters. True/False

7. The MDRD equation is the recommended method of estimating renal function for use in modifying drug doses in patients at extremes of weight. True/False

8. Dosing of opiates should be adjusted in renal impairment due to their narrow therapeutic index and method of elimination from the body. True/False

9. Potassium-sparing diuretics are the diuretic of choice in patients with renal impairment. True/False

10. A reduction in kidney function due to ramipril could be described as an idiosyncratic reaction. True/False

REFERENCES

British National Formulary (online). BMJ Group and Pharmaceutical Press, London. https://bnf.nice.org.uk/.

FURTHER READING

Ashley, C. and Dunleavy, A. (eds) (2018) *The Renal Drug Handbook: The ultimate prescribing guide for renal practitioners*, 5th edn. CRC Press, Boca Raton.

Department of Health Management of Medicines (2004) *A Resource Document for Aspects Specific to the National Service Framework for Renal Services*. Department of Health, London.

Devaney, A. and Thompson, C. (2006) Chronic kidney disease – new approaches to classification. *Hosp Pharm* 13:406–410.

Khan, S., Loi, V. and Rosner, M.H. (2017) Drug-induced kidney injury in the elderly. *Drugs Aging* 34(10):729–741.

Kwiatkowska, E., Domański, L., Dziedziejko, V., Kajdy, A., Stefanska, K. and Kwiatkowska, S. (2021) The mechanism of drug nephrotoxicity and the methods for preventing kidney damage. *Int J Mol Sci* 22(11):6109.

Levey, A.S., Bosch, J.P., Breyer-Lewis, J.B., et al. (1999) A more accurate method to estimate the glomerular filtration rate from serum creatinine: a new prediction equation. *Ann Intern Med* 130:461–470.

National Kidney Foundation (2002) K/DOQI clinical practice guidelines for chronic kidney disease: evaluation, classification and stratification. *Am J Kidney Dis* 39(Suppl 1):S1–S266.

Pannu, N. and Nadim, M.K. (2008) An overview of drug-induced acute kidney injury. *Crit Care Med* 36 (4 Suppl):S216–S223.

Perazella, M.A. (2018) Pharmacology behind common drug nephrotoxicities. *Clin J Am Soc Nephrol* 13(12):1897–1908.

Taber, S.S. and Pasko, D.A. (2008) The epidemiology of drug-induced disorders: the kidney. *Expert Opin Drug Saf* 7:679–690.

USEFUL WEBSITES

NICE guidance NG28 (2015) *Type 2 diabetes in adults: management*. Published 2 December 2015, updated 29 June 2022. https://www.nice.org.uk/guidance/ng28.

| REUSABLE |
| LEARNING |
| OBJECTS |

Kidney anatomy. www.nottingham.ac.uk/nursing/ sonet/rlos/bioproc/kidneyanatomy/index.html.

Physiology of the kidneys. www.nottingham.ac.uk/ nursing/sonet/rlos/bioproc/kidneyphysiology/ index.html.

The Respiratory System

Richard Roberts

LEARNING OUTCOMES

By the end of this chapter the reader should be able to:

- understand the nature of the regulation of the airways

- understand the role of inflammation in respiratory disease

- understand the mechanism of action, clinical uses and major adverse effects of the following bronchodilators:

  o β-adrenoceptor agonists (short- and long-acting)

  o muscarinic receptor antagonists (short- and long-acting)

  o phosphodiesterase inhibitors (e.g., methylxanthines)

- understand the mechanism of action, clinical uses and major adverse effects of the following anti-inflammatory agents:

  o corticosteroids

  o leukotriene receptor antagonists

  o biologics (e.g., omalizumab)

- describe the different routes of administration used for drugs which affect the respiratory system

- understand drugs which should be used with caution or are contraindicated

- critically apply current clinical guidelines for respiratory conditions.

THE REGULATION OF AIRWAY TONE

Air enters the lungs through the trachea, which branches into the main bronchi to feed air into the two main lobes of the lungs (Figure 20.1). Further branching into smaller bronchi and then bronchioles allows for increased surface area for gas exchange at the terminal alveoli. The lumen of the airways is lined by epithelial cells, which, in turn, are surrounded by smooth muscle cells. Contraction and relaxation of the smooth muscle cells allows alteration of the diameter of the lumen of the airways, thus altering airway resistance and air flow.

The airways are innervated by the parasympathetic nervous system through vagal inputs. Parasympathetic nerves release acetylcholine as a neurotransmitter, which acts on muscarinic acetylcholine receptors. The main subtype on airway smooth muscle cells is the muscarinic M_3 receptor (Ikeda et al. 2012). M_3 receptors are coupled to Gq proteins, leading to increases in intracellular calcium, which results in contraction of the smooth muscle. Pre-synaptic M_2 receptors are present on vagal nerve terminals, which, when activated by acetylcholine, inhibit the release of further acetylcholine from the nerve endings as a negative feedback mechanism (Pincus et al. 2021).

The New Prescriber: An Integrated Approach to Medical and Non-medical Prescribing, Second Edition.
Edited by Joanne Lymn, Alison Mostyn, Roger Knaggs, Michael Randall, and Dianne Bowskill.
© 2024 John Wiley & Sons Ltd. Published 2024 by John Wiley & Sons Ltd.

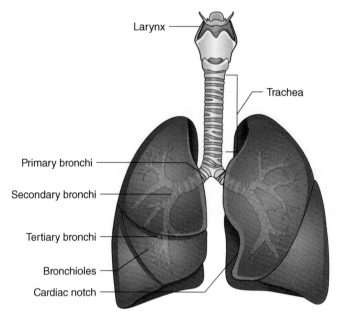

FIGURE 20.1   The human airways or bronchial tree created using Biorender.

Muscarinic receptors are also present on mucus-secreting goblet cells located in the epithelial layer (Rogers 2001). Activation of these receptors leads to increased mucus production and secretion into the lumen. Mucus plays an important role in trapping particles and pathogens breathed in with the air.

Airway smooth muscle cells also contain β-adrenoceptors, which are activated by circulating adrenaline released by the adrenal glands. The β_2-adrenoceptor is the most densely expressed subtype, although β_1-adrenoceptors are found in lung parenchyma (Ikeda et al. 2012). Activation of β_2-adrenoceptors leads to relaxation of airway smooth muscle. β-adrenoceptors are coupled to Gs proteins, resulting in activation of adenylyl cyclase and subsequent production of (cyclic adenosine monophosphate (cAMP). cAMP leads to activation of protein kinase A, which mediates the relaxation response.

β-adrenoceptors are also associated with goblet cells, but whether β-adrenoceptors increase or decrease mucus secretion is unclear (Bennett 2002). β_2-adrenoceptor agonists increase the clearance of mucus in healthy humans, which could be due to a combination of reduced mucus secretion and increased frequency of beating of cilia on the surface of the epithelial cells (Bennett 2002). However, whether this also occurs in patients with airway disease is less clear.

Airways are also innervated by the sensory nervous system, which plays a role in local reflex responses to inhaled irritants, as well as endogenous mediators (Gu and Lee 2021). Sensory nerves appear to play an important role in the cough reflex, as well as airway constriction, and receptors on sensory nerves, such as transient receptor potential (TRP) receptors, are potential targets for treatment of chronic cough, as well as exercise and cold-induced asthma (Gu and Lee 2021).

THE ROLE OF INFLAMMATION IN RESPIRATORY DISEASE

Airway inflammation underlies many chronic respiratory diseases, including asthma, chronic obstructive pulmonary disease (COPD) and cystic fibrosis.

Asthma is characterised by reversible increases in airway resistance, leading to wheezing and shortness of breath. On spirometry there are reversible decreases in the forced expiratory volume in the first second to forced vital capacity ratio (FEV_1:FVC) of less than 70–80%. There are also variations in peak expiratory flow, which improve with a β_2 agonist or treatment with cortiosteroids.

Allergic asthma occurs because of allergen-induced degranulation of mast cells, leading to release of inflammatory mediators such as histamine and leukotrienes (LTC_4 and LTD_4). These cause contraction of airway smooth muscle, leading to increased resistance in the airways and hence a reduced flow of air into the lungs, giving the symptom of breathlessness common in an asthma attack. Histamine also causes mucus secretion, which also increases airway resistance, as well as airway oedema. This phase of an asthma attack is known as the immediate phase. Although histamine is a major mediator of asthma attacks, histamine receptor antagonists (antihistamines) are not effective in treating asthma owing to the complexity of the immune response.

Chemokines released from the mast cells lead to recruitment of other immune cells to the site of inflammation, including eosinophils, neutrophils and T-cells. These cells exacerbate the inflammatory response, releasing other inflammatory mediators, which are associated with airway remodelling (including increased growth of smooth muscle cells) and hyperresponsiveness of the airways, so that the next time the patient is exposed to the allergen there is a greater contractile response.

The underlying pathogenesis of exercise and cold-induced asthma is less understood. However, the sensory nervous system is likely to be involved in these responses. Inflammation leads to increased sensitivity of the sensory neurons so that susceptible individuals see an increased response at relatively low stimuli. Sensory nerve endings contain cold-sensing receptors such as transient receptor potential melastatin 8 (TRPM8) receptors, which might be involved in the response to cold-induced asthma (Gu and Lee 2021). Patients with airway inflammation such as asthma and COPD are also susceptible to chronic cough, which is also mediated by sensory nerves. Capsaicin, which activates transient receptor potential vanilloid 1 (TRPV1) receptors on sensory nerve endings to release sensory neuropeptides (Caterina et al. 1997), induces cough in humans. Patients with asthma or COPD are more sensitive to this capsaicin-induced cough reflex, an indication of the sensitisation of the sensory nerves in inflammatory airways disease (Doherty et al. 2000).

PRACTICE APPLICATION

Bronchodilator therapies are based on two mechanisms:

- activation of β_2-adrenoceptors in airway smooth muscle
- inhibition of muscarinic receptors.

COPD is a term describing emphysema (destruction of the parenchyma), chronic bronchitis and small airways disease. Small airways disease (relating to airways of <2 mm in diameter) is caused by narrowing of the airways due to thickening of the smooth muscle layer, as well as hypersecretion of mucus and loss of elasticity of the lungs (Barnes 2019). COPD is associated with chronic inflammation, which is thought to lead to increased mucus production and remodelling of the airways. Smoking is the major cause of COPD. It is a progressive disease, with lung function decreasing over time. Unlike asthma, in which the decrease in lung function is readily reversed by bronchodilators, the decrease in lung function with COPD is not readily reversible.

Lung function can be assessed using spirometry, which measures the volume of air expelled from the lungs by forced expiration in 1 second (forced expiratory volume in 1 second, FEV_1) and the total volume of air expelled from the lung (forced vital capacity, FVC). Both asthma and COPD lead to a decrease in FEV_1 and the ratio between FEV_1 and FVC. However, in asthma, a bronchodilator will result in an increase in FEV_1, whereas in patients with COPD there is little or no change in FEV_1. The severity of COPD can be graded by the level of FEV_1 after treatment with a bronchodilator. Mild COPD is classed as an FEV_1 of ≥80% of the predicted FEV_1 (predicted FEV_1 for someone of the same age, sex and build), moderate COPD is when the FEV_1 is between 50% and 80% of predicted, severe COPD between 30% and 50% of predicted, and very severe less than 30% of predicted (GOLD 2021).

Cystic fibrosis is a genetic condition in which patients present with numerous conditions, including impaired lung function and a predisposition to respiratory infections. Cystic fibrosis is caused by an impairment of a chloride channel (cystic fibrosis transmembrane conductance regulator [CFTR]), which leads to reduced secretion of fluid into the lumen of the lungs and thus increased thickness of the mucus in the lumen. The mucus is therefore harder to clear from the lungs, leading to impaired airflow and breathlessness. Bronchodilators are often used in patients with cystic fibrosis to improve lung function, as well as other drugs such as mucolytics to break down mucus.

BRONCHODILATORS

A bronchodilator is a term for any drug that causes relaxation of the airway smooth muscle to increase air flow into the lungs. Bronchodilators can be split into three main families of drugs:

- β-adrenoceptor agonists
- muscarinic receptor antagonists
- methylxanthines.

β-ADRENOCEPTOR AGONISTS

β_2-adrenoceptor agonists act on β_2-adrenoceptors present on airway smooth muscle to relax the airways (Figure 20.2 and Table 20.1). Short-acting β_2-adrenoceptor agonists (SABAs) are used as required to reverse the bronchoconstriction and relieve breathlessness. They also reduce the release of inflammatory mediators from mast cells. Common SABAs include salbutamol and terbutaline. Long-acting β_2-adrenoceptor agonists (LABAs, e.g., salmeterol) are used as preventative treatments. These drugs have long, lipophilic side chains in their structure which are thought to interact with the lipid membranes of cells. This means that the LABAs are not as readily excreted from the body and are able to interact with the receptors for longer.

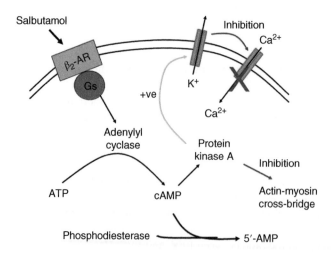

FIGURE 20.2 Stimulation of bronchodilation by β_2-adrenoceptor agonists and the role of phosphodiesterase inhibition. 5′-AMP, 5′-adenosine monophosphate; cAMP, cyclic adenosine monophosphate; ATP, adenosine triphosphate; β_2-AR, β_2-adrenoceptor.

Table 20.1 Examples of short- and long-acting bronchodilators commonly used to treat asthma and COPD

	Selective β_2-adrenergic receptor agonists	Muscarinic receptor antagonists
Short-acting	Salbutamol	Ipratropium
	Terbutaline	
Long-acting	Salmeterol	Tiotroprium
	Formoterol	Aclidinium bromide

SABAs are the drugs of first choice for asthma and COPD, and can be used in the diagnosis of asthma compared to COPD. In asthma, the FEV_1 should improve after treatment with a SABA, whereas the decrease in airway function in COPD is less readily reversed with a SABA. LABAs, such as salmeterol and formoterol, are used as add-on therapy for patients with difficult to treat asthma. The long-acting nature of the drugs means that they also prevent asthma attacks by preventing the release of inflammatory mediators from mast cells.

Side effects

β_2-adrenoceptor agonists are commonly delivered through inhalers, enabling direct delivery to the site of action. This allows lower concentrations to be given, thus reducing the incidence of side effects. In acute, severe asthma, β_2-adrenoceptor agonists might be delivered in higher doses using a nebuliser, or orally for those patients who are unable to use an inhaler. In these cases, β_2-adrenoceptor agonists are more likely to produce side effects such as arrhythmias (through interaction with β_1-adrenoceptors in the heart), tremor (through interaction with β_2-adrenoceptors on skeletal muscle) and hypokalaemia (through stimulation of K^+ uptake into skeletal muscle) (Moratinos and Reverte 1993).

STOP AND THINK

Apart from the increase in adverse effects, what else makes the oral route less suitable for salbutamol administration?

STOP AND THINK

Why is tachycardia a side effect of β_2-adrenoceptor agonist use?

β-BLOCKERS AND ASTHMA

β-adrenoceptor antagonists, even agents with selectivity for β_1-adrenoceptors over β_2-adrenoceptors are contraindicated in asthma. β-adrenoceptor antagonists will block adrenaline-induced bronchodilation and this can lead to bronchoconstriction; they will also oppose the effects of β_2-adrenoceptor agonists. β-adrenoceptor antagonists are used with caution in COPD.

MUSCARINIC RECEPTOR ANTAGONISTS

Muscarinic receptors on airway smooth muscle cause bronchoconstriction. Muscarinic receptor antagonists bind to muscarinic receptors, preventing the endogenous ligand acetylcholine from activating the receptor, thereby allowing the sympathetic stimulation of β_2-adrenoceptors to induce relaxation. Muscarinic receptor antagonists are often given with β_2-adrenoceptors agonists, particularly in COPD or difficult to treat asthma.

Ipratropium is a short-acting muscarinic receptor antagonist, whereas tiotropium is a long-acting muscarinic receptor antagonist. Ipratropium's duration of action is 3–6 hours and it is usually given three times a day, whereas tiotropium is given once a day (Moulton and Fryer 2011). None of the muscarinic receptor antagonists used clinically are selective for muscarinic receptor subtypes, although tiotropium exhibits some functional selectivity for M_3 receptors over M_2 receptors because it dissociates more readily from M_2 receptors (Moulton and Fryer 2011).

Side effects

Muscarinic antagonists have a slower onset of action than β_2-adrenoceptor agonists and are only given by inhalation. Inhaled muscarinic receptor antagonists exhibit fewer systemic side effects as the drug is delivered locally to the lungs. However, all muscarinic receptor antagonists have numerous side effects owing to their non-selective nature, but particularly when given by nebuliser. These include dry mouth due to inhibition of salivation, tachycardia due to antagonism of cardiac muscarinic receptors and constipation due to reduction of gastrointestinal smooth muscle contraction.

METHYLXANTHINES

Theophylline is a key example that is usually given orally as a modified release tablet. Aminophylline is an injectable version of theophylline; a combination of theophylline with ethylenediamine which increases the water solubility of the drug. This is used in emergency treatment of asthma to induce a rapid reversal of the bronchoconstriction.

Methylxanthines such as theophylline and related compounds are inhibitors of the intracellular enzyme phosphodiesterase. Phosphodiesterases metabolise the cyclic nucleotide signalling compounds cAMP and cyclic guanosine monophosphate (cGMP). Inhibition of phosphodiesterase activity prevents this metabolism, thereby increasing the levels of cyclic nucleotides in the cell. In the airways, cAMP mediates relaxation of airway smooth muscle downstream of activation of β_2-adrenoceptors, and so an increase in cAMP within the smooth muscle cells will enhance bronchodilation (Figure 20.2). cAMP also inhibits the release of mediators from mast cells, therefore inhibition of phosphodiesterase will also inhibit further the release of inflammatory mediators. Although theophylline does inhibit phosphodiesterase, whether this is the mechanism underlying its clinical effect is not clear. Studies indicate that the concentration of theophylline required to inhibit phosphodiesterase is far higher than that used clinically (Boswell-Smith et al. 2006).

Other proposed mechanisms include antagonism of adenosine receptors (Ito et al. 2002). Both theophylline and enprophylline antagonise adenosine receptors, but doxophylline does not, suggesting that this may not be the mechanism underlying the effects of these methylxanthines (van Mastbergen et al. 2012). Lower doses of theophylline used clinically have anti-inflammatory effects, and this may be the main effect of these compounds. Theophylline induces histone deacetylase activity, leading to a decrease in inflammatory gene expression (Ito et al. 2002), which could underlie many of its clinical effects. Interestingly, theophylline may reduce steroid resistance in COPD and severe asthma due to these effects on histone deacetylase.

Theophylline's use is limited by its narrow therapeutic index and drug interactions. Many of the unwanted side effects of theophylline, including central nervous system hyperactivity, cardiac arrhythmias and gastro-oesophageal reflux, could be due to inhibition of phosphodiesterases and/or antagonism of adenosine receptors (Matera et al. 2017). Doxophylline does not display these side effects, which may be due to a lack of effect at adenosine receptors. Plasma levels of theophylline should be monitored and dose adjusted accordingly. This also applies to aminophylline, as theophylline is the active ingredient in this drug.

STOP AND THINK

Why should theophylline levels be monitored?

Table 20.2 Some important potential interactions of methylxanthines with other drugs through modulation of cytochrome P450 activity

Drug	Action on CYP450 isoform	Possible effect on plasma theophylline levels
Alcohol	Induction of CYP2E1	Decreased
Ciprofloxacin	Inhibition of CYP1A2	Increased
Clarithromycin	Inhibition of CYP3A4	Increased
Erythromycin	Inhibition of CYP3A4	Increased
Carbamazepine	Induction of CYP3A4	Decreased
Phenytoin	Induction of CYP3A4	Decreased
Disulfiram	Inhibition of CYP2E1	Increased
Rifampicin	Induction of CYP3A4	Decreased
St John's wort	Induction of CYP3A4	Decreased

Theophylline metabolism is induced by cigarette smoke and alcohol, therefore if patients give up smoking, a dose reduction might be required to prevent any unwanted side effects. Theophylline also has numerous interactions with other drugs due to effects on drug metabolism (Table 20.2). The side effects and drug interactions limit the use of theophylline, particularly with newer drugs available.

ANTI-INFLAMMATORY AGENTS

Both asthma and COPD are associated with airway inflammation. In asthma, inflammation leads to remodelling of the airways and is associated with airway hyperresponsiveness, therefore reducing inflammation is a key therapeutic aim and so patients with newly diagnosed asthma are given an inhaled corticosteroid. Corticosteroids are less effective in COPD and some forms of severe asthma. This may be due to modification of the glucocorticoid receptor that corticosteroids act on, increased efflux of the drug or reduced translocation of the drug to the nucleus. Decreased levels of histone deacetylase 2 (HDAC2) are thought to be a major contributor to steroid resistance in COPD (Jiang and Zhu 2016), and combined treatment with theophylline, which increases histone deacetylase activity, might help reverse steroid resistance.

CORTICOSTEROIDS

Corticosteroids, commonly referred to just as steroids, activate the intracellular glucocorticoid receptor. Steroids are lipophilic and therefore can cross the plasma membrane into the cytosol, where they interact with two glucocorticoid receptors to form a dimer. This dimer then crosses the nuclear membrane into the nucleus, where it interacts with glucocorticoid response elements (GREs) on genes to alter gene transcription. Trans-activation of GREs leads to an increase in expression of anti-inflammatory genes such as annexin A1 and IκB, as well as β_2-adrenoceptors (Barnes 2006). This latter effect is beneficial in that it can help prevent desensitisation of β_2-adrenoceptors during treatment with β_2-adrenoceptor agonists. Co-prescribing of a steroid alongside a β_2-adrenoceptor agonist therefore helps maintain β_2-adrenoceptor function.

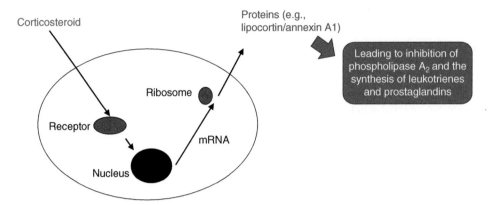

FIGURE 20.3 Schematic diagram summarising the action of corticosteroids acting via intracellular receptors to influences gene transcription, leading to mRNA coding for modulators of the inflammatory response. mRNA, messenger ribonucleic acid.

Annexin A1 is an endogenous inhibitor of phospholipase A_2, which breaks down phospholipids in the cell membrane to release arachidonic acid (Figure 20.3). Arachidonic acid is subsequently metabolised to leukotrienes and prostaglandins by lipoxygenase and cyclooxygenase, respectively. Leukotrienes and prostaglandins are involved in the inflammatory response, therefore reducing the production of these mediators helps to reduce inflammation. Annexin A1 also acts through the formyl peptide receptor to inhibit the release of histamine from mast cells (Sinniah et al. 2021). As well as the changes in gene transcription, more recently more rapid, non-genomic effects of steroids have been noted (Panettieri et al. 2019).

Activation of glucocorticoid receptors also recruits HDAC2 to the site of transcription, resulting in a decrease in gene transcription of inflammatory genes such as cytokines, chemokines, adhesion molecules and a number of enzymes (Barnes 2006; Nicolaides et al. 2010). These changes in gene transcription take time, and steroids need to be taken daily to maintain their anti-inflammatory effect. Furthermore, patients treated with oral steroids for longer than 3 weeks should have a step-down in the dose of steroid if the steroid treatment is to be stopped. This is because of the changes in gene transcription and suppression of the hypothalamus-pituitary–adrenal (HPA) axis, leading to reduced cortisol secretion, with chronic treatment with a steroid. If a patient stops taking a steroid abruptly, then this may lead to adrenal insufficiency (Gurnell et al. 2021). Adrenal crisis can have effects on the patient's wellbeing, including fatigue, weight loss and gastrointestinal disturbances, and can be life-threatening. The mnemonic HIGH STAKES can be used to identify adrenal insufficiency (Table 20.3). Long-term use of oral corticosteroids should be avoided in asthma, and use of steroid-sparing drugs, which can be given to control the inflammation as an alternative to steroids, should be considered.

HPA suppression is more likely with oral corticosteroid use and, in general, is dose dependent (Gurnell et al. 2021). Delivery of steroids direct to the lungs using an inhaler allows for delivery of lower doses of steroid, thus reducing the risk of systemic side effects, such as HPA suppression. Inhaled corticosteroids are therefore the drugs of first choice for preventing asthma attacks and should be taken on a daily basis.

Practice applications and side effects

Corticosteroids are associated with several side effects due to suppression of the immune response and suppression of the HPA axis. Inhaled corticosteroids can lead to mouth or throat infections such as oral thrush, as well as a hoarse voice (dysphonia), and patients should rinse their mouth with water after using their steroid inhaler (Hanania et al. 1995).

Table 20.3   The HIGH STAKES mnemonic for identifying adrenal insufficiency

---
Hypotension with dizziness

Inability to mount acute stress response

Generalised aches and pains, back and leg cramps or spasms

Hypoglycaemia

Shock and fever in intercurrent illness

Tiredness or fatigue and weakness

Abdominal pain, anorexia, weight loss, nausea and vomiting, and gastrointestinal upset

sKin hyperpigmentation

Electrolyte disturbance (hyponatraemia)

Somnolence, confusion, delirium or coma

Chronic use of high-dose steroids increases the risk of hypertension (>30% of patients; Rice et al. 2017) possibly due to fluid retention (Goodwin and Geller 2012). Long-term use of steroids is also associated with bone demineralisation leading to osteoporosis (Rice et al. 2017). Patients should maintain an adequate intake of calcium in the diet and patients on high doses of steroids, or at higher risk of osteoporosis, may need to take a calcium supplement.

Long-term use of oral steroids is also associated with an increased risk of gastrointestinal bleeding due to suppression of the production of prostaglandins. Prostaglandins reduce the secretion of acid from parietal cells in the stomach and increase the production of bicarbonate ions and mucus (Chapter 16), therefore inhibition of prostaglandin synthesis due to the production of annexin A1 increases the risk of ulcer formation due to excess acid secretion. As a result, patients on long-term steroids who are consider at risk of a gastric ulcer should also be given a proton pump inhibitor to monitor the increased acid production (NICE 2020).

HPA suppression and effects on bone mineralisation in children can lead to impairment of growth and so children on steroids should be monitored for height and weight (NICE 2020). Long-term use of inhaled corticosteroids is thought to reduce the rate of growth of the child, but the effect on the overall adult height gained may be slight (Zhang et al. 2014).

STOP AND THINK

Why might patients be reluctant to take inhaled steroids? What advice should you give patients?

NON-STEROIDAL ANTI-INFLAMMATORY DRUGS AND ASTHMA

About 15% of patients with asthma are sensitive to non-steroidal anti-inflammatory drugs (NSAIDs), which may cause a worsening of the condition. An explanation of this adverse event is that through cyclo-oxygenase inhibition, NSAIDs cause a diversion of arachidonic acid down the lipoxygenase pathway, increasing the production of inflammatory and bronchoconstrictor leukotrienes (Figure 20.4).

CYSTEINYLLEUKOTRIENE RECEPTOR ANTAGONISTS

The cysteinylleukotrienes LTC_4, LTD_4 and LTE_4 are produced by eosinophils, basophils and mast cells. LTC_4 and LTD_4 act on Cysteinylleukotriene Receptor 1 (CysLT1) on smooth muscle cells to cause bronchoconstriction. The CysLT1 receptor also increases the permeability of endothelial

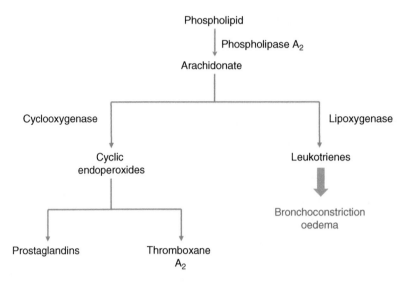

FIGURE 20.4   Production and consequences of leukotrienes in the airways.

cells in the microvasculature, leading to tissue oedema, as well as increased mucus production. Cysteinylleukotrienes are also involved in attraction of immune cells to the site of inflammation and stimulate the release of inflammatory mediators, including interleukins, from immune cells such as eosinophils, therefore cysteinylleukotrienes play a role in both the early phase of the asthma response and the late phase. Montelukast and zafirlukast are CysLT1 receptor antagonists (LTRAs) licensed for use in asthma. National Institute for Health and Care Excellence (NICE) guidelines indicate that LTRAs should be used as add-on therapy for adult patients for whom a LABA does not provide adequate control. For children under 5 years of age, an LTRA is the recommended first-line preventative treatment instead of an inhaled corticosteroid, whereas in children 5 or over, an LTRA can be used as an additional therapy for children on very-low-dose inhaled corticosteroid (NICE 2019). LTRAs are administered orally. Montelukast is given once a day in the evening, whereas zafirlukast is given twice a day.

Side effects

Gastrointestinal pain or disturbances are common, as are headaches.

PHOSPHODIESTERASE INHIBITORS

Phosphodiesterase enzymes (PDEs) metabolise the intracellular signalling compounds cAMP and cGMP. There are 12 isoforms of these enzymes, each having different selectivity for either cAMP or cGMP, or metabolising both. PDE IV is selective for breakdown of cAMP and therefore inhibition of PDE IV leads to an increase in intracellular levels of this compound. cAMP levels are raised by activation of β-adrenoceptors and mediate the effects of β_2-adrenoceptor agonists on both smooth muscle and mast cells. Roflumilast is an inhibitor of PDE IV which is licensed for use in COPD. It has been shown to reduce inflammatory responses within COPD (Rabe 2011). Roflumilast also improves the FEV_1 of patients with COPD both before and after bronchodilator treatment, indicating that it also has bronchodilator activity (Rabe 2011).

BIOLOGICS

The development of monoclonal antibodies for treatment of inflammation has opened up the possibility of new treatments for severe or difficult to treat asthma, or for steroid-sparing regimens. Omalizumab is a monoclonal antibody against immunoglobulin E (IgE) that binds to free IgE in the plasma and prevents it from binding to mast cells. Binding of allergen to the IgE bound to mast cells leads to mast cell degranulation, therefore omalizumab effectively reduces the amount of IgE able to bind to mast cells and so reduces allergen-induced mast cell degranulation.

Monoclonal antibodies are peptides and so have to be given by subcutaneous injection. The dose is adjusted based on the concentration of IgE in the patient's plasma, as well as the patient's body weight. Injections are given every 4 weeks.

Benralizumab and mepolizumab target interleukin 5, which is required for recruitment of eosinophils to the lungs and underlies hypersensitivity, increased bronchoconstriction, airway remodelling and increased mucus production (Tan et al. 2020). They are used under specialist care for patients with severe, eosinophilic asthma. Benralizumab is a monoclonal antibody that binds to the interleukin-5 (IL-5) receptor on eosinophils, preventing IL-5 binding. Mepolizumab, on the other hand, binds to IL-5 itself, thus preventing it from interacting with its receptor. Benralizumab also reduces the number of eosinophils present by inducing cell death (Tan et al. 2020).

Dupilumab binds to the IL-4 receptor, which prevents both IL-4 signalling and IL-13 signalling. This appears to be more effective than targeting either IL-4 or IL-13 separately (Tan et al. 2020). Dupilumab is used for patients with severe eosinophilic asthma not controlled with other medications and can lead to a reduction in the use of oral corticosteroids (Tan et al. 2020).

MUCOLYTICS AND RELATED COMPOUNDS

Airway inflammation or respiratory infection leads to an increase in mucus production. Excess mucus production contributes to increased airway resistance, particularly in chronic bronchitis and cystic fibrosis. Mucolytics aim to reduce the build up of mucus and increase clearance of the mucus from the airways. Mucus is produced by goblet cells in the epithelium and is made up of glycoproteins (Balsamo et al. 2010).

N-acetylcysteine

This is a reducing agent that leads to a breakdown of disulphide bonds in the mucus, thus reducing the thickness of the mucus and making it easier to clear from the lungs. It also has antioxidant properties, which may help reduce inflammation (Balsamo et al. 2010). Erdosteine and carbocisteine are similar compounds that also have antioxidant effects.

Dornase alfa

This is recombinant human DNase that breaks down DNA released from leukocytes during respiratory infections, which contributes to the increased viscosity of mucus (Shak 1995). It is used to reduce mucus viscosity, and hence improve mucus clearance, in patients with cystic fibrosis.

Ivacaftor

This is used for treatment of cystic fibrosis patients who have a G551D mutation in the gene encoding the CFTR (Condren and Bradshaw 2013). The CFTR regulates the secretion of chloride ions and in patients with cystic fibrosis there is reduced activity of this channel. Ivacaftor increases the time that the channel remains open, thus increasing secretion of chloride ions. This in turn increases the amount of fluid secreted into the lumen, thus helping to reduce the viscosity of the mucus (Van Goor et al. 2009).

GUIDANCE

Both NICE and the British Thoracic Society (BTS) have produced guidance on the management of asthma (NICE 2017; BTS/SIGN 2019) and COPD (NICE 2019). Whilst there are some differences between NICE and BTS guidance for the management of asthma, they both emphasise the stepped care approach. The usual initial management of asthma involves both low-dose inhaled corticosteroids and a short-acting β_2-adrenoceptor agonist as required (up to three times a week). If there is increased use of the short-acting β_2-adrenoceptor agonist, that is a signal to step up therapy.

SUMMARY

- Short-acting β_2-adrenoceptor agonists are important bronchodilators used in asthma and chronic obstructive pulmonary disease (COPD).

- Inhaled corticosteroids are the mainstay of therapy for asthma as preventive drugs and are effective with limited side effects. Inhaled corticosteroids are used in COPD, but many patients have a limited response.

- Long-acting β_2-adrenoceptor agonists are used as preventers in asthma (usually in addition to inhaled corticosteroids) and in COPD.

- Muscarinic receptors are coupled to bronchoconstriction and both short- and long-acting antimuscarinic drugs are used in the management of COPD.

- Leukotriene receptor antagonists are used in asthma.

- β-adrenoceptor antagonists are contraindicated in asthma and used with caution in COPD. Some patients with asthma are sensitive to non-steroidal anti-inflammatory drugs, which can worsen asthma.

ACTIVITY

1. Which ONE of the following is part of the second messenger system associated with activation of β_2-adrenoceptors?

   (a) Activation of adenylyl cyclase

   (b) Decrease in cAMP

   (c) Increase in calcium

   (d) Increase in cGMP

   (e) Opening of calcium channels

2. Which ONE of the following is a feature of inhaled corticosteroids?

   (a) An initial response is delayed by a few days

   (b) Standard doses are associated with significant suppression of the hypothalamus-pituitary–adrenal axis

   (c) They act via G-protein-coupled receptors

   (d) They are contraindicated in hypertension

   (e) They are used to relieve asthmatic attacks

3. Which ONE of the following drugs should be avoided in asthma?

   (a) ACE inhibitors (e.g., ramipril)

   (b) β_2-adrenoceptor agonists (e.g., salbutamol)

   (c) β_1-adrenoceptor antagonists (e.g., bisoprolol)

   (d) Muscarinic receptor antagonists (e.g., tiotropium)

   (e) Phosphodiesterase inhibitors (e.g., theophylline)

REFERENCES

Balsamo, R., Lanata, L. and Egan, C.G. (2010) Mucoactive drugs. *Eur Respir Rev* 116:127–133.

Barnes, P.J. (2006) How corticosteroids control inflammation: Quintiles Prize Lecture 2005. *Br J Pharmacol* 148:245–254.

Barnes, P.J. (2019) Small airway fibrosis in COPD. *Int J Biochem Cell Biol* 116:105598.

Bennett, W.D. (2002) Effect of beta-adrenergic agonists on mucociliary clearance. *J Allergy Clin Immunol* 110(6 Suppl):S291–S297.

Boswell-Smith, V., Cazzola, M. and Page, C.P. (2006) Are phosphodiesterase 4 inhibitors just more theophylline? *J Allergy Clin Immunol* 117:1237–1243.

BTS/SIGN (2019) British guideline on the management of asthma. SIGN158.

Caterina, M.J., Schumacher, M.A., Tominaga, M., Rosen, T.A., Levine, J.D. and Julius, D. (1997) The capsaicin receptor: a heat-activated ion channel in the pain pathway. *Nature* 389:816–824.

Condren, M.E. and Bradshaw, M.D. (2013) Ivacaftor: a novel gene-based therapeutic approach for cystic fibrosis. *J Pediatr Pharmacol Ther* 18:8–13.

Doherty, M.J., Mister, R., Pearson, M.G. and Calverley, P.M. (2000) Capsaicin responsiveness and cough in asthma and chronic obstructive pulmonary disease. *Thorax* 55:643–49.

GOLD (2021) Global Initiative for Chronic Obstructive Lung Disease. https://goldcopd.org/wp-content/uploads/2020/11/GOLD-REPORT-2021-v1.1-25Nov20_WMV.pdf.

Goodwin, J.E. and Geller, D.S. (2012) Glucocorticoid-induced hypertension. *Pediatr Nephrol* 27:1059–1066.

Gu, Q. and Lee, L.Y. (2021) TRP channels in airway sensory nerves. *Neurosci Lett* 748:135719.

Gurnell, M., Heaney, L.G., Price, D. and Menzies-Gow, A. (2021) Long-term corticosteroid use, adrenal insufficiency and the need for steroid-sparing treatment in adult severe asthma. *J Intern Med* 290:240–256.

Hanania, N.A., Chapman, K.R. and Kesten, S. (1995) Adverse effects of inhaled corticosteroids. *Am J Med* 98:196–208.

Ikeda, T., Anisuzzaman, A.S.M., Yoshiki, H., et al. (2012) Regional quantification of muscarinic acetylcholine receptors and β-adrenoceptors in human airways. *Br J Pharmacol* 166:1804–1814.

Ito, K., Lim, S., Caramori, G., et al. (2002) A molecular mechanism of action of theophylline: Induction of histone deacetylase activity to decrease inflammatory gene expression. *Proc Natl Acad Sci USA* 99:8921–8926.

Jiang, Z. and Zhu, L. (2016) Update on molecular mechanisms of corticosteroid resistance in chronic obstructive pulmonary disease. *Pulm Pharmacol Ther* 37:1–8.

Matera, M.G., Page, C. and Cazzola, M. (2017) Doxofylline is not just another theophylline! *Int J Chron Obstruct Pulmon Dis* 12:3487–3493.

Moratinos, J. and Reverte, M. (1993) Effects of catecholamines on plasma potassium: the role of alpha- and beta-adrenoceptors. *Fun Clin Pharmacol* 7:143–153.

Moulton, B.C. and Fryer, A.D. (2011) Muscarinic receptor antagonists, from folklore to pharmacology; finding drugs that actually work in asthma and COPD. *Br J Pharmacol* 163:44–52.

NICE (2017) Asthma: diagnosis, monitoring and chronic asthma management. NICE guidance NG80.

NICE (2019) Chronic obstructive pulmonary disease in over 16s: diagnosis and management. NICE Guidance NG115.

NICE (2020) https://cks.nice.org.uk/topics/corticosteroids-oral/.

Nicolaides, N.C., Galata, Z., Kino, T., Chrousos, G.P. and Charmandari, E. (2010) The human glucocorticoid receptor: molecular basis of biologic function. *Steroids* 75:1–12.

Panettieri, R.A., Schaafsma, D., Amrani, Y., Koziol-White, C., Ostrom, R. and Tliba, O. (2019)

Non-genomic effects of glucocorticoids: an updated view. *Trends Pharmacol Sci* 40:38–49.

Pincus, A.B., Fryer, A.D. and Jacoby, D.B. (2021) Mini review: Neural mechanisms underlying airway hyperresponsiveness. *Neurosci Lett* 751:135795.

Rabe, K.F. (2011) Update on roflumilast, a phosphodiesterase 4 inhibitor for the treatment of chronic obstructive pulmonary disease. *Br J Pharmacol* 163:53–67.

Rice, J.B., White, A.G., Scarpati, L.M., Wan, G. and Nelson, W.W. (2017) Long-term systemic corticosteroid exposure: a systematic literature review. *Clin Ther* 39:216–229.

Rogers, D.F. (2001) Motor control of airway goblet cells and glands. *Respir Physiol* 125:129–144.

Shak, S. (1995) Aerosolized recombinant human DNase I for the treatment of cystic fibrosis. *Chest* 107(2 Suppl):65S–70S.

Sinniah, A., Yazid, S. and Flower, R.J. (2021) From NSAIDs to glucocorticoids and beyond. *Cells* 10:3524.

Tan, R., Liew, M.F., Lim, H.F., Leung, B.P. and Wong, W.S.F. (2020) Promises and challenges of biologics for severe asthma. *Biochem Pharmacol* 179:114012.

Van Goor, F., Hadida, S., Grootenhuis, P.D., et al. (2009) Rescue of CF airway epithelial cell function in vitro by a CFTR potentiator, VX-770. *Proc Natl Acad Sci USA* 106:18825–18830.

van Mastbergen, J., Jolas, T., Allegra, L. and Page, C.P. (2012) The mechanism of action of doxofylline is unrelated to HDAC inhibition, PDE inhibition or adenosine receptor antagonism. *Pulm Pharmacol Ther* 25:55–61.

Zhang, L., Prietsch, S.O.M. and Ducharme, F.M. (2014) Inhaled corticosteroids in children with persistent asthma: effects on growth. *Evid Based Child Health* 9:829–830

FURTHER READING

Ritter, J.M., Flower, R., Henderson, G., et al. (2023) *Rang and Dale's Pharmacology*, 10th edn. Elsevier, Amsterdam.

CLINICAL GUIDELINES

BTS/SIGN (2019). British guideline on the management of asthma. SIGN158.

NICE (2017) Asthma: diagnosis, monitoring and chronic asthma management. NICE guidance NG80.

NICE (2019). Chronic obstructive pulmonary disease in over 16s: diagnosis and management. NICE Guidance NG115.

NICE (2020) https://cks.nice.org.uk/topics/corticosteroids-oral/.

Introduction to the Central Nervous System

CHAPTER 21

Yvonne Mbaki

LEARNING OUTCOMES

By the end of this chapter the reader should be able to:

- describe the major areas of the brain and their associated functions

- demonstrate an understanding of the basic properties of nerve cells such as the action potential, graded potential and the chemical synapse

- identify the principal neurotransmitters in the central nervous system and their physiological effects

- identify examples of illnesses that are based on alterations in these neuro-transmitters

CENTRAL NERVOUS SYSTEM

The nervous system can be divided into two components, namely the peripheral nervous system and the central nervous system (CNS). The CNS can be further divided into the spinal cord and the brain. The spinal cord conducts signals to and from the brain: sensory information is conducted from the peripheral nervous system to the brain while motor information is transferred from the brain to effector systems throughout the body. The brain receives sensory input from the spinal cord as well as from its own nerves, which are the olfactory and optic nerves. Most of the power of the brain is devoted to processing these sensory inputs and initiating and co-ordinating the appropriate motor outputs.

PARTS OF THE BRAIN

The brain can be divided into three major areas known as the hindbrain, midbrain and forebrain, which are themselves divided into different regions (Figure 21.1) and are all responsible for regulating different functions.

THE HINDBRAIN

The hindbrain is at the top of the spinal cord and consists of three separate structures:

- *Medulla oblongata*: responsible for maintaining basic homeostatic functions such as breathing and heart rate.

- *Pons*: involved in movement control, sensory analysis and arousal.

- *Cerebellum*: involved in movement regulation and balance.

The New Prescriber: An Integrated Approach to Medical and Non-medical Prescribing, Second Edition.
Edited by Joanne Lymn, Alison Mostyn, Roger Knaggs, Michael Randall, and Dianne Bowskill.
© 2024 John Wiley & Sons Ltd. Published 2024 by John Wiley & Sons Ltd.

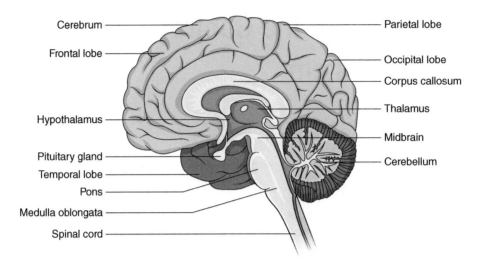

FIGURE 21.1   The major anatomical areas of the brain.

THE MIDBRAIN

The midbrain is the smallest processing region of the brain, but it has a vital role in relaying sensory information and connects the hindbrain to the forebrain. The key anatomical regions are as follows:

- *Tectum*: involved with visual and auditory processing.
- *Cerebral peduncle*: contains the large axon bundles involved in voluntary movement.
- *Substantia nigra*: neural pathways associated with initiation of movement. Dysfunction of these pathways occurs in Parkinson's disease (Chapter 22).

THE FOREBRAIN

The forebrain is the largest part of the brain and is where conscious thought and action are initiated. Anatomically it is made up of the following parts:

- *Cerebrum*: the outer layers forming the cerebrum are responsible for the control of perception, memory and all higher cognitive functions.
- *Thalamus*: relays sensory information to the cerebral cortex.
- *Hypothalamus*: involved in the regulation of the homeostatic function of the body.
- *Limbic system*: important in memory, emotion and decision making.

    This neuroanatomy has fascinated scientists and clinicians for generations and there are many online resources for this topic (e.g., CNS Forum).

NEURONAL STRUCTURE AND FUNCTION

The basic structural unit of the brain and spinal cord is the nerve cell or neuron. However, for these nerve cells to function normally, the support of glial cells is required.

GLIAL CELLS

These cells do not directly take part in the electrical communication in the CNS but are nonetheless critically important because they provide the neurons with nutrients, form the myelin insulation around neurons, provide anatomical support for brain structures, destroy pathogens and recycle dead neurons. Taking this together, glia can modulate neuronal function. Motor neuron disease is an example of a glial disorder that leads to dysfunction of the control of voluntary muscles.

ANATOMY AND PHYSIOLOGY OF NERVE CELLS

The neuron is one of the cornerstone concepts of neurophysiology, so much so that it is worth extending your knowledge of its function a bit further. In Chapter 14 we looked at the basic structure of the neuron and discussed its function; it is important here to think about this in more detail (Figure 21.2).

The principal communication medium of the nervous system is electrical charge. In our journey from the input to the output of a neuron, we will look at these events and by reviewing the function of the neuron, you can learn a great deal about how the whole nervous system functions.

INTEGRATION OF INPUTS VIA THE DENDRITES

The electrical events at the input end of the neuron are small and are called graded potentials. These graded potentials can be excitatory post synaptic potentials (EPSPs) or inhibitory post synaptic potentials (IPSPs). It is the addition of these postsynaptic potentials that determines what information the neuron will transmit.

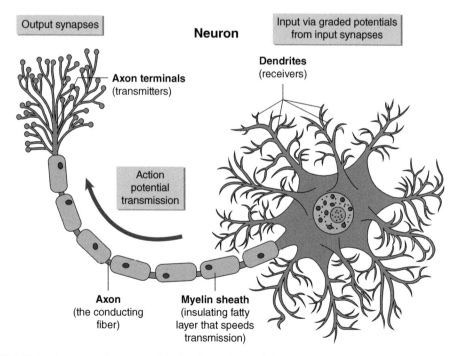

FIGURE 21.2 Anatomy of a neuron showing the pathway of electrical transmission.

EXCITATORY POSTSYNAPTIC POTENTIAL

An EPSP is a local depolarisation of the membrane of the receiving neuron (the postsynaptic neuron) due to release of transmitters from the input neuron (presynaptic). This transmitter binds to receptors on the membrane of the postsynaptic neuron, opening sodium (Na^+) and/or calcium (Ca^{2+}) channels as well as closing chloride (Cl^-) and/or potassium (K^+) channels.

INHIBITORY POSTSYNAPTIC POTENTIAL

An IPSP is a local hyperpolarisation of the membrane of a postsynaptic neuron due to release of transmitter from the presynaptic terminal. This transmitter binds to receptors on the membrane of the postsynaptic neuron, closing sodium (Na^+) and/or calcium (Ca^{2+}) channels as well as opening chloride (Cl^-) and/or potassium (K^+) channels.

The combination of IPSPs and EPSPs provides electrical stimulation to the neuron for it to filter out stray information and add together (summate) the information that needs to be transmitted. There are two categories of summation: one to do with the frequency of stimulation (temporal) and the other to do with the anatomical position of the input synapses (spatial).

- *Temporal summation*: adding together of EPSPs generated by firing of the same presynaptic terminal at high frequency to generate an action potential in the postsynaptic neuron (Figure 21.3b).

- *Spatial summation*: adding together of EPSPs generated by the firing of two or more presynaptic neurons simultaneously to generate the action potential in the postsynaptic neuron (Figure 21.3c).

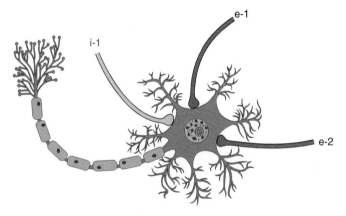

Nerve cell showing two excitatory inputs (e-1 and e-2) and one inhibitory input (i-1). The resultant electrical activity is recorded below.

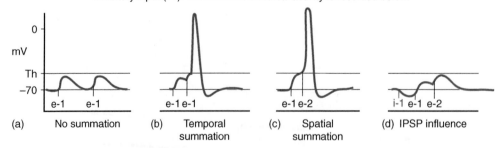

FIGURE 21.3 The influence of excitatory and inhibitory inputs on a nerve cell as measured by electrodes in nerve cells (21.3a-d). 21.3a 'no summation' - EPSPs do not summate effectively due to week synaptic input or longer time interval between EPSPs. 21.3d 'IPSP influence' - counters the summation of EPSPs generated. EPSP, excitatory postsynaptic potential, IPSP, inhibitory post synaptic potential; Th, threshold for action potential generation; mV, millivolt (membrane potential). http://www.bio.miami.edu/~cmallery/150/neuro/c7.48.18.summation.jpg

ACTION POTENTIAL TRANSMISSION

The combination of EPSPs and IPSPs when summed at the axon hillock (the site where the axon meets the cell body) can produce a depolarising threshold electrical stimulus that generates the propagating 'all or none' electrical signal for transmission over distance. The evoked spike of electrical activity is the action potential (Figure 21.4) and it is this that is propagated along the axon to the output synapse. The speed at which the action potential travels is dependent on the size of the axon (larger diameter is faster) and the amount of myelin insulation (longer nerves have more myelin wrapped around the axon). In some of the very long nerves involved in controlling skeletal muscle function, the speed of transmission can be as much as 25 m/s. The properties of myelin insulation produce an effect called saltatory conduction, where the electrical signal jumps along the nerve following the path of least resistance (gaps in the myelin). This transmission can be effectively blocked by local anaesthetic agents as they disrupt nerve membrane channel function (Chapter 26). The failure of this insulation is a component of several neuromuscular disorders, including motor neuron disease.

OUTPUT SYNAPSES

This is a physical gap between neurons and their target cells (e.g., neurons, muscles and glands) that promotes a primarily unidirectional flow of information (pre to post). In the next section, we will look at the chemical transmitters produced by the body to cross this gap.

STOP AND THINK

Why do you think the majority of transmission from one neuron to another occurs by chemical rather than electrical transmission?

PRINCIPAL NEUROTRANSMITTERS OF THE CNS

Understanding the basic functions of these neurotransmitters in the CNS allows you to apply that knowledge to drugs that interact with these systems. An agonist will mimic or enhance the 'normal' physiological response and an antagonist will stop or reduce the 'normal' response and may even

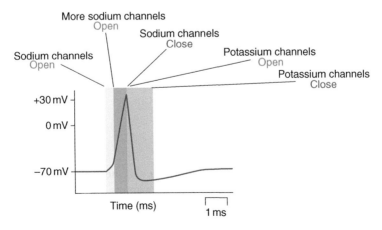

FIGURE 21.4   Ionic components of the action potential showing the roles of sodium (Na^+) and potassium (K^+) in its formation. ms, millisecond; mV, millivolt (membrane potential). http://faculty.washington.edu/chudler/ap3.gif

Table 21.1 Principal neurotransmitters in the central nervous system and the receptor classes they interact with to produce an excitatory or inhibitory response

Neurotransmitter	Post synaptic excitation (receptor labels)	Post synaptic inhibition (receptor labels)
Acetylcholine	nAChR, M1, M3, M5	M2, M4
Noradrenaline	α1, β	α2
Dopamine	D1	D2
Serotonin (5HT)	5HT2, 5HT3, 5HT4, 5HT6, 5HT7	5HT1, 5HT5,
γ-amino butyric acid		GABA-A, GABA-B, GABA-C
Glutamate	AMPA, Kainate, NMDA	
Opioids		Mu (μ), delta (δ), kappa (k), ORL

5HT1, serotonin 1 receptor; 5HT2, serotonin 2 receptor; 5HT3, serotonin 3 receptor; 5HT4, serotonin 4 receptor; 5HT5, serotonin 5 receptor; 5HT6, serotonin 6 receptor; 5HT7, serotonin 1 receptor; α1, alpha 1; α2, alpha 2; AMPA, α-amino-3-hydroxy-5-methyl-4-isoxazole propionic acid; β, beta; D1, dopamine 1 receptor; D2, dopamine 1 receptor; GABA-A, γ-aminobutyric acid type A; GABA-B, γ-aminobutyric acid type B; GABA-C, γ-aminobutyric acid type C; M1, muscarinic acetylcholine receptor M1; M2, muscarinic acetylcholine receptor M2; M3, muscarinic acetylcholine receptor M3; M4, muscarinic acetylcholine receptor M4; M5, muscarinic acetylcholine receptor M5; nAChR, nicotinic acetylcholine receptor; NMDA, N-methyl-D-aspartate receptor; ORL, opioid receptor like 1

promote the opposite effect. The following brief overview of the neurotransmitters listed in Table 21.1 highlights their main effects (primarily within the CNS).

ACETYLCHOLINE

There are two receptor subtypes associated with acetylcholine (ACh): the nicotinic (nAChR) and muscarininc (M) receptors. Both subtypes are found in the CNS and just as in the autonomic nervous system, acetylcholine is broken down in the synaptic cleft by the enzyme acetylcholinesterase. In the CNS, acetylcholine is involved with:

- motor co-ordination pathways
- arousal
- short-term memory and cognition
- central pain perception
- central breathing control.

The link between acetylcholine and the motor co-ordination pathways suggests a link between acetylcholine signalling and Parkinson's disease while the association with short-term memory and cognition suggests a link to Alzheimer's disease (Chapter 22).

NORADRENALINE

Noradrenaline (called norepinephrine in North America and most of Europe) is a monoamine neurotransmitter that has a similar synthesis pathway to dopamine. This means that drugs affecting dopamine synthesis (e.g., L-dopa) will also modify noradrenaline production. There are two receptor subtypes associated with noradrenaline: alpha- and beta-receptors. The actions of noradrenaline in the synaptic cleft are ended by reuptake mechanisms (noradrenaline transporters) and subsequent cellular metabolism by monoamine oxidase (MAO) enzymes (MAO-A). Noradrenaline is associated with the following:

- ascending tracts involved with mood, behaviour, stress, depression and reward reinforcement
- blood pressure and sympathetic tone in the brainstem
- control of sleep/wake cycle and levels of arousal in the locus coeruleus
- temperature regulation, sleep and arousal in the hypothalamus
- 'fight and flight' reactions and anxiety.

The link between noradrenaline and mood, behaviour and sleep/wake cycle points to the involvement of this neurotransmitter in depression and anxiety.

DOPAMINE

Dopamine, also a monoamine neurotransmitter, has a similar synthetic pathway to noradrenaline. There are two dopamine receptor subtypes, namely D_1 and D_2 receptors. Drugs affecting the autonomic nervous system may modulate actions of the dopaminergic system. As is seen with noradrenaline, the action of dopamine in the synaptic cleft is ended by the removal of dopamine by reuptake mechanisms (dopamine transporters), and subsequent cellular metabolism by MAO-B. It is worth noting that the monoamine oxidase involved in the breakdown of dopamine is not the same isoform as that involved in the breakdown of noradrenaline. In the brain dopamine is involved in:

- ascending tracts from the ventral tegmental area to the mesolimbic/mesocortical regions, controlling mood, behaviour and stress
- ascending tracts from the substantia nigra to the corpus striatum associated with control of movement
- communication between the hypothalamus and the pituitary gland.

As a consequence, a side effect of some antipsychotic agents is prolactin-induced subfertility. It is the involvement of dopamine pathways in the mesolimbic/mesocortical regions of the brain that suggests that alteration to dopamine transmission may be important in depression, addiction and schizophrenia. Similarly, the involvement of dopamine pathways in the substantia nigra, which is associated with movement control, suggests a major role for dopamine in Parkinson's disease (Chapter 22).

PRACTICE APPLICATION

Drugs of abuse, including heroin, amphetamines, cocaine, marijuana, alcohol, nicotine and caffeine, trigger release and/or increase the effective levels of dopamine in the CNS.

SEROTONIN (5-HYDROXYTRYPTAMINE OR 5HT)

Serotonin is widely distributed both within and outside the CNS (including mast cells, platelet and enterochromafin cells of the digestive tract). In fact, more serotonergic cells are located in the digestive tract (98%) than in the brain. The action of serotonin in the synapse is curtailed by the reuptake of serotonin into the presynaptic neuron and the subsequent cellular metabolism by monoamine oxidase enzymes. The monoamine oxidase involved in the breakdown of serotonin is MAO-A, the same isoform involved in the breakdown of noradrenaline.

Within the CNS, serotonin:

- suppresses appetite: drugs that increase 5HT levels are appetite suppressants (e.g., D-fenfluramine)

- interacts with hormonal systems and the CNS, for example oestrogen can modify presynaptic 5HT levels

- is found at low levels in depressed people and is linked with the aetiology of many mental health disorders such as depression, anxiety, schizophrenia, eating disorders, obsessive compulsive disorder and panic disorders.

Outside the CNS, 5HT is a potent vasoconstrictor and modulates the clotting cascade.

PRACTICE APPLICATION

Serotonin syndrome is a potentially fatal effect that can be precipitated by a combination of serotonergic agents (such as a selective serotonin reuptake inhibitor with a triptan) that may produce euphoria, drowsiness, sustained rapid eye movement, over-reaction of reflexes, rapid muscle contraction, shivering, diarrhoea, loss of consciousness and death.

GAMMA-AMINO BUTYRIC ACID

Gamma-amino butyric acid (GABA) is the primary inhibitory neurotransmitter of the CNS, with cell bodies that are widespread throughout the CNS. There are a substantial number of short projections and local pathways in the CNS and spinal cord. One of the best-described effects of GABA receptor function is the desensitisation that occurs with prolonged exposure to GABA or GABA stimulants (such as barbiturates or benzodiazepines). These drugs become less effective with prolonged exposure in a dose-dependent way.

Within the CNS, GABA is involved with:

- motor control, vision, sensory processing, epilepsy, arousal, Huntington's disease, Alzheimer's disease, psychoses, endocrine regulation, catatonia, memory loss, brown adipose tissue regulation, analgesia, anaesthesia and gastric motility

- promoting sedation, which can be useful in a variety of mental health conditions.

STOP AND THINK

Why do you think the GABAergic system is the drug target for some hypnotic and anxiolytic medications?

GLUTAMATE

Glutamate is the major fast-acting neuroexcitatory agent in the CNS and its effects may be linked to its widespread distribution in the CNS. Glutamate is involved with:

- cell death processes (necrosis and apoptosis), either as a causative agent or promoter of the effect. Hence glutamate plays an important role in neurodegenerative disorders, including Alzheimer's disease, stroke and amyotrophic lateral sclerosis

- reflex pathways in the spinal cord

- long-term potentiation (memory) in the hippocampus

- sensory processing, motor co-ordination and movement disorders.

ENDOGENOUS OPIOIDS

All currently recognised opioid receptors (four classes: mu, kappa, delta and opioid receptor like 1) are found both in opioid-specific pathways and scattered throughout the CNS. Analysis of the distribution of neurons that contain or respond to opioids in the CNS suggests that these neurotransmitters are involved with:

- analgesia: reducing intensity of pain by inhibiting the release of pain-signalling transmitters

- euphoria, addiction and drug reinforcement

- sedation

- respiratory depression: respiration is reduced with all doses, with the respiratory centres in the brainstem becoming less sensitive to higher levels of CO_2

- cough suppression (antitussive)

- nausea and vomiting: stimulating receptors in the area postrema

- reduced gastrointestinal motility.

Via their activation of mu receptors in the mesolimbic dopamine system, opioids reduce the inhibition exerted by GABAergic neurons on dopaminergic neurons in the ventrotegmental area, releasing more dopamine and reinforcing this pathway. The presence of opioid receptors in the hypothalamus means that they have an effect on temperature regulation and hormone secretion.

Further information on the clinical use of opioids as analgesics can be found in Chapter 26.

SUMMARY

- The brain can be divided into three major areas: the hindbrain, midbrain and forebrain.

- The basic structural unit of the brain and spinal cord is the nerve cell or neuron.

- The combination of inhibitory post synaptic potentials and excitatory post synaptic potentials provides electrical stimulation to the neuron for it to filter stray information and add together (summate) the information that needs to be transmitted.

- There are two categories of summation, one concerned with the frequency of stimulation (temporal) and the other concerned with the anatomical position of the input synapses (spatial).

- Transmission across the synapse is chemical rather than electrical.

- Acetylcholine is broken down in the synaptic cleft by the enzyme acetylcholinesterase.

- Acetylcholine is associated with both motor co-ordination and short-term memory and cognition.

- The actions of monoamines in the synaptic cleft are ended by their removal by uptake mechanisms and subsequent cellular metabolism by monoamine oxidase enzymes.

- Alterations in dopamine are associated with neurodegenerative disorders.

- Gamma-amino butyric acid is the primary inhibitory neurotransmitter of the central nervous system.

- Glutamate is the major fast-acting neuroexcitatory agent in the central nervous system.

ACTIVITY

1. The brain is divided into three major areas (hindbrain, midbrain and forebrain).   True/False

2. The tectum is only involved with auditory processing.

    True/False

3. The limbic system is important in emotion and decision making.

    True/False

4. Glial cells take no direct part in electrical communication in the CNS.

    True/False

5. An EPSP is a local hyperpolarisation of the membrane of the receiving neuron.   True/False

6. A small-diameter axon has the fastest transmission of action potentials.

    True/False

7. Noradrenaline and dopamine have different synthesis pathways.

    True/False

8. Serotonin is more prevalent in the CNS than in any other part of the body.

    True/False

9. Dopamine and serotonin are broken down by the same monoamine oxidase enzyme.   True/False

10. Glutamate is the major excitatory neurotransmitter in the CNS.

    True/False

FURTHER READING

Aidley, D.J. (1998) *The Physiology of Excitable Cells*, 4th edn. Cambridge University Press, Cambridge.

Barker, R.A. (1993) *Neuroscience: An Illustrated Guide*. Ellis Horwood, New York.

Ross, J. (2015) *Crash Course Nervous System*, 4th edn. Elsevier Health Sciences.

Kruk, Z.L. and Pycock, C.J. (1991) *Neurotransmitters and Drugs*, 3rd edn. Chapman and Hall, London.

Kester, M., Karpa, K.D. and Vrana, K.E. (2011) *Elsevier's Integrated Review Pharmacology E-Book: with Student Consult Online Access*. https://books.google.co.uk/books?hl=en&lr=&id=kU6gilUvb SkC&oi=fnd&pg=PP1&dq=Kester+,+M.,+Karpa,+K.+D.+and,+%26+Vrana,+K.+E.+(2011)&ots=YdC5lOyxpp&sig=5mub9rGWRewavr43dhdMw3Hyo_s&redir_esc=y#v=onepage&q&f=false.

Ritter, J.M., Flower, R., Henderson, G., et al. (2023) *Rang and Dale's Pharmacology*, 10th edn. Elsevier, Amsterdam.

Webster, R. (Ed.). (2001) *Neurotransmitters, Drugs and Brain Function*. John Wiley & Sons, Chichester.

Zimmermann, H. (ed.) (2013) *Cellular and Molecular Basis of Synaptic Transmission*, Vol. 21. Springer Science & Business Media, Berlin.

USEFUL WEBSITE

CNS Forum. http://www.cnsforum.com/educational resources/imagebank

Neurodegenerative Disorders

David Kendall

LEARNING OUTCOMES

By the end of this chapter the reader should be able to:

- describe the clinical features and diagnosis of Parkinson's disease

- state the pathogenesis and risk factors in the development of Parkinson's disease

- understand the mechanisms of action and major adverse effects of drugs used to treat Parkinson's disease

- describe the clinical features and diagnosis of Alzheimer's disease

- give an account of the pathophysiology of Alzheimer's disease

- understand the mechanism of action and major adverse effects of drugs used to treat Alzheimer's disease.

PARKINSON'S DISEASE

EPIDEMIOLOGY

Parkinson's disease (PD) was first described in the modern context by James Parkinson in 1817, but it has been known for centuries, with one of the first written accounts given by Galen in the second century AD. It is a chronic, progressive and currently incurable disease. PD is common, with approximately 6·1 million people affected worldwide in 2016. For reasons that are not yet fully understood, the incidence and prevalence of PD have risen rapidly in recent years (Dorsey et al. 2018). There is about a 1:500 chance of developing the disease in the over-60s, although it can also affect younger people. PD affects both men and women, but the incidence is lower in women and their age at onset is higher.

CLINICAL FEATURES AND DIAGNOSIS

PD is typically characterised by a combination of motor disturbances, particularly bradykinesia and tremor, and non-motor features, including depression, constipation and disturbed sleep. The non-motor symptoms can precede the onset of the motor syndrome.

In practice, diagnosis is clinical, based on history taking and neurological examination and, except for genetic testing in specific cases, a definitive diagnosis can only be established by post-mortem identification of neuropathological changes in the brain.

PATHOGENESIS

PD results in accelerated death primarily of dopaminergic neurons of the substantia nigra pathway in the midbrain, but multiple other motor and non-motor circuits are affected. Loss of nigrostriatal dopamine-containing cells causes striatal dopamine depletion, resulting in an

The New Prescriber: An Integrated Approach to Medical and Non-medical Prescribing, Second Edition.
Edited by Joanne Lymn, Alison Mostyn, Roger Knaggs, Michael Randall, and Dianne Bowskill.
© 2024 John Wiley & Sons Ltd. Published 2024 by John Wiley & Sons Ltd.

imbalance between direct (facilitatory) and indirect (inhibitory) pathways through the basal ganglia, resulting in bradykinesia. Patients can lose 70–80% of these neurons before any obvious symptoms are detected. Dopamine would normally inhibit acetylcholine release from the corpus striatum but in PD the loss of dopamine means less inhibition of acetylcholine release and hence greater activity of these cholinergic neurons. Hence PD is associated, to some extent, with an imbalance in the activity of dopamine-containing and acetylcholine-containing neurons.

PD neuropathology is highly heterogeneous, but the pathological hallmark is the Lewy body, which contains aberrant accumulation of the protein α-synuclein along with dysfunction of mitochondria, lysosomes or vesicle transport, synaptic transport issues and neuroinflammation (Armstrong and Okun 2020).

GENETICS AND OTHER RISK FACTORS

In most populations, only 3–5% of PD is fully explained by genetic causes linked to known PD genes (monogenic PD), whereas 90 genetic variants collectively explain 16–36% of the heritable risk of non-monogenic PD. Most interest is focused on mutations in the genes SNCA, LRRK2, PRKN, PINK1 and GBA (Trin et al. 2018).

Persuasive non-genetic risk factors include exposure to environmental toxins, such as pesticides, and traumatic head injury. There are negative associations with coffee drinking, anti-inflammatory drug use, high plasma urate levels, physical activity and, counterintuitively, smoking. The possible causal nature of these associations is uncertain.

ANTI-PARKINSONIAN THERAPY

In PD, the principal aim is to increase the levels of dopamine in the surviving neurons in the central nervous system (CNS), or to mimic its actions. Increasing neuronal dopamine can be achieved by supplying more substrate for its synthesis (levodopa) or reducing its breakdown by inhibiting catechol-O-methyl transferase (COMT) and monoamine oxidase B (MAO-B) (Figure 22.1). Various dopamine receptor agonists can be used to mimic the actions of the neurotransmitter. Dopamine itself cannot be given as it would be rapidly metabolized in the periphery, and it is excluded from the brain by the blood–brain barrier. A secondary aim is to reduce the effect of acetylcholine, whose activity counteracts, to some extent, that of dopamine in motor pathways. There are no validated disease-modifying drugs and therapy is based on the treatment of symptoms.

TREATMENT OF MOTOR SYMPTOMS

Levodopa

In the early stages of PD, patients whose motor symptoms decrease their quality of life should be offered levodopa combined with the decarboxylase (aromatic L-amino acid decarboxylase) (DOPA) inhibitors carbidopa (co-careldopa) or benserazide (co-beneldopa). In the absence of the decarboxylase inhibitors, levodopa would be converted in the periphery to dopamine, which is excluded from the brain (as are the inhibitors) by the blood–brain barrier (Figure 22.2).

Levodopa is the gold standard of anti-Parkinsonian therapy and nearly every patient with PD will eventually receive this drug treatment (LeWitt 2009). However, efficacy reduces over time, requiring increased dose level and frequency, with an associated increase in side effects, which include dyskinesia and painful dystonia. Levodopa has many side effects due to it being a component of the noradrenaline and adrenaline routes of synthesis. This goes some way to explain

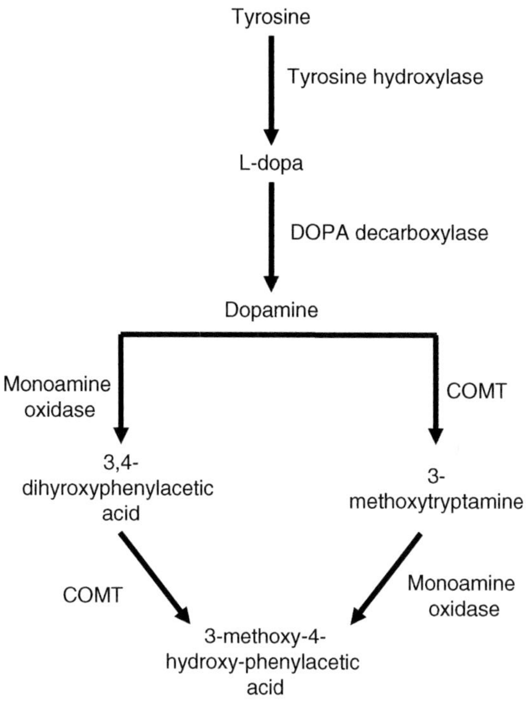

FIGURE 22.1 Synthesis and breakdown of dopamine. COMT, catechol–O-methyltransferase; L-DOPA, L-3,4-dihydroxyphenylalanine

why drugs used to treat PD symptoms can have cardiovascular side effects. Other common side effects include nausea, depression, confusion, psychoses and dyskinesia.

The 'on-off' phenomenon, which is an end-of-dose reduction in response leading to immobility, is common in long-term PD patients (50% occurrence after 6 years).

Early-stage patients, in whom motor symptoms do not affect their quality of life, may be prescribed a choice of levodopa, a non-ergot-derived dopamine-receptor agonist or an MAO-B inhibitor.

Dopamine agonists

Dopamine agonists mimic the action of dopamine in the brain but do not affect neuronal dopamine availability. They activate a variety of dopamine receptor subtypes (Table 22.1).

The older ergot-derived agonists (bromocriptine, cabergoline, pergolide) are associated with pulmonary, retroperitoneal and pericardial fibrotic reactions, and should only be prescribed as an adjunct therapy in patients who are poorly controlled by levodopa or a non-ergot-derived agonist.

Non-ergot-derived agonists (pramipexole, ropinirole, rotigotine) can be used alone to delay levodopa administration or to lower levodopa dosage in the early stages of PD.

The weak dopamine receptor agonist amantadine hydrochloride could be considered in patients in whom dyskinesias are inadequately controlled by other drugs.

The main side effects of all dopamine agonists include nausea and vomiting, through stimulation of dopamine receptors in the chemoreceptor trigger zone (Chapter 16), and a lowering of blood pressure caused by changes in posture (orthostatic hypotension). They all can produce impulse control disorders, including pathological gambling, binge eating and hypersexuality.

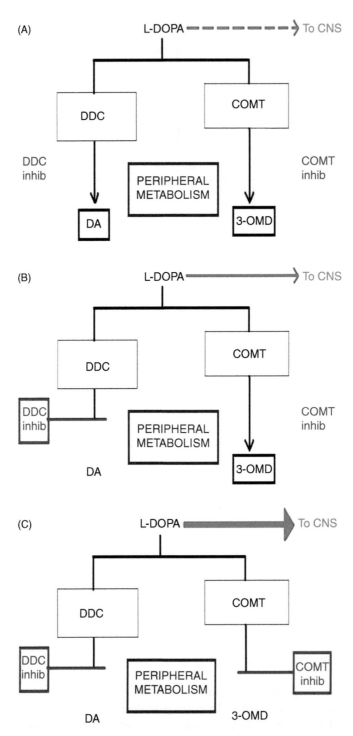

FIGURE 22.2 The role of peripheral DA metabolism inhibitors in raising dopamine levels in the CNS. Without enzyme inhibitors very little L-DOPA reaches the CNS (A). The use of DDC inhibitors (B) and then COMT inhibitors (C) increases the available L-DOPA from any given oral dose. CNS, central nervous system; COMT, catechol–O-methyltransferase; DA, dopamine; DDC, DOPA decarboxylase; L-DOPA, L-3,4-dihydroxyphenylalanine; 3-OMD, 3-O-methyldopa; inhib, inhibitor

Table 22.1 Dopamine agonists

Generic name	Primary receptor targets	Secondary receptor target
Pergolide	D_2	D_1, D_3, D_4, D_6
Bromocriptine	D_2, α_{1A}-antagonist	D_3, 5-HT$_{1A}$, α_{2A}-antagonist
		(D_1, D_4, D_6)
Cabergoline	D_2	
Apomorphine	D_4	D_2, D_3, D_6 (D_1, 5-HT$_{1A}$, α_{2A}-antagonist)
Ropinirole	D_3	(D_2, D_4, 5-HT$_{1A}$)
Rotigotine	D_3, D_4, D_6	D_1, D_2, 5-HT$_{1A}$ (α_{1A}, α_{2A})
Pramipexole	D_3	(D_2, D_4, 5-HT$_{1A}$)

D_1, D_2, D_3, D_4, D_6 are dopamine receptors, 5-HT$_{1A}$ is a serotonin receptor, and α_{1A} and α_{2A} are adrenergic receptors.

Monoamine oxidase-B inhibitors

MAO-B inhibitors reduce dopamine metabolism (predominantly in the presynaptic neuron) and prolong the effect of naturally released dopamine. MAO-B is distinct from monoamine oxidase-A, which is responsible for the neuronal metabolism of noradrenaline and serotonin (Chapter 21). MAO-A inhibitors can be used for the treatment of depression (Chapter 23) but not PD.

MAO-B inhibitors (rasagiline, selegiline) are alternatives to dopamine receptor agonists as an adjunct therapy in early PD. They carry a risk of cardiovascular side effects, including postural hypotension and atrial fibrillation.

COMT inhibitors

COMT is one of several enzymes that metabolise catecholamines (dopamine, adrenaline, noradrenaline). It is largely neuronal membrane-bound, unlike MAOs that are bound to the outer membrane of mitochondria. Tolcapone is the only truly efficacious COMT inhibitor (clinical evidence for entacapone is poor), but it can cause liver damage and treatment requires specialist monitoring. Levodopa is a substrate for COMT and tolcapone can be used in combination to reduce levodopa metabolism and lessen the 'off' time in those PD patients suffering from end-of-dose dyskinesia.

STOP AND THINK

Antischizophrenic medications inhibit dopamine D_2 receptors. How would adding an antipsychotic to the drug list of someone with PD affect their treatment?

Muscarinic antagonists (anticholinergics)

Muscarinic antagonists are not widely used in PD therapy and have only a limited effect. Benzhexol or orphenadrine can reduce tremor, but the anticholinergic side effects (dry mouth, dizziness, visual impairment, urinary retention, memory loss, insomnia) are troublesome, and they enhance confusion, particularly in PD patients suffering dementia.

TREATMENT OF NON-MOTOR SYMPTOMS

Excessive daytime sleepiness/sudden sleep onset: modafinil (dopamine reuptake inhibitor) can be effective.

Nocturnal akinesia: rotigotine patches can be considered if oral levodopa and dopamine receptor agonists are ineffective.

Postural hypotension: the sympathomimetic (α_1-adrenoceptor agonist) midodrine can be considered.

Depression: antidepressant therapy (serotonin reuptake inhibitors first line) can be appropriate.

Psychotic symptoms: hallucinations and delusions, which can be side effects of anti-Parkinsonian drugs, need not be treated if they are well tolerated and reducing dosage carries the risk of withdrawal effects and reduced anti-PD efficacy. Quetiapine (although unlicensed) could be considered, but other antipsychotic medicines (such as phenothiazines and butyrophenones) can worsen the motor features of PD by blocking dopamine receptors (Chapter 24).

ADVANCED PARKINSON'S DISEASE

Apomorphine can be prescribed as intermittent injections or continuous subcutaneous infusion, although nausea and vomiting are serious side effects.

Levodopa-carbidopa (Duodopa) intestinal gel, administered with a pump directly into the duodenum or upper jejunum, is used for PD patients with severe motor fluctuations and hyperkinesia or dyskinesia.

STOP AND THINK

Why are dry mouth, mydriasis, tachycardia, constipation and urinary retention side effects of muscarinic antagonists in the treatment of PD?

PRACTICE APPLICATION

Drugs which increase the effect of neurotransmitters, such as tricyclic antidepressants or serotonin reuptake inhibitors, may interact with selegiline, resulting in an increased risk of hypertension and serotonin syndrome (Chapter 23).

ALZHEIMER'S DISEASE

EPIDEMIOLOGY

Alzheimer's disease (AD) is the most common cause of dementia (Burne and Iliffe 2009). It is defined as a progressive, irreversible, degenerative neurological disease that begins insidiously and is characterized by a gradual loss of cognitive function and disturbances in behaviour and mood. Dementia can also be caused by other neurodegenerative or cerebrovascular pathologies, particularly in older patients, and its worldwide prevalence is expected to increase from 50 million in 2010 to 113 million by 2050 (Brodaty et al. 2011).

AD affects about 6% of the population over 65 (Burns and Iliffe 2009). Prevalence doubles every 5 years after 65 so that by 85+, one in three people is likely to have AD. Life expectancy for AD from diagnosis is generally between 8 and 12 years. Taking the gender difference in all-cause mortality into account, there is little or no sex-related bias in dementia prevalence.

PATHOPHYSIOLOGY

AD is a synaptic dysfunction disorder resulting in failures in neuronal circuitry, most marked in the cerebral cortices, with a loss of neurons, particularly of the cholinergic type, resulting in reduced brain volume that is observable in MRI scans and on postmortem examination.

AD brains contain extracellular neuritic plaques (composed of a protein, amyloid-beta [Aβ]), which are found throughout the cerebral cortex, and intracellular neurofibrillary tangles containing hyperphosphorylated tau protein. There is microglial cell proliferation, especially in association with the plaques, suggesting that inflammatory processes and free radicals also play a role in the disease process.

Aβ peptides are derived from amyloid precursor protein (APP) by β-secretase and γ-secretase enzymes. Aβ is secreted into the extracellular space as a monomer but Aβ42 in particular has a high propensity to aggregate. The resulting Aβ oligomers are thought to be toxic to surrounding neurons, possibly due to interaction with metabotropic glutamate and N-methyl-D-aspartate (NMDA) receptors, and others including nicotinic acetylcholine and insulin receptors.

Tau is a protein that is normally present in the cytoplasm of axons, where its main function is microtubule stabilization. Post-translational modification can cause tau to aggregate in a hyperphosphorylated form and to be released into the extracellular space from where it is taken up into surrounding neurons and glia. The precise mechanisms whereby tau contributes to AD neurotoxicity are still unclear.

Another key protein player in AD pathophysiology is apolipoprotein E (ApoE). ApoE (formed in glia) normally complexes with Aβ monomers and transports them into the perivascular spaces around arterioles and venules for removal. Malfunction in this pathway can therefore contribute to Aβ aggregation and neuritic plaque formation.

RISK FACTORS

Age is the most important risk factor for AD.

More than 600 genes have been investigated as susceptibility factors for AD. Of these, apolipoprotein E (APOE) polymorphism is the most important genetic risk factor for AD occurring after 65 years (Table 22.2). There are rare, dominantly inherited, mutations in APP, PSEN1 and PSEN2 genes, but overall the genetic contribution to AD development is modest.

Several non-genetic, modifiable risk factors, occurring in midlife, include diabetes mellitus, hypertension, obesity and low high-density lipoprotein cholesterol, hearing loss, traumatic brain injury and alcohol abuse.

DIAGNOSIS

AD has memory loss as a key feature of its diagnosis, with CNS damage occurring primarily in the cerebral cortex. There are other dementias that also have features of AD that can lead to misdiagnosis, such as vascular dementia, dementia with Lewy body and frontotemporal dementia, but since there are no specific treatments for AD or the other dementias, the importance of this is debatable.

Clinical diagnosis for dementia involves the use of either the Bayer Activities of Daily Living (Bayer-ADL) scale or the Neuropsychiatric Inventory with Caregiver Distress (NPI-D)

Table 22.2 Genetic predisposition (familial risk) and gene linkage in relation to Alzheimer's disease

Gene name	Chromosome	Other information
Amyloid precursor protein	Ch 21	Link to Down's syndrome
Presenilin 1	Ch 14	Autosomal dominant
Presenilin 2	Ch 1	
Apolipoprotein E4	Ch 19	Expression suggests an increased risk
Apolipoprotein E2	Ch 19	Expression suggests a decreased risk

Table 22.3 Stages of dementia

Stage 1: Mild (early)	Stage 2: Moderate	Stage 3: Late (terminal)
Routine loss of recent memory	Chronic loss of recent memory	Mixes up past and present
Mild aphasia or word-finding difficulty	Moderate aphasia	Expressive and receptive aphasia
Seeks familiar and avoids unfamiliar places	Gets lost at times even inside home	Misidentifies familiar persons and places
Some difficulty writing and using objects	Repetitive actions, apraxia	Parkinsonism and falls risk
Apathy and depression	Possible mood and behavioral disturbances	More mood and behavioral disturbances
Needs reminders for some ADLs	Needs reminders and help with most ADLs	Needs help with all ADLs, incontinent

ADLs, activities of daily living.

scale. Amongst the diagnostic criteria needed are an indication of multiple cognitive deficits with both memory impairment (plus one or more of aphasia, apraxia, agnosia and executive function) and impaired abstraction and/or judgement. This usually coincides with impaired social or occupational function. With these criteria, care must be taken to check that the cognitive deficits are not due to other processes (e.g., substance abuse, systemic processes, delirium and other acute conditions). Patients will be classified as having one of three stages of dementia (Table 22.3).

More technical approaches to antemortem, AD-specific diagnosis have been developed and the assay of biomarkers in the cerebrospinal fluid is used clinically. The best validated and widely accepted CSF biomarkers for AD are decreases in Aβ42 and increases in phosphorylated tau (p-tau181). Fully developed blood-based biomarkers would be a significant diagnostic advancement. Quantitative Aβ-positron emission tomography (PET) imaging can provide evidence on the extent and location of amyloid deposition and several tau-PET ligands have been developed.

Although the technology can help, diagnosis rests primarily on the ability of the physician to integrate information from the patient, their family and the mental status and neurological examination results.

PHARMACOLOGICAL INTERVENTIONS IN AD

These are limited to three acetylcholinesterase inhibitors and the NMDA receptor antagonist memantine.

Acetycholinesterase inhibitors

The acetycholinesterase inhibitors donepezil, rivastigmine and galantamine are approved for use with people who have been assessed as having mild to moderate AD (Table 22.4). Donepezil is also approved for severe dementia but only in the USA. These drugs have a wide range of side effects due to an increase in the available acetylcholine in the autonomic nervous system. The adverse effects include nausea, vomiting, loose stools or loss of appetite in a minority of individuals and, less commonly, muscle cramps, headaches and unpleasant dreams. Once a person starts on a drug regimen, the following cycles of treatment are often based on the monitoring of acetylcholinesterase inhibitor efficacy by caregiver report, quantified mental status examination, effects on activities related to daily living and effects on behaviour.

Table 22.4 Available acetylcholinesterase inhibitors

Year available	1996	2000	2001
Drug generic	Donepezil	Rivastigmine	Galantamine
Reversible	Yes	Pseudo-irreversible	Yes
AchE	Yes	Yes	Yes
BuChE	Minimal	Yes	Minimal

ACh E, acetylcholinesterase; BuChE, butylcholinesterase.

Donepezil preferentially inhibits acetylcholinesterase (as opposed to peripheral butyrylcholinesterase), which might explain why it has a lower incidence of gastrointestinal-related side effects than the other inhibitors.

Rivastigmine has fewer drug interactions compared to the other acetylcholinesterase inhibitors, but it has been shown that discontinuation can lead to a more rapid decline in cognitive function.

STOP AND THINK

Why might the use of acetylcholinesterase inhibitors result in diarrhoea?

Memantine

Memantine is a glutamate (NMDA) receptor antagonist that reduces glutamate excitotoxicity and neuronal cell death. It might also inhibit the interaction of Aβ with NMDA receptors (see above).

Memantine is used in moderate to severe AD and may be combined with donepezil as this targets a different receptor system. Side effects include hallucinations, confusion and dizziness, and it should be used with caution in patients with renal impairment.

Neither the cholinesterase inhibitors nor memantine have any relevant effects on the underlying pathophysiology of AD.

PRACTICE APPLICATION

Patients with moderate AD should be assessed every 6 months and drug treatment should normally continue only if the Mini-Mental State Examination score remains at or above 10 points and if treatment is considered to have a worthwhile effect on global, functional and behavioural condition (NICE 2006).

OTHER APPROACHES TO TREATMENT

A number of pharmaceutical companies have produced monoclonal antibodies targeting Aβ, but most have failed to produce benefits in clinical trials. However, one drug, aducanumab (a monoclonal antibody that targets Aβ protofibrils), has shown some slowing of decline on the Clinical Dementia Rating scale in phase III trials and this strategy is continuing to evolve. Prevention studies for AD with passive Aβ immunization are in process.

TREATMENT OF NEUROPSYCHIATRIC SYMPTOMS IN AD

Neuropsychiatric symptoms in AD typically emerge in three phases: (1) irritability, depression and nighttime behaviour changes; (2) anxiety, appetite changes, agitation and apathy; and (3) elation, motor disturbances, hallucinations, delusions and disinhibition (Masters et al. 2015). Second-generation antipsychotics, such as risperidone, olanzapine, quetiapine and aripiprazole, have been used for the treatment of psychosis in dementia, but they have minimal efficacy and are associated with many adverse effects. There is little evidence of efficacy for any of the approved antidepressant drugs in depressed AD patients and psychosocial interventions such as exercise, increasing social contact and reminiscent therapy are more appropriate.

SUMMARY

- Parkinson's disease (PD) is strongly associated with the degeneration of the dopamine-containing neurons of the substantia nigra.
- The principal strategy in PD is to increase the levels of dopamine in the central nervous system and less importantly to reduce the effect of increased cholinergic receptor activity.
- Levodopa is the gold standard of therapy for PD.
- Levodopa is usually given combined with the DOPA decarboxylase inhibitors benzerazide or carbidopa.
- Drugs used to treat PD symptoms commonly have cardiovascular side effects.
- Alzheimer's disease (AD) is a progressive, irreversible, degenerative disease characterised by gradual losses of cognitive function and disturbances in behaviour.
- AD is characterised by a decrease in the number of neurons, particularly cholinergic.
- The mainstay of treatment for AD symptoms is the use of acetylcholinesterase inhibitors.
- The neuropsychiatric features of AD sometimes require other drugs to suppress them, leading to complex polypharmacy.

ACTIVITY

1. Parkinson's disease is associated with a loss of dopaminergic neurons in the substantia nigra.   True/False

2. Parkinson's disease is associated with decreased acetylcholine activity.   True/False

3. Monoamine oxidase-B inhibitors inhibit the metabolism of all monoamines.   True/False

4. Dopamine agonists act to replenish the body's supply of dopamine.   True/False

5. Levodopa has fewer side effects if administered with a decarboxylase inhibitor.   True/False

6. Levodopa can exhibit cardiovascular side effects due to the nature of its synthesis path.   True/False

7. Age does not play a contributory role in the development of Alzheimer's disease.   True/False

8. Acetylcholinesterase inhibitors have only limited side effects as their effects are restricted to the central nervous system.   True/False

9. Memantine is a NMDA receptor antagonist.   True/False

10. All drugs used to treat Alzheimer's disease increase acetylcholine levels.   True/False

REFERENCES

Armstrong, M.J. and Okun, M.S. (2020) Diagnosis and treatment of Parkinson disease: a review. *JAMA* 323:548–560.

Brodaty, H., Breteler, M.M.B., Dekosky, S.T., et al. (2011). The world of dementia beyond 2020. *J Am Geriatr Soc* 59:923–927.

Dorsey, E.R., Sherer, T., Okun, M.S. and Bloem, B.R. (2018) The emerging evidence of the Parkinson pandemic. *J Parkinsons Dis* 8:S3–S8.

Burne, A. and Iliffe, S. (2009) Alzheimer's disease. *BMJ* 338:467–471.

LeWitt, P.A. (2009) Levodopa therapeutics for Parkinson's disease: new developments. *Parkinsonism Relat Disord* 15(Suppl 1):S31–S34.

Masters, M.C., Morris, J.C. and Roe, C.M. (2015) 'Noncognitive' symptoms of early Alzheimer disease: a longitudinal analysis. *Neurology* 84:1–6.

Trinh, J., Zeldenrust, F.M.J., Huang, J., et al. (2018) Genotype-phenotype relations for the Parkinson's disease genes SNCA, LRRK2, VPS35: MDSGene systematic review. *Mov Disord* 33:1857–1870.

FURTHER READING

Bertram, L. and Tanzi, R.E. (2008) Thirty years of Alzheimer's disease genetics: the implications of systematic meta-analysis. *Nat Rev Neurosci* 9:768–778.

Bloem, B.R., Okun, M.S. and Klein, C. (2021). Parkinson's disease. *Lancet* 397:2284–2303.

Cowan, W.M. and Kandel, E.R. (2001) Prospects for neurology and psychiatry. *JAMA* 285:594–600.

Knopman, D.S., Amieva, H., Petersen, R.C., Chételat, G., Holtzman, D.M., Hyman, B.T., Nixon, R.A. and Jones, D.T. (2021) Alzheimer disease. *Nature reviews. Disease primers* 7(1):33.

Lanctôt, K.L., Amatniek, J., Ancoli-Israel, S., et al. (2017) Neuropsychiatric signs and symptoms of Alzheimer's disease: New treatment paradigms. *Alzheimers Dement (N Y)* 3:440–449.

Miller, D.B. and O'Callaghan, J.P. (2008) Do early-life insults contribute to the late-life development of Parkinson and Alzheimer diseases? *Metabolism* 57(Suppl 2):S44–S49.

Nomoto, M., Nishikawa, N., Nagai, M., et al. (2009) Inter- and intra-individual variation in L-dopa pharmacokinetics in the treatment of Parkinson's disease. *Parkinsonism Relat Disord* 15(Suppl 1):S21–S24.

Ritter, J.M., Flower, R., Henderson, G., et al. (2023) *Rang and Dale's Pharmacology*, 10th edn. Elsevier, Amsterdam.

USEFUL WEBSITES

British National Formulary (online). https://bnf.nice.org.uk/

Health Institute of Australia. https://www.healthdirect.gov.au/alzheimers-disease

NICE guidance on Alzheimer's disease. https://www.nice.org.uk/guidance/ng97; https://www.nice.org.uk/guidance/ta217

CHAPTER 23

Depression and Anxiety

Yvonne Mbaki

LEARNING OUTCOMES

By the end of this chapter the reader should be able to:

- demonstrate an understanding of the nature of depressive illness and the monoamine theory

- demonstrate an understanding of the mechanisms of action of the major groups of antidepressants

- describe the common adverse reactions associated with antidepressant use

- identify the main groups of anxiolytic drugs

- demonstrate an understanding of the mechanisms of action of anxiolytic drugs

- describe the adverse effects associated with anxiolytic use.

Both depression and anxiety are mental health states that are associated with imbalances of excitatory and inhibitory neural pathways within the central nervous system (CNS) (Chapter 21). Depression is thought to occur due to underactivity of monoamine neurotransmitter pathways, principally noradrenaline and serotonin (5-hydroxytryptamine,5-HT). Anxiety-related disorders are generally the reverse of this, due primarily to the overactivity of monoamine pathways (dopamine and noradrenaline).

This chapter will initially consider depression and its treatment, then move on to anxiety disorders. It is worth remembering that overmedication for depression can produce anxiety-related side effects and overmedication for anxiety can produce depression as a side effect, and sometimes both depression and anxiety may be present in the same patient.

DEPRESSION

Globally, depression is a common mental illness, with the World Health Organization (WHO) indicating an estimated 280 million people known to be afflicted (World Health Organization 2020; Institute of Health Metrics and Evaluation 2022). Most people have experienced the short-term effects of a 'bad day' and 'feeling down', but for our needs, we must consider the differentiation of this from depression. A diagnosis of major depression requires a patient to exhibit either depressed mood and/or anhedonia (an inability to experience pleasure) on most days, most of the time for at least 2 weeks, combined with several other physical and psychological symptoms (Box 23.1).

The causes of depression are multifaceted, with no singular origin identified. For example, stress/stressful event may trigger depression but is unlikely to be the singular cause. Indeed, there is evidence that some people are vulnerable to depression due to their personality, hence an interest by researchers to identify 'at risk' individuals or the appropriate therapeutic interventions (Klein et al. 2011). Whilst depression has a complex aetiology due to the multiple contributing factors, the consensus is that there are clues provided of developmental, genetic and biological components of depression.

The New Prescriber: An Integrated Approach to Medical and Non-medical Prescribing, Second Edition.
Edited by Joanne Lymn, Alison Mostyn, Roger Knaggs, Michael Randall, and Dianne Bowskill.
© 2024 John Wiley & Sons Ltd. Published 2024 by John Wiley & Sons Ltd.

BOX 23.1   HOW DO I DIAGNOSE DEPRESSION?

Persistent sadness or low mood
Loss of interest/pleasure in normal activities
Fatigue/low energy
Difficulty sleeping/waking early
Poor/increased appetite
Poor concentration/indecisiveness

Loss of self-confidence
Guilt/self-blame
Agitation or slowing of movements
Thinking about suicide

Source: NICE (2022).

Developmental influences linked to socio-economic disadvantage during childhood and adolescence may potentially result in poor mental health in adulthood due to exposure to multiple stressful life situations (Reiss et al. 2019). However, the neural pathways through which socio-economic factors may exert a developmental influence on mental health remain the subject of debate and investigation.

The genetic influence on disorders is assessed by concordance rates (probability that if one twin has the disorder, the other one does too). When the concordance rate for identical twins is high and is significantly higher than that for fraternal twins, a disorder has a large genetic component. The concordance rates for major depression are 20% for identical twins and 14% for fraternal twins, highlighting a genetic component. That said, whilst there is this indication of a familial contribution, the investigatory paradigm is a limiting factor when considering depression as an entity (Parker 2021).

MONOAMINE THEORY OF DEPRESSION

Evidence from neurobiology and pharmacology studies seeking an understanding of depression led to the inception of the monoamine theory of depression (Schildkraut 1965; Coppen et al. 1967). This theory of depression suggested that disruptions in the serotonergic, dopaminergic and noradrenergic systems result in depressive illness, with evidence inferred from the mechanism of action of relevant antidepressant drugs. The prevailing notion is that these disruptions are associated with insufficient or poorly utilised noradrenaline and/or serotonin in brain synapses, which may in turn be due to insufficient production, overly rapid reabsorption and/or insensitive receptors. Notably, areas of the brain that use noradrenaline and serotonin have links to endocrine glands that regulate metabolism, sleep/wake cycles, alertness, sex drive and appetite, all of which are disturbed in depressive illness. Indeed, this association between antidepressant drugs and the monoamine theory of depression reveals therapeutic targets that function to restore monoamines to normal levels.

ANTIDEPRESSANT DRUGS

There are a number of groups of drugs used to treat depression and these are categorised into:

- selective serotonin reuptake inhibitors (SSRIs)

- tricyclic antidepressants (TCAs)

- serotonin and noradrenaline reuptake inhibitors (SNRIs)

- monoamine oxidase inhibitors (MAOIs)

- reversible inhibitors of monoamine oxidase A (RIMAs)

- herbal products.

Whilst the drug chosen is based on individual patient requirements, SSRIs are better tolerated and safer in overdose than other drug groups and are therefore first line for the treatment of depression.

To show an improvement in mood, there needs to be a prolonged enhancement of noradrenaline and serotonin levels within the synapse and hence it takes several weeks for antidepressant drugs to exert a meaningful clinical effect.

Selective serotonin reuptake inhibitors

The SSRIs inhibit the reuptake of serotonin (5-HT) into the presynaptic neuron, thus increasing the amount of serotonin in the synapse and prolonging serotonin signalling. SSRIs do what their name suggests and have a much greater affinity for the serotonin transporter than the noradrenaline or dopamine transporters. The intended aim of developing SSRIs was to reduce the number of side effects caused by other antidepressant groups, particularly the TCAs and MAOIs.

SSRIs can, however, interact with other receptors, such as the muscarinic acetylcholine receptor, to a limited degree and affect liver enzyme systems (Figure 23.1). The degree of interaction depends on the specific SSRI and therefore one cannot assume that they all have the same level of effect. Moreover, this class of drugs can present with an increased suicide risk in adolescents.

Fluoxetine is the prototypical SSRI. Used predominantly as an antidepressant, it serves as a treatment for obsessive-compulsive disorder and bulimia nervosa. It is the drug of first choice in children (5–11 years) and young people (12–18 years) if depression is unresponsive to psychological therapy (NICE 2022a).

Common side effects of SSRIs can be categorized into cardiac (e.g., palpitations), gastrointestinal (e.g., diarrhoea and nausea), nervous system (e.g., headaches and dizziness) and psychiatric (e.g., insomnia), amongst other adverse effects (NICE 2022b).

SSRIs may also cause hyponatremia (low plasma sodium concentration), which can be problematic in the elderly.

Tricyclic antidepressants

TCAs produce non-selective inhibition of noradrenaline and serotonin reuptake systems in the CNS. These drugs have the effect of raising noradrenaline and serotonin levels throughout the body, including the CNS.

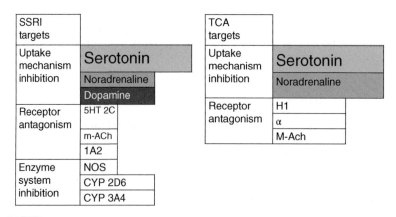

FIGURE 23.1 Target sites for selective serotonin reuptake inhibitors and tricyclic antidepressants. The size of the bar is an indication of the level of interaction. 5HT 2C, serotonin type 2C receptor; CYP 2D6, cytochrome P450 2D6; CYP 3A4, cytochrome P450 3A4; H1, histamine type 1 receptor; α, α-adrenoceptor; m-Ach, muscarininc acetylcholine receptors; 1A2, adenosine A2 receptor; NOS, nitric oxide synthetase.

TCAs exhibit substantially more side effects than SSRIs, with these effects related to their antagonist action at other receptors in the body, including the muscarinic acetylcholine and histamine H_1 receptors (Figure 23.1). In clinical practice, one of the major problems associated with the use of TCAs is that patients may notice side effects of these drugs within a very short space of time, long before the therapeutic effects are apparent, thus potentially affecting compliance.

STOP AND THINK

What side effects can you predict given that TCAs act as antagonists at muscarinic acetylcholine, histamine H_1 and α-adrenergic receptors?

Many TCAs have pharmacologically active metabolites. For example, nortriptyline, which is a drug in its own right, is actually a metabolite of amitriptyline. The presence of active metabolites may increase the severity of side effects. TCAs have a higher rate of Q-T interval prolongation than SSRIs, especially at higher doses and in overdose. They also have a narrow therapeutic index, which means that when used together with drugs that inhibit cytochrome P450 activity, the severity of side effects may be increased, possibly leading to increased toxicity. On the other hand, when used with drugs that induce cytochrome P450 activity this interaction may diminish the therapeutic effect.

Serotonin and noradrenaline reuptake inhibitors

Two SNRIs in clinical use are venlafaxine and duloxetine. These drugs work by selectively inhibiting the reuptake of serotonin and noradrenaline in much the same way that TCAs do. However, they do not show antagonist activity at other receptors, therefore diminishing their side effect profile.

SNRIs are sympathomimetic and at high doses venlafaxine has been associated with hypertensive crisis. On the other hand, hypertensive crisis is considered to be 'rare' or 'very rare' with duloxetine.

Monoamine oxidase inhibitors

Some MAOIs, such as phenelzine, isocarboxazid and tranylcypromine, produce a non-selective irreversible inhibition of the mitochondrial enzyme monoamine oxidase. By inhibiting the enzyme responsible for monoamine metabolism, they inhibit the breakdown of monoamines (e.g., serotonin and noradrenaline), resulting in enhanced levels of monoamines available in the presynaptic neuron. MAOIs use is mainly within the context of treating patients who are refractory to at least three or four trials of other antidepressant drugs (Suchting et al. 2021).

PRACTICE APPLICATION

Foods rich in the essential amino acid tyramine, such as mature cheese, pickled herring, broad bean pods, meat or yeast extract products (Bovril®, Marmite® and Oxo®), may cause a potentially fatal rise in blood pressure if taken together with an MAOI.

Reversible inhibitors of monoamine oxidase type A

The only RIMA used in clinical practice is moclobemide, which produces reversible inhibition of monoamine oxidase type A (Figure 23.2). Due to this reversible effect, the dietary restrictions of irreversible MAOIs are not required. Moreover, there is a reduced incidence of hypertensive crisis following the use of moclobemide. However, an important consideration for moclobemide as a therapeutic agent is that its use should be followed by a washout period before starting other antidepressant therapy.

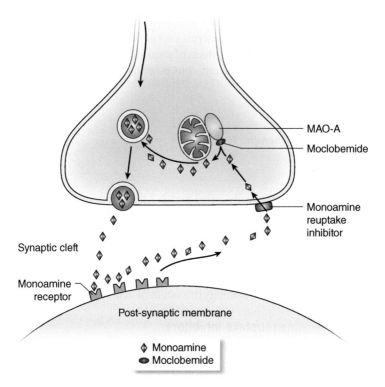

FIGURE 23.2 Mechanism of action of moclobemide (from http://www.cnsforum.com/imagebank/item/ MAOB_inhib/default.aspx).

STOP AND THINK

When switching from sertraline, why must you wait a period of 2 weeks before starting mo-clobemide therapy?

Herbal preparations

The most common use of St John's wort preparations (*Hypericum perforatum*) is to relieve symptoms associated with mild to moderate depression. Whilst there is conflicting evidence of St John's wort use as a therapeutic agent, various clinical trials have reported efficacy that is comparable to fluoxetine (Behnke et al. 2002), sertraline (Brenner et al. 2000) and imipramine (Philipp et al. 1999; Woelk 2000). Moreover, other clinical trials have demonstrated the superiority of St John's wort when compared to placebo (Gastpar et al. 2006; Kasper et al. 2006). However, the active constituents of St John's wort may increase or decrease the activity of specific cytochrome P450 enzymes, thus rendering its use a challenge due to its pharmacokinetic interaction with other drugs. There are also concerns over its pharmaceutical purity and quality control in relation to doses.

ANXIETY DISORDERS

Experience of some anxiety is an expected, normal, transient response to day-to-day stress and, indeed, it is likely to be a necessary cue for adaptation and coping. Our interest in this chapter is pathological anxiety, which can manifest by the continued presence of:

Table 23.1 Some pathological anxiety disorders

Pathological anxiety disorder	Portrait of disorder
Panic disorder (with or without agoraphobia)	Recurrent, unexpected panic attacks, sudden onset, limited duration
Generalised anxiety disorder (GAD)	Excessive and persistent worry (over several months) revolving around everyday events, considered to be disproportionate
Obsessive-compulsive disorder (OCD)	Intrusive, recurrent, unwanted thoughts, impulses, images or compulsive behaviours or rituals that cause marked anxiety or distress
Post-traumatic stress disorder (PSD)	Triggered by exposure to a traumatic event, for example natural or manmade disasters, serious accident, unexpected violent manner etc.
Social phobia	A marked and persistent fear of social or performance situations in which the person is distressed due to perceived scrutiny from others
Specific phobia	This is a marked, persistent fear of circumscribed situations or objects

Adapted from ICD-11 for Mortality and Morbidity Statistics (2022).

- affective symptoms: feelings of edginess, 'losing control', 'going to die'
- physiological symptoms: tachycardia, tachypnoea, diarrhoea, diaphoresis (excessive sweating), dizziness, lightheadedness
- behavioural alterations: avoidance, compulsions
- cognitive symptoms: apprehension, worry, obsessions.

The basis for classifying pathological anxieties is the signs and symptoms exhibited by a patient. Diagnosing pathological anxiety is a specialist area, as the diagnosing clinician has to differentiate the patient's condition from a number of pathological anxiety disorders (Table 23.1).

ANXIOLYTIC THERAPY

The medications used in controlling some of the symptoms of pathological anxiety fall principally into the following four categories:

1. benzodiazepines
2. azapirones
3. antidepressants
4. β-adrenoceptor antagonists.

Benzodiazepines

Benzodiazepines are widely prescribed for all anxiety disorders (except obsessive-compulsive disorder) as they are effective and generally more rapid acting than other anxiolytic treatments.

All benzodiazepines act via the γ-aminobutyric acid-a ($GABA_a$) receptor (Figure 23.3) by producing changes that increase the effectiveness of the naturally produced (endogenous) GABA. Increased GABA interaction leads to an increase in chloride influx and thus prolonged hyperpolarisation (brain suppression). Benzodiazepines only work in the presence of endogenous GABA.

The speed of action and elimination of individual benzodiazepines varies. These differences are primarily due to variations in pharmacokinetic properties such as absorption, lipid solubility (if high then rapid onset of action), presence or absence of active metabolites, hepatic metabolism

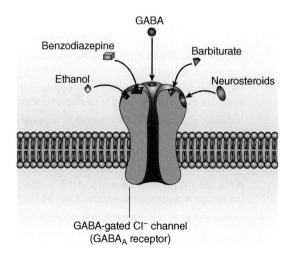

FIGURE 23.3 The GABA$_A$ receptor with representations of the exogenous drugs targeting the receptor.

and elimination half-life. Some benzodiazepines have many active metabolites, which complicates an understanding of their pharmacokinetic profile. Fast-acting benzodiazepines have higher lipid solubility and therefore cross cell membranes, including the blood–brain barrier, more easily than more water-soluble (hydrophilic) drugs. They are also much more addictive.

PRACTICE APPLICATION

In generalised anxiety disorder (GAD), the National Institute for Health and Care Excellence (NICE) discourages the prescription of benzodiazepines with the exception of short-term use during a crisis, as directed by the *British National Formulary*.

Benzodiazepines have side effects that can potentially be difficult for patients to deal with. Amongst these are disinhibition (especially in children and the elderly), CNS depression, rebound insomnia, anxiety (especially for short-acting benzodiazepines such as midazolam) and respiratory depression. As well as onset of adverse reactions, benzodiazepines have a complex series of withdrawal signs and symptoms that can mimic the conditions for which the drug was initially prescribed, such as 'rebound anxiety' or panic attacks. Discontinuation of benzodiazepines therefore requires tapering of the dose, which allows the body to adjust to a reduction in GABAergic output in a way that does not precipitate rebound sympathomimetic effects, such as anxiety.

Some benzodiazepines alter the activity of cytochrome P450 enzymes in the liver and this may alter the pharmacokinetics and effects of the benzodiazepine or other drugs prescribed concomitantly. If given with other drugs that are CNS depressants, such as TCAs, anticonvulsants or antipsychotic drugs, there will be enhanced sedation.

PRACTICE APPLICATION

Caution is advised when midazolam is administered concomitantly with drugs that are known to inhibit the hepatic CYP3A4 enzyme system (e.g., cimetidine, erythromycin and verapamil) as these drug interactions may result in prolonged sedation due to a decrease in the plasma clearance of midazolam.

Apart from their anxiolytic properties, benzodiazepines are also used in other clinical areas, including:

- sedation/insomnia
- agitation
- anaesthesia induction
- akathisia (motor restlessness due to antipsychotics)
- seizures, including status epilepticus.

An awareness of these other uses is necessary as one may encounter patients who receive benzodiazepines as part of other treatments.

Azapirones

Azapirones are a group of drugs that are agonists on the $5HT_{1A}$ receptor and display effectiveness in treating GAD. The only example of this type of drug used clinically is buspirone.

Buspirone acts as a partial agonist at the $5HT_{1A}$ receptor. $5HT_{1A}$ receptors are predominantly autoinhibitory presynaptic receptors and activation produces decreased firing of the serotonergic neurons on which they occur. Buspirone is effective in treating GAD and the relief of symptoms of anxiety with or without accompanying depression. Additionally, buspirone's use is to augment the effect of antidepressants.

Side effects of buspirone are less problematic than those of benzodiazepines, and include nausea, nervousness, restlessness and lightheadedness. Buspirone has less abuse potential than benzodiazepines and as such presents with a low risk of lethality in overdose for a person with a substance abuse disorder.

STOP AND THINK

What is meant by the term partial agonist? How does the efficacy of a partial agonist compare to that of a full agonist?

Antidepressants

Antidepressants are a key component in first-line treatment for anxiety disorders (especially SSRIs). Treatments for anxiety using antidepressants usually start at low doses, which can cause initial 'edginess', and it can take several weeks before benefit is appreciated. In more severe cases of anxiety, the antidepressant augmentation with other drugs, for example benzodiazepine, may be considered. As a process over time, the antidepressant dose should be increased, with the benzodiazepine dose tapered off.

Whilst SSRIs are commonly prescribed in anxiety (see earlier in this chapter), trazadone (which shares properties of the SSRIs) may be useful in elderly patients with dementia to reduce anxiety, agitation and aggression. TCAs can also be used in anxiety management but there is a higher risk of lethality in overdose as they are cardiotoxic.

β-Adrenoceptor antagonists

The normal function of the adrenergic β-receptors, when stimulated by noradrenaline (and/or adrenaline), is to produce an increase in heart rate, blood pressure and respiratory rate. Blocking these receptors with a β-adrenoceptor antagonist reduces the severity of the symptoms occurring in anxiety, although these drugs are contraindicated in patients with asthma (Chapter 20). A classic example of a β-adrenoceptor antagonist used in the treatment of anxiety is propranolol, which is primarily indicated for use in performance anxiety (e.g., for musicians and those involved in public speaking) as it acts to dull sympathetic symptoms such as palpitations and tremor.

SUMMARY

- Depression is primarily due to underactivity of monoamine neurotransmitter pathways, principally noradrenaline and serotonin.

- Mild depression may be triggered by stressful life events.

- Current drug therapy for depression aims to increase levels of serotonin and noradrenaline.

- Selective serotonin reuptake inhibitors interact with other receptors and liver enzyme systems.

- Many tricyclic antidepressants are more active as a metabolite of the parent drug and this can lead to problems with the cardiovascular system.

- Monoamine oxidase inhibitors produce a non-selective irreversible inhibition of the mitochondrial enzyme monoamine oxidase.

- The active constituents of St John's wort can induce and inhibit drug metabolising enzymes.

- Pathological anxiety can be manifested by the continued presence of affective symptoms, physiological symptoms, behavioural alterations and cognitive symptoms.

- All benzodiazepines act via the $GABA_a$ receptor by producing changes that increase the effectiveness of the endogenous GABA.

- Some benzodiazepines alter the activity of cytochrome P450 enzymes in the liver and this may alter the pharmacokinetics of other drugs prescribed concomitantly.

- Antidepressants are a key component in first-line treatment for anxiety disorders and are often augmented by buspirone.

- β-adrenoceptor antagonists reduce the severity of the symptoms which may occur in anxiety, but their effect on lung smooth muscle can be a problem for asthmatics.

ACTIVITY

1. Stressful life events are a trigger for major depression.   True/False

2. The monoamine theory suggests that depression is associated with an increase in serotonin levels.   True/False

3. SSRIs preferentially inhibit the reuptake of serotonin into the presynaptic neuron.   True/False

4. Tricyclic antidepressants exhibit antimuscarinic side effects.   True/False

5. Tricyclic antidepressants have a wide therapeutic index and are safe to use across a wide range of doses.   True/False

6. Venlafaxine is a widely used selective serotonin reuptake inhibitor.   True/False

7. Serotonin and noradrenaline reuptake inhibitors and tricyclic antidepressants both inhibit noradrenaline and serotonin reuptake.   True/False

8. Serotonin and noradrenaline reuptake inhibitors are sympathomimetic. True/False

9. Moclobemide exhibits the same dietary restrictions as phenelzine. True/False

10. St John's wort affects cytochrome P450 enzymes. True/False

11. Anxiety is associated with increased glutamate. True/False

12. Fast-acting benzodiazepines have high lipid solubility. True/False

13. Buspirone is a full agonist. True/False

14. β-blockers are useful in treating the underlying cause of anxiety. True/False

REFERENCES

Behnke, K., Jensen, G.S., Graubaum, H.J. and Gruenwald, J. (2002) Hypericum perforatum versus fluoxetine in the treatment of mild to moderate depression. *Adv Ther* 19:43–52.

Brenner, R., Azbel, V., Madhusoodanan, S. and Pawlowska, M. (2000) Comparison of an extract of hypericum (LI 160) and sertraline in the treatment of depression: a double-blind, randomized pilot study. *Clin Ther* 22:411–419.

British National Formulary 1800 (online) BMJ Group and Pharmaceutical Press, London. https://bnf.nice.org.uk/.

Coppen, A., Shaw, D.M., Herzberg, B. and Maggs, R. (1967) Tryptophan in the treatment of depression. *Lancet* 2:1178–1180

Gastpar, M., Singer, A. and Zeller, K. (2006) Comparative efficacy and safety of a once-daily dosage of hypericum extract STW3-VI and citalopram in patients with moderate depression: a double-blind, randomised, multicentre, placebo-controlled study. *Pharmacopsychiatry* 39:66–75.

ICD-11 for Mortality and Morbidity Statistics (2022). 06 Mental, behavioural or neurodevelopmental disorders. https://icd.who.int/browse11/l-m/en#/http%3a%2f%2fid.who.int%2ficd%2fentity%2f334423054.

Institute of Health Metrics and Evaluation. 1800 Global Health Data Exchange (GHDx). https://www.who.int/news-room/fact-sheets/detail/mental-disorders (accessed May 2022).

Kasper, S., Anghelescu, I.G., Szegedi, A., Dienel, A. and Kieser, M. (2006) Superior efficacy of St John's wort extract WS® 5570 compared to placebo in patients with major depression: a randomized, double-blind, placebo-controlled, multi-center trial [ISRCTN77277298]. *BMC Med* 4(1):1–13.

Klein, D.N., Kotov, R. and Bufferd, S.J. (2011) Personality and depression: explanatory models and review of the evidence. *Ann Rev Clin Psychol* 7:269–295.

NICE (2022a) When should I suspect a diagnosis of depression? NICE Clinical Knowledge Summaries. https://cks.nice.org.uk/topics/depression/diagnosis/diagnosis/ (accessed May 2022).

NICE (2022b) Antidepressant drugs. https://bnf.nice.org.uk/treatment-summary/antidepressant-drugs.html (accessed May 2022).

Parker, G. (2021) Clinical depression: the fault not in our stars? *Australas Psychiatry* 29(6):652–654.

Philipp, M., Linde, K., Kohnen, R., Hiller, K.O. and Berner, M. (1999) Hypericum extract versus imipramine or placebo in patients with moderate depression: randomised multicentre study of treatment for eight weeks. *BMJ* 319(7224):1534–1539.

Reiss, F., Meyrose, A.K., Otto, C., Lampert, T., Klasen, F. and Ravens-Sieberer, U. (2019) Socioeconomic status, stressful life situations and mental health problems in children and adolescents: Results of the German BELLA cohort-study. *PloS One* 14(3):e0213700.

Schildkraut, J.J. (1965) The catecholamine hypothesis of affective disorders: a review of supportive evidence. *Am J Psychiatry* 122:509–522.

Suchting, R., Tirumalaraju, V., Gareeb, R., et al. (2021) Revisiting monoamine oxidase inhibitors for the treatment of depressive disorders: a systematic review and network meta-analysis. *J Affect Disorders* 282:1153–1160.

Woelk, H. (2000) Comparison of St John's wort and imipramine for treating depression: randomised controlled trial. *BMJ* 321(7260):536–539.

World Health Organization (2020) Depressive disorder (depression). https://www.who.int/news-room/fact-sheets/detail/depression (accessed May 2022).

FURTHER READING

Bazire, S. (2020/21) *Psychotropic Drug Directory*. Lloyd-Reinhold Publications Ltd, Shaftesbury.

CNS Forum. 1800 http://www.cnsforum.com/educationalresources/imagebank/.

Gianaros, P.J., Horenstein, J.A., Hariri, A.R., et al. (2008) Potential neural embedding of parental social standing. *Soc Cogn Affect Neurosci* 3:91–96.

Ritter, J.M., Flower, R., Henderson, G., et al. (2023) *Rang and Dale's Pharmacology*, 10th edn. Elsevier, Amsterdam.

Stahl, S.M. (2021) *Stahl's Essential Psychopharmacology: Prescriber's guide*, 7th edn. Cambridge University Press, Cambridge.

Zemrak, W.R. and Kenna, G.A. (2008) Association of antipsychotic and antidepressant drugs with Q-T interval prolongation. *Am J Health Syst Pharm* 65: 1029–1038.

CLINICAL GUIDELINES

NICE (2022) Depression in adults: treatment and management. NICE Guideline NG222.

NICE (2019) Depression in children and young people: identification and management. NICE Guideline NG134.

NICE (2011) Generalised anxiety disorder and panic disorder in adults: management. Clinical guideline CG113.

CHAPTER 24

Schizophrenia

David Kendall

LEARNING OUTCOMES

By the end of this chapter the reader should be able to:

- describe the symptoms and diagnosis of schizophrenia

- identify risk factors that influence the development of schizophrenia

- understand the neurochemical basis of schizophrenia

- state the recommended therapies for schizophrenia

- understand the mechanisms of action of antischizophrenic drugs

- describe the adverse effects associated with antischizophrenic drugs.

DESCRIPTION AND EPIDEMIOLOGY

Schizophrenia is a psychotic disorder that involves characteristic distortions of thinking and perception. It is a severe, disabling condition associated with social and occupational dysfunction resulting in a major reduction in the sufferer's quality of life. Up to a third of people with schizophrenia experience complete remission of symptoms, others have a cycle of worsening and remission periodically throughout their lives, while others experience a gradual worsening of symptoms over time (Harrison et al. 2001).

Although it is not as common as many other mental health disorders, schizophrenia affects approximately 1 in 300 people (0.32% or 20 million) worldwide. Onset is most often during late adolescence or in the 20s. Although onset tends to happen earlier among men than among women, overall there is no significant gender bias.

The characteristic symptoms of schizophrenia are, somewhat inappropriately, labelled positive (Table 24.1) and negative (Table 24.2). The negative symptoms include apathy, speech paucity and blunted or incongruous emotional responses (e.g., laughing at bad news) often with social withdrawal. Cognitive deficiency is not uncommon.

A diagnosis of schizophrenia should only be made if the subject has one very clear positive symptom, either delusions or hallucinations, or at least two, if less clear cut, positive or negative symptoms. Because many people have brief psychotic-like episodes, schizophrenia should only be diagnosed if symptoms last for at least 6 months and are present, for most of the time, for at least 1 month and there is significant impairment of social and/or work function.

Structural magnetic resonance imaging in schizophrenia shows that both whole-brain volume and grey matter volume are reduced. White matter abnormalities have also been reported and may be one of the key findings consistent with the dissociative thinking and cognitive defects observed in this illness (Keshavan et al. 2008). However, such observations are not sufficiently robust to be considered as a potential diagnostic factor.

The New Prescriber: An Integrated Approach to Medical and Non-medical Prescribing, Second Edition.
Edited by Joanne Lymn, Alison Mostyn, Roger Knaggs, Michael Randall, and Dianne Bowskill.
© 2024 John Wiley & Sons Ltd. Published 2024 by John Wiley & Sons Ltd.

Table 24.1 Positive psychotic symptoms

Symptom/sign	Description
Delusional thinking	Firmly held beliefs are untrue and contrary to a person's educational and cultural background. This may include elements of persecution, jealousy, sin/guilt, grandiosity, religion, somatic, reference, control, mind reading, broadcasting, thought insertion and withdrawal.
Hallucinations	Perceptions experienced without external stimuli and can be auditory (including commands and commentary), visual, tactile, olfactory and gustatory
Disorganized speech/thought disturbances	Associative loosening, illogical thinking, over-inclusive thinking, poverty of speech, poverty of content of speech, tangential replies, perseveration, distractibility, clanging, neologisms, echolalia and blocking. This leads to problems in organizing ideas and speaking so that a listener can understand. Key amongst these are loose associations (cognitive slippage) with continual shifting from topic to topic without any apparent or logical connection between thoughts.
Disorganized or bizarre behaviour	Catatonic stupor, catatonic excitement, stereotypy, echopraxia, inappropriate mannerisms, automatic obedience, negativism. Deterioration of grooming, dress, abode, social behaviour (public masturbation, shouting obscenities, etc.). Incongruity of affect (e.g., inappropriate smiling), motor disturbances, extreme activity levels (unusually high or low), peculiar body movements or postures (e.g., catatonic schizophrenia), strange gestures and grimaces.

Table 24.2 Negative psychotic symptoms

Symptom/sign	Description
Anhedonia	An inability to feel pleasure along with a lack of interest or enjoyment in activities or relationships.
Avolition	An inability or lack of energy to engage in routine (e.g., personal hygiene) and/or goal-directed activities (e.g., work, school)
Alogia	A lack of meaningful speech. May take several forms, including poverty of speech (reduced amount of speech) and/or poverty of content of speech (little information is conveyed, vague, repetitive).
Asociality	Impairments in social relationships; few friends, poor social skills, little interest in being with other people.
Flat affect	No stimulus can elicit an emotional response. Patient may stare vacantly, with lifeless eyes and expressionless face. Voice may be toneless. Flat affect refers only to outward expression, not necessarily internal experience.

AETIOLOGY OF SCHIZOPHRENIA

Schizophrenia is a multifactorial disorder, with interactions between multiple susceptibility genes, epigenetic processes and environmental factors. It is at least partly heritable, with genetic factors accounting for around 80% of disease liability (Tandon et al. 2008).

GENETIC FACTORS

Epidemiological studies indicate that the lifetime risk of developing schizophrenia in the general population is 0.5–1%, although it increases considerably if a family member is schizophrenic. The risk is approximately 2% for third-degree relatives, 9% for first-degree relatives, 27% for children of two affected parents and 50% for monozygotic twins (Ng et al. 2009).

Genome-wide association studies have indicated a number of genes possibly associated with schizophrenia, including the zinc finger protein 804 A gene, the transcription factor 4 gene, the neurogranin gene and the major histocompatibility complex region. However, it is abundantly clear that no single gene mutation is the cause of schizophrenia (Trifu et al. 2020) and interactions of many of these genetic influences with other risk factors are the key to understanding the disease.

Large studies on common and rare variants of the disorder have indicated potential causal factors, including disruption of glutamate pathways, particularly N-methyl-D-aspartate (NMDA) receptor signalling, postsynaptic density integrity, calcium channels, targets of micro-RNA miR-137 and other processes related to neurogenesis and synaptic function (Trifu et al. 2020) but none of these is a single culprit.

OTHER RISK FACTORS

A variety of other factors are also involved in schizophrenia (Kelly and Murray 2000).

Place and time of birth: Urban births and late-winter births have been shown to increase schizophrenic risk, and the bigger the town the greater the risk.

Obstetric complications: Children with significant evidence of perinatal brain damage (especially hypoxia-associated) are seven times more likely to develop schizophrenia than controls.

Social risk factors: Migration, poor mothering and single living status.

Substance abuse: More common in schizophrenic patients than the general population and there has been a particular focus on cannabis use in adolescence as a significant risk factor. However, cause and effect are far from straightforward, and a persuasive hypothesis is that there is a commonality in the genetic determinants of schizophrenia and substance abuse disorder making them, in essence, comorbidities rather than one causing the other (Khokhar et al. 2018).

PATHOGENESIS OF SCHIZOPHRENIA

THE DOPAMINE HYPOTHESIS

Dopamine excess is, perhaps, the most well-established theory with regard to the pathophysiology of schizophrenia, although most of the evidence for this theory is indirect. Key factors in the supporting evidence include:

- the hyperactivity found in the mesolimbic dopaminergic system, particularly dopamine D_2 receptor-linked pathways
- the use of antipsychotics can produce tardive dyskinesia due to dopamine blockade
- dopamine receptor hypersensitivity (D_2 receptor population is upregulated by approximately 20–40%)
- antipsychotic drug efficacy is correlated to D_2 receptor blocking activity
- D_2 receptor agonists, such as amphetamine, worsen symptoms.

However, dopamine malfunction cannot be the only explanation of schizophrenia. For example, the newer 'atypical' antipsychotics have a broader range of activity, including interactions with dopamine D_1, dopamine D_4 and 5-hydroxytryptamine (5HT)$_2$ receptors in the frontal cortex and striatum. First-generation antipsychotic drugs have fewer extrapyramidal effects (similar to the effects of Parkinson's disease) because of less D_2 receptor activity. Additionally, the complete blockade of D_2 receptors does not completely alleviate all schizophrenic symptoms.

THE GLUTAMATE HYPOTHESIS

In the search for other explanations for neurochemical imbalance leading to schizophrenia, researchers found decreased activity and concentration of glutamate in schizophrenic brains. This was particularly notable in drug abusers taking phenylcyclohexylpiperidine and ketamine, which are NMDA receptor antagonists whose use causes negative schizophrenic-like symptoms and can exacerbate chronic schizophrenia. Postmortem studies have reported reduced expression of NMDA glutamate receptors in a variety of brain regions (Keshavan et al. 2008). Subsequent investigations revealed that first-generation antipsychotics increase NMDA receptor activity by acting through the D_2 receptors.

PRACTICE APPLICATION

Many schizophrenics are avid smokers, but nicotine increases NMDA receptor activity and they may, in fact, be self-medicating.

THE SEROTONIN HYPOTHESIS

The serotonin hypothesis is closely linked with the glutamate hypothesis. This hypothesis arose from studies on interactions between the hallucinogenic drug LSD and 5HT. Both the major classes of psychedelic hallucinogens, the indoleamines (e.g., LSD) and phenethylamines (e.g., mescaline), produce their central effects through an action on $5HT_{2A}$ receptors in the locus coeruleus and the cerebral cortex, which enhances glutamatergic transmission. Many first-generation antipsychotic drugs show a greater affinity for $5HT_{2A}$ than D_2 receptors and the role of serotonergic antagonism in mitigating the extrapyramidal effects of antipsychotics is well established (Keshavan et al. 2008).

What is clear is that the neurochemistry involved with schizophrenia is complex and multifactorial.

TREATMENT OF SCHIZOPHRENIA

The aims of treatments for schizophrenia are to minimise the impairment and achieve the best level possible of mental functioning. Although a range of social and psychological therapies is used in the management of schizophrenia, appropriate and timely drug treatment is also essential.

There are two main types of antipsychotic drugs: the older first-generation (previously called 'typical') antipsychotic drugs (such as chlorpromazine and haloperidol) and the second-generation (previously called 'atypical') antipsychotic drugs (like olanzapine and respiridone).

FIRST-GENERATION (TYPICAL) ANTIPSYCHOTICS

The first-generation antipsychotic drugs are predominately D_2 receptor antagonists and are most effective in the management of the positive symptoms of schizophrenia. The therapeutic effect of antipsychotic drugs is thought to be the result primarily of D_2 receptor blockade. This does not mean, however, that they act only to block D_2 receptors. Indeed, these drugs act as antagonists at other dopamine receptors and muscarinic, adrenergic, histamine H_1 and serotonergic receptors (Table 24.3), which may account for the side-effect profiles seen with these drugs.

Side effects

Interaction with D_2 receptors in other neuronal pathways in the brain results in the so-called movement associated 'extrapyramidal' side effects of antipsychotic drugs. These can be acute or

Table 24.3 Receptor targets of typical antipsychotic drugs

Antipsychotic	Confirmed receptor targets
Haloperidol	D_2, D_3 and D_4 receptor antagonist (primarily D_2 receptor)
Loxapine	D_2/D_4 antagonist
	$5HT_{2A/2B}$ and $5HT_7$ antagonist
Chlorpromazine	D_2 antagonist
	H_1 antagonist
Fluphenazine	D_1/D_2 antagonist
	H_1 antagonist
Thioridazine	D_2 receptor antagonist, with reduced extrapyramidal side effects
	Ca^{2+} channel blocker

D, dopamine; 5HT, 5-hydroxytryptamine; H, histamine; Ca^{2+}, calcium.

chronic. They include acute Parkinson's disease-like rigidity and bradykinesia (slowness of movement and initiation of movement), but also effects that appear to be the opposite of Parkinsonian symptoms, including akathisia (motor restlessness) and tardive dyskinesia (repetitive tic-like movements). The latter might be due to hypersensitivity of dopamine receptors as a reaction to long-term blockade.

Because dopamine usually increases the secretion of prolactin from the pituitary gland, blockade with first-generation antipsychotics can lead to gynaecomastia in men and galactorrhoea.

STOP AND THINK

What side effects of first-generation antipsychotic drugs does antagonism at the α_1-adrenoceptor, muscarinic acetylcholine receptor and histamine H_1 receptor produce?

Neuroleptic malignant syndrome is a rare but potentially fatal side effect of antipsychotic drugs. It is characterised by hyperthermia, muscle rigidity and autonomic instability. Discontinuation of the antipsychotic drug is essential as there is no known wholly successful treatment.

Typical antipsychotics may potentiate the effects of central nervous system depressants such as anaesthetics, opioids and alcohol. All first-generation antipsychotic drugs should be administered with caution to patients with cardiovascular disorders because of the possibility of transient hypotension and/or precipitation of angina pain.

Interactions

While there are many drug interactions listed in the *British National Formulary* (BNF) for antipsychotic drugs, relatively few are of clinical significance. Propranolol increases the plasma concentrations of chlorpromazine, and carbamazepine increases the metabolism of haloperidol.

STOP AND THINK

Can you describe the mechanism by which carbamazepine increases the metabolism of haloperidol?

PRACTICE APPLICATION

Many patients with schizophrenia struggle to remember to take medication on a regular basis. Some antipsychotic medicines have been formulated as long-acting depot injections that need only be given every 2–4 weeks by deep intramuscular injection. Following injection of the drug, it is slowly released from the vehicle over a period of 2–4 weeks.

SECOND-GENERATION (ATYPICAL) ANTIPSYCHOTICS

Second-generation antipsychotic drugs, like the first-generation antipsychotics, block dopaminergic pathways but also block the serotonergic pathways from the raphe nucleus to the basal ganglia, limbic structures and the entire cortex (Table 24.4). This results in fewer extrapyramidal side effects and more effective treatment of the negative symptoms of schizophrenia. Aripiprazole differs from all other typical and atypical antipsychotic drugs by acting as a partial agonist at D_2 receptors, distinguishing its action from the full antagonist profile of other antipsychotics (Mamo et al. 2007).

Side effects

Second-generation antipsychotics are not, however, without side effects. There are important differences in terms of the side effects they produce and these side effects are often dose-related and can be affected by patient age and gender (Haddad and Sharma 2007).

It is important, therefore, to have a clear idea of the potential adverse reactions before starting treatment.

- The risk of developing acute extrapyramidal symptoms is particularly high for risperidone, with the highest risk being with high doses.

Table 24.4 Receptor targets of atypical antipsychotic drugs

Antipsychotic	Confirmed receptor targets
Risperidone	Antagonist with high affinity for D_2 and weak affinity for D_1
	Antagonist with high affinity for $5HT_2$, α_1 and α_2, and H_1. Lower affinity for $5HT_{1C}$, $5HT_{1D}$ and $5HT_{1A}$. Weak affinity for haloperidol-sensitive sigma site.
Quetiapine	Antagonist at D_1 and D_2
	Antagonist at $5HT_{1A}$ and $5HT_2$, H_1, plus α_1 and α_2
Olanzapine	Antagonist with high-affinity binding to D_{1-4}
	Antagonist with high-affinity binding to $5HT_{2A/2C}$, M_{1-5}, H_1 and α_1 receptors. Binds weakly to $GABA_A$, BZD and β adrenergic receptors.
Aripiprazole	Agonist/antagonist with high affinity for D_2 and D_3, and moderate affinity for D_4. Partial agonist at D_2.
	Agonist/antagonist with high affinity for $5HT_{1A}$ and $5HT_{2A}$ receptors, moderate affinity for $5HT_{2C}$, $5HT_7$, α_1 and H_1 receptors, and moderate affinity for the serotonin reuptake site. Partial agonist at the $5HT_{1A}$ receptor and antagonist at $5HT_{2A}$ receptor.
Clozapine	Selective antagonist for D_4 receptor
	Antagonist at $5\text{-}HT_{2A}$, $5\text{-}HT_{2C}$, $5\text{-}HT_3$, $5\text{-}HT_6$ and $5\text{-}HT_7$ receptors

D, dopamine receptor; 5HT, 5-hydroxytryptamine receptor; α, alpha adrenoceptor; H, histamine receptor.

- Risk of agranulocytosis, particularly with clozapine. Patients being treated must have a baseline white blood cell and differential count before initiation of treatment as well as regular white blood cell counts during treatment and for 4 weeks after discontinuation.

- Seizures have been associated with the use of atypical antipsychotics, with a greater likelihood at higher doses; this is particularly true for clozapine.

- Prolongation of the ECG QTc interval; highest risk with ziprasidone and sertindole.

- Significant weight gain; highest risk with olanzapine and clozapine.

- Hyperprolactinaemia; highest risk with risperidone.

Interactions

There are a large number of potential drug interactions with second-generation antipsychotic drugs listed in the BNF, many of which are associated with modulation of cytochrome P450 activity, including:

- fluoxetine and paroxetine increase the plasma concentration of risperidone

- plasma concentration of aripiprazole is decreased by St. John's wort

- metabolism of olanzapine, quetiapine, risperidone and sertindole is accelerated by carbamazepine and phenytoin

- metabolism of aripiprazole is inhibited by ketoconazole.

Second-generation antipsychotics are currently more expensive than the older first-generation drugs and are not necessarily associated with higher quality-adjusted life-years (Davies et al. 2007). The variability in terms of pharmacodynamics and tolerability of second-generation antipsychotics also suggests that it might be a mistake to regard them as being a uniform drug class. Instead, selection of an antipsychotic should be on an individual patient basis.

PRACTICE APPLICATION

Second-generation antipsychotics should be considered when choosing first-line treatment of newly diagnosed schizophrenia (NICE 2009).

CHOICE OF ANTIPSYCHOTIC TREATMENT

There is no clear evidence that any antipsychotic medication is more efficacious than any other for first-episode schizophrenia (Barnes et al. 2020). Treatment resistance is a common problem, and this is defined as the failure of two trials of an antipsychotic at an optimal dose for an adequate period of time. Risperidone is often regarded as one of the two agents appropriate for an initial trial, whereas olanzapine is specifically excluded as a recommended initial choice because of the issue of metabolic side effects and weight gain (Keating et al. 2017).

Clozapine is the only medicine licensed for treating refractory schizophrenia (Flanagan et al. 2020) but has a long list of adverse side effects, the most important being the relatively uncommon incidence of agranulocytosis, and clinical therapeutic monitoring is essential (Kar et al. 2016).

Once remission has been achieved, maintenance treatment with the chosen antipsychotic medication, at a standard dose, will substantially reduce the risk of relapse for at least 2 years.

OTHER USES OF ANTIPSYCHOTIC MEDICINES

Many antipsychotic drugs have clinical uses other than controlling symptoms of schizophrenia (Table 24.5).

SUMMARY

- Schizophrenia is a psychotic disorder in which thinking and emotion are impaired, and the individual has trouble with social and occupational function.

- Schizophrenia is heritable, with a greater incidence in males.

- Environmental risk factors for developing schizophrenia include urbanicity and migration.

- Genetic, developmental and biological factors all contribute to the development of schizophrenia.

- The three main biological hypotheses underlying schizophrenia involve alteration in dopamine, glutamate and serotonin function in the midbrain and frontal cortex.

- Antipsychotic drugs are currently classified as first-generation 'typical' (e.g., chlorpromazine, haloperidol) or second-generation 'atypical' (e.g., olanzapine, rispiridone).

- First-generation antipsychotic drugs all act as dopamine receptor antagonists.

- First-generation antipsychotic drugs have more significant antagonist effects on muscarinic, histamine H_1 and α-1-adrenergic receptors.

- Second-generation antipsychotics block the first-generation antipsychotic pathways plus the serotonergic pathways from the raphe nucleus to the basal ganglia, limbic structures and the entire cortex.

- Second-generation antipsychotics have fewer extrapyramidal side effects.

Table 24.5 Other uses of antipsychotic drugs

Drug	Other prescribed uses
Haloperidol	Control of motor tics, including verbal tics linked with Tourette's disorder
	Nausea and vomiting
	Control of violent behaviour in children failing to respond to psychotherapy or other drugs
Chlorpromazine	Treatment of mania in bipolar disorder
	Control of violent behaviour in children
	Control nausea and vomiting, to relieve hiccups lasting 1 month or longer, and to relieve restlessness and nervousness that may occur just before surgery
	Treatment of acute intermittent porphyria
	Used along with other medications to treat tetanus
Risperidone	Used to treat episodes of mania or mixed episodes in adults and in teenagers and children 10 years of age and older with bipolar disorder
	Used to treat behaviour problems such as aggression, self-injury and sudden mood changes in teenagers and children 5-16 years of age who have autism
Aripiprazole	Used with an antidepressant to treat depression when symptoms cannot be controlled by the antidepressant alone

- Second-generation antipsychotics exhibit variations in tolerability and side effects, and should be considered individually.

- Clozapine is the only antipsychotic licensed for treatment-resistant schizophrenia.

ACTIVITY

1. The more closely related a person is to someone with schizophrenia, the more likely they are to show psychoses associated with schizophrenia. True/False

2. Risk factors for schizophrenia include environmental factors such as urbanicity. True/False

3. Antipsychotic drug efficacy is correlated to D_2 blocking activity. True/False

4. The complete blockade of D_2 receptors completely alleviates all schizophrenic symptoms. True/False

5. First-generation antipsychotic drugs are most effective in managing positive symptoms of schizophrenia. True/False

6. First-generation antipsychotics do not antagonise muscarinic, histaminergic or adrenergic receptors. True/False

7. First-generation antipsychotics do not potentiate the action of opioids. True/False

8. Second-generation antipsychotics have fewer extrapyramidal side effects. True/False

9. Weight gain can be a major side effect of atypical antipsychotics. True/False

10. All second-generation antipsychotics act as full antagonists at D_2 receptors. True/False

REFERENCES

Barnes, T.R., Drake, R., Paton, C., et al. (2020). Evidence-based guidelines for the pharmacological treatment of schizophrenia: Updated recommendations from the British Association for Psychopharmacology. *J Psychopharmacol* 34:3–78.

Davies, L.M., Lewis, S., Jones, P.B., et al., on behalf of the CUtLASS Team (2007). Cost-effectiveness of first- v. second-generation antipsychotic drugs: results from a randomised controlled trial in schizophrenia responding poorly to previous therapy. *Br J Psychiatry* 191:14–22.

Flanagan, R.J., Lally, J., Gee, S., Lyon, R. and Every-Palmer, S. (2020). Clozapine in the treatment of refractory schizophrenia: a practical guide for healthcare professionals. *Br Med Bull* 135:73–89.

Haddad, P.M. and Sharma, S.G. (2007). Adverse effects of atypical antipsychotics: differential risk and clinical implications. *CNS Drugs* 21:911–936.

Harrison, G., Hopper, K., Craig, T., Laska, E., Siegel, C. and Wanderling, J. (2001) Recovery from psychotic illness: a 15- and 25-year international follow-up study. *Br J Psychiatry* 178:506–517.

Kar, N., Barreto, S. and Chandavarkar, R. (2016) Clozapine monitoring in clinical practice: beyond the mandatory requirement. *Clin Psychopharmacol Neurosci* 14:323–329.

Keating, D., McWilliams, S., Schneider, I., et al. (2017) Pharmacological guidelines for schizophrenia: a systematic review and comparison of recommendations for the first episode. *BMJ Open* 7:e013881.

Kelly, J. and Murray, R.M. (2000) What risk factors tell us about the causes of schizophrenia and related psychoses. *Curr Psychiatry Rep* 2:378–385.

Keshavan, M.S., Tandon, R., Boutros, N.N. and Nasrallah, H.A. (2008) Schizophrenia, 'Just the Facts'. What we know in 2008. Part 3: Neurobiology. *Schizophr Res* 106:89–107.

Khokhar, J.Y., Dwiel, L.L., Henricks, A.M., Doucette, W.T. and Green, A.I. (2018) The link between schizophrenia and substance use disorder: A unifying hypothesis. *Schizophr Res* 194:78–85.

Mamo, D., Graff, A., Shammi, C.M., et al. (2007) Differential effects of aripiprazole on D2, 5-HT2 and 5-HT1A receptor occupancy in patients with schizophrenia: a triple tracer PET study. *Am J Psychiatry* 164:1411–1417.

Ng, M.Y., Levinson, D.F., Faraone, S.V., et al. (2009) Meta-analysis of 32 genome-wide linkage studies of schizophrenia. *Mol Psychiatry* 14:774–785.

NICE (2009) *Clinical Guideline 82: Schizophrenia*. Core Interventions in the Treatment and Management of Schizophrenia in Adults in Primary and Secondary Care. National Institute for Health and Clinical Excellence, London.

Tandon, R., Keshavan, M.S. and Nasrallah, H.A. (2008) Schizophrenia, 'Just the Facts'. What we know in 2008. Part 2: Epidemiology and etiology. *Schizophr Res* 102:1–18.

Trifu, S.C., Kohn, B., Vlasie, A. and Patrichi, B.E. (2020) Genetics of schizophrenia (Review). *Exp Ther Med* 20:3462–3468.

FURTHER READING

Bennett, P.N. and Brown, MJ. (2003) *Clinical Pharmacology*, 9th edn. Churchill Livingstone, Edinburgh.

Collier, J., Longmore, M., Turmezel, T. and Mafi, A.R. (2009) *Oxford Handbook of Clinical Specialities*. Oxford University Press, Oxford, pp 356–361.

Kruk, Z.L. and Pycock, C.J. (1991) *Neurotransmitters and Drugs*, 3rd edn. Chapman and Hall, London.

Ritter, J.M., Flower, R., Henderson, G., et al. (2023) *Rang and Dale's Pharmacology*, 10th edn. Elsevier, Amsterdam.

Wagner, H. and Silber, K. (2004) *Instant Notes: Physiological Psychology*. BIOS Scientific Publishers, Oxford.

World Health Organization (2001) *Mental Health Report 2001. Mental Health: New Understanding, New Hope*. World Health Organization, Geneva.

USEFUL WEBSITES

BNF treatment summary. Psychoses and related disorders. https://bnf.nice.org.uk/treatment-summaries/psychoses-and-related-disorders/

Psychosis and schizophrenia in adults. NICE guideline on treatment and management. https://www.nice.org.uk/guidance/cg178/evidence/full-guideline-490503565.

WHO Fact sheet. Schizophrenia. https://www.who.int/news-room/fact-sheets/detail/schizophrenia

Epilepsy and Antiseizure Drugs

Michael F O'Donoghue and Christina Giavasi

CHAPTER 25

LEARNING OUTCOMES

By the end of this chapter the reader should be able to:

- appreciate how knowledge of the diverse types of seizure and epilepsy influence clinical management

- understand the process of decision-making in the most common scenarios: a patient presenting with a first seizure or new epilepsy, a follow-up outpatient consultation and advising following an emergency admission to hospital with seizures

- understand the special considerations in women with epilepsy, people with intellectual disability, young people in transition from paediatric services and the elderly

- deliver evidence-based care for people with epilepsy using the clinical pharmacology of the commonly used antiseizure medications (ASMs): lamotrigine, levetiracetam, brivaracetam, carbamazepine, oxcarbazepine, eslicarbazepine, sodium valproate, ethosuximide, topiramate, zonisamide, lacosamide, gabapentin, pregabalin, perampanel, clobazam, and cenobamate

- propose other options for people with intractable epilepsy (third-line ASM, vagal nerve stimulation, epilepsy surgery and ketogenic diet)

- practice holistic care for people with epilepsy, considering common comorbidities.

INTRODUCTION AND DEFINITIONS

This introduction to the treatment of epilepsy assumes the prescriber is working as part of a multidisciplinary team including a neurologist. It is focused on epilepsy in adults and young people (approximately 12 years and older) as infantile and childhood epilepsies have complexities beyond the scope of the chapter.

A seizure is defined as 'a transient occurrence of signs and/or symptoms due to abnormal excessive or synchronous neuronal activity in the brain' (Fisher et al. 2005). The pattern of signs and symptoms during the seizure will depend on which brain regions or networks are engaged by the epileptic brain rhythms. A careful history from the patient and witnesses of the sequence of symptoms from start to recovery allows a precise diagnosis.

Epilepsy is defined as 'a disorder of the brain characterised by an enduring predisposition to generate epileptic seizures and by the neurobiologic, cognitive, psychological, and social consequences of this condition' (Fisher et al. 2005). This implies more than one seizure has occurred and excludes isolated seizures triggered by a metabolic or toxic insult (such as alcohol). It emphasises that seizures are only part of the disorder, and that psychological and cognitive effects are important.

The New Prescriber: An Integrated Approach to Medical and Non-medical Prescribing, Second Edition.
Edited by Joanne Lymn, Alison Mostyn, Roger Knaggs, Michael Randall, and Dianne Bowskill.
© 2024 John Wiley & Sons Ltd. Published 2024 by John Wiley & Sons Ltd.

Practically speaking, epilepsy is two epileptic seizures in a 5-year period or one seizure with risk factors indicating at least a 60% risk of a second seizure (Fisher et al. 2014). Antiseizure medications reduce the risk of seizure occurrence if taken regularly, but do not change the natural history of the disorder.

SEIZURE TYPES AND EPILEPSIES

Seizures can be classified according to whether epileptic activity starts within a restricted network of neurons in one hemisphere (focal seizures) or engages both cerebral hemispheres from the onset (generalised seizures) or the origin is unknown (Fisher et al. 2017). Seizures can further be classified according to whether awareness is lost or not, and to the presence of motor and other behavioural signs (Figure 25.1). The common generalised seizures are absences, myoclonus and tonic-clonic seizures. The most common focal seizures arise from the temporal or frontal lobes. These clinical distinctions are crucial to the approach to patient investigation (focal epilepsy often has underlying lesions on magnetic resonance imaging [MRI]), treatment (seizure type influences drug choice) and prognosis (generalised seizures more often remit on treatment). The precise type of epilepsy can also be classified. This process starts with seizure type and uses other clinical features such as age of onset, electroencephalogram (EEG) results, MRI, and clinical and genetic features to arrive at a precise epilepsy syndrome and aetiology (Scheffer et al. 2017).

Epilepsy is common, with a prevalence of about 1% of the population (Thijs et al. 2019). The cause will often depend on age of onset. Epilepsy in infancy is caused by genetic disorders, brain malformations and insults to the prenatal or infant cortex. In young adults and midlife, the common causes are idiopathic generalised epilepsy (also known as genetic generalised epilepsy, although the gene may not be known), trauma, brain tumours and infection (Thijs et al. 2019). In later life, stroke and dementia are important factors (Sen 2020).

The evaluation of a patient with epilepsy starts with a comprehensive assessment of seizures, epilepsy syndrome, aetiology and comorbidities (both physical and mental health). All of this is the prelude to deciding treatment (Figure 25.2). It is vital to exclude the common mimics of epileptic seizures: syncope and dissociative seizures at an early stage (Smith 2012).

Classification of Seizure Types			
	Onset	Awareness	First prominent sign or symptom
	Focal: Originating in networks limited to one hemisphere	Aware or impaired awareness	Motor signs	Automatisms, atonic, clonic, epileptic spasms, hyperkinetic, myoclonic[1], tonic
			Non-motor signs	Autonomic, behavioural arrest, cognitive, emotional, sensory
	Generalised: Originating within bilateral networks	Awareness impaired	Motor signs	Tonic-clonic, clonic, tonic, myoclonic, myoclonic-tonic-clonic, myoclonic-atonic, atonic, epileptic spasms
			Absence	typical, atypical, myoclonic, eyelid myoclonic
	Unknown: Onset was unobserved	Awareness impaired	Motor	Tonic-clonic, other motor
			Non-motor	Behavioural arrest

[1] Myoclonic seizures are so short that awareness is not lost.

FIGURE 25.1 Classification of seizure types.

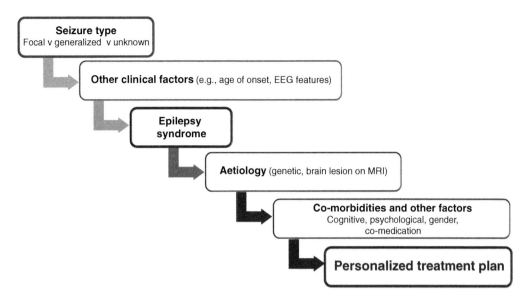

FIGURE 25.2   The decision-making process in epilepsy. EEG, electroencephalogram; MRI, magnetic resonance imaging.

COMMON ANTISEIZURE MEDICATIONS: MECHANISMS AND USE

Neurons are excitable cells that depend on voltage-gated ion channels (e.g., sodium, potassium, calcium channels) to send electrical signals around the nervous system. Neurons communicate with each other at excitatory synapses (using the neurotransmitter glutamate) and at inhibitory synapses (using γ-aminobutyric acid [GABA]) (Chapter 21). This is an oversimplification but is sufficient for our purposes. Epileptic hyperexcitability arises because of disturbances in ion channels and synaptic function (amongst other influences). Antiseizure medication (ASM) targets these processes (Sills and Rogawski 2020). The most important targets are ion channels (especially the sodium and calcium channels), the inhibitory transmitter GABA and mechanisms regulating transmitter release using synaptic vesicle protein 2a (SV2a) (see Table 1 for a list of ASMs and postulated targets).

The choice of ASM is guided by seizure type (Löscher and Klein 2021). Absences respond well to sodium valproate and ethosuximide, and to some extent to benzodiazepines, lamotrigine and topiramate. Myoclonus responds well to valproate, levetiracetam, brivaracetam and benzodiazepines. Absences and myoclonus can be worsened by carbamazepine and related drugs, phenytoin, gabapentin, pregabalin, vigabatrin, tiagabine and sometimes lamotrigine (Chaves and Sander 2005; Gayatri and Livingston 2006). Tonic-clonic seizures respond to most drugs except ethosuximide. There is a clinical impression of a spectrum of potency partly supported by trial evidence. Valproate, topiramate and perampanel are more potent, and gabapentin and pregabalin are less potent. Focal seizures respond to all drugs except ethosuximide with a similar gradation in efficacy.

ASMs differ in their tolerability, in both the severity and the nature of side effects. Lamotrigine is amongst the best tolerated ASMs (apart from an incidence of rash) and valproate, topiramate and perampanel have a higher incidence of side effects. A complete description of the efficacy and tolerability of ASMs should be sought in the authoritative review by Shorvon et al. (2015).

Large randomised pragmatic trials (the SANAD trials) have considered the combination of efficacy and tolerability to arrive at recommendations for the initial treatment of generalised and focal epilepsies (Marson et al. 2007a,b, 2021a,b). Following the SANAD I and II trials lamotrigine was found to be superior for focal epilepsy when considering combined efficacy and tolerability

Table 25.1 The mechanisms of action and uses of the most important antiseizure medication

Drug	Mechanism/target	Effective for seizure type	Comments
Valproate	Multiple targets, including GABA and sodium channel	A, M, TC, focal	The most effective drug for generalized seizures. Also used in status epilepticus. Cannot be used in women of child-bearing age without specialist advice
Lamotrigine	Sodium channel	Focal, TC	First line for focal and generalized seizures
Carbamazepine	Sodium channel	Focal, TC (worsens A, M)	Second line for focal seizures. Sometimes used for tonic-clonic seizures, but risk of worsening absences and myoclonus
Oxcarbazepine	Sodium channel	Focal, TC (worsens A, M)	Second line for Focal seizures
Eslicarbazepine	Sodium channel	Focal, TC (worsens A, M)	Second line for focal seizures
Lacosamide	Sodium channel	Focal, TC	Second line for focal seizures and tonic-clonic seizures
Phenytoin	Sodium channel	Focal, TC (worsens A, M)	Second line for focal seizures and sometimes tonic-clonic seizures, but risk of worsening absences and myoclonus
Topiramate	Sodium channel and GABA, glutamate and carbonic anhydrase	Focal, TC (A, M)	Second line for focal and generalized seizures
Zonisamide	Sodium channel and carbonic anhydrase	Focal, TC (A, M)	Second line for focal and generalized seizures
Rufinamide	Sodium channel	TC, tonic, atonic seizures	Third line in intractable generalized syndromes, including Lennox–Gastaut syndrome
Cenobamate	Sodium channel and GABA$_a$	Focal	Novel drug. Third line for focal seizures
Ethosuximide	T type calcium channel	A (M)	Used especially in childhood absence epilepsy
Levetiracetam	SV2a	Focal, M, TC (A)	First line in focal and generalized seizures
Brivaracetam	SV2a	Focal, M, TC (A)	First line in focal and generalized seizures, especially if levetiracetam not well tolerated
Benzodiazepines (clobazam, diazepam, clonazepam, lorazepam, midazolam)	Modulators of GABA$_a$ receptor	Effective in all seizure types	Useful for terminating seizures acutely. First line for prolonged or clustering seizures. Clobazam used add-on long term for intractable focal and generalized seizures
Phonobarbital	Modulator of GABA$_a$	Focal, TC, (M)	Mainly used in infancy and developing countries (due to lack of access to modern drugs)

Table 25.1   (Continued)

Drug	Mechanism/target	Effective for seizure type	Comments
Tiagabine	Blocks GAT1 GABA transporter enhancing GABA levels	Focal (worsens A M)	Used rarely
Vigabatrin	Blocks GABA transaminase enhancing GABA levels	Focal and infantile spasms (worsens A, M)	Used mainly in infancy
Stiripentol	GABA	Dravet syndrome	Exclusive use in Dravet syndrome
Perampanel	Blocks AMPA (glutamate) receptor	Focal, TC (M)	Second line for focal and generalized seizures
Gabapentin	$\alpha 2 \Delta$ calcium channel subunit	Focal (may worsen A, M)	Third line for focal seizures
Pregabalin	$\alpha 2 \Delta$ calcium channel subunit	Focal (may worsen A, M)	Third line for focal seizures
Cannabidiol	Unknown	Tonic, TC and atonic seizures	Exclusively in Dravet and Lennox–Gastaut syndromes and seizures related to tuberous sclerosis

A, absence seizures; M, myoclonic seizures; TC, Tonic clonic. Less consistent effects are shown in parentheses.

compared with levetiracetam, carbamazepine, oxcarbazepine, topiramate, zonisamide and gabapentin (Marson et al. 2007b, 2021). The benefits of lamotrigine over levetiracetam, carbamazepine, topiramate and zonisamide mainly relate to lamotrigine's better tolerability. Similarly, the SANAD I and II trials found sodium valproate to be superior to lamotrigine, topiramate and levetiracetam in generalised or unclassifiable epilepsy, mainly due to sodium valproate being more effective (Marson et al. 2007b, 2021a). Until 2023, the SANAD trial findings informed ASM choice (NICE 2022). In late 2023 the UK Medicines and Healthcare products Regulatory Authority (MHRA) issued warnings about the reproductive safety of sodium valproate in men and women that complicates decision making. This is discussed further below.

PRACTICE APPLICATIONS WITH COMMON SCENARIOS

We will discuss the treatment approach to the most common situations the prescriber will face. It is emphasised that this is necessarily multidisciplinary.

NEW EPILEPSY

When someone presents with new-onset epilepsy it is essential the diagnosis is correct before starting treatment. The non-medical prescriber should work as part of a team to ensure the mimics of epilepsy have been excluded following a detailed history of the seizures and review of home videos, and all patients should have an electrocardiogram (as a basic screen for cardiac abnormalities). Investigations (MRI and often EEG) provide more information about the cause of the epilepsy (Smith 2012). The underlying causes of epilepsy (e.g., stroke or tumour) need to be managed in parallel.

The risk of a second seizure following a first is assessed by looking for risk factors for recurrence. The presence of a neurological deficit, focal seizures and an abnormal EEG carry an increased risk of recurrence (Bonnett et al. 2022). People at elevated risk may be offered ASMs after the first seizure. A second seizure increases the risk for a third seizure (Kim et al. 2006; Berg 2008). Hence, most neurologists would recommend ASM treatment once a second seizure has occurred. Treating a first seizure reduces the risk of a second seizure, but the benefits may be marginal in low-risk patients and the impact on quality of life equivocal once treatment-related side effects are considered (Marson et al. 2005).

All these factors should be discussed with the patient before starting treatment. There is a general principle of starting at a low dose and gradually titrating over a few weeks to a modest target dose in non-emergency settings. This helps minimise side effects and maximise adherence. Written instructions should be given to optimise adherence. Adults, regardless of their sex, with focal epilepsy should start on lamotrigine, starting at 25 mg per day and titrating over 8–16 weeks. As part of safety-netting, the person should be warned about lamotrigine-associated rashes and given a point of contact for urgent review due to the risk of serious morbidity. Lamotrigine should be stopped after any significant rash. Women should be warned that the combined oral contraceptive lowers the plasma level of lamotrigine, therefore a higher dose may be required.

Men with generalised epilepsy should be offered a choice of lamotrigine and/or levetiracetam or sodium valproate following a detailed discussion of the benefits and potential risks of sodium valproate. Sodium valproate is more likely than lamotrigine and levetiracetam to provide prolonged remission of generalised seizures, particularly if myoclonic seizures and/or absences are present. Sodium valproate, however, has been associated with cases of reversible impaired male fertility due to reduced sperm count and motility (MHRA 2023). Sodium valproate may be associated with a small increase in neuro-developmental delay, although at the time of writing (April 2024) the evidence is inadequate for a definitive statement and decision making is difficult and controversial (Berkovic and Perucca 2024). In the UK, as of February 2024, two specialists must agree that sodium valproate is necessary for any male or female of childbearing potential under the age of 55 before the drug is started. For men with generalised epilepsy it will be important to undertake a careful individualised appraisal of personal risk from tonic-clonic seizures versus potential fertility and developmental risks. Women with generalised epilepsy under the age of 55 and of childbearing potential should be offered either lamotrigine or levetiracetam after careful appraisal of the syndrome type and patient-specific factors (e.g., risk of mood disorder with levetiracetam). Patients should be advised about the importance of good adherence to the AED regimen and the importance of avoiding alcohol excess and sleep deprivation.

In the UK, epilepsy prescriptions are free of charge by signing a medical exception certificate (FP92a). Safety (e.g., discouraging unsupervised bathing) and driving rules should be discussed, and patients directed to reliable information about epilepsy (e.g., www.epilepsy.org.uk and www.epilepsysociety.org.uk). When appropriate, sudden unexpected death in epilepsy (SUDEP) and how to mitigate the risk of this should be discussed (Giussani et al. 2023). Follow-up appointments should be arranged and patients encouraged to keep a seizure diary.

The treatment approach in patients presenting with serial seizures or status epilepticus is different. The priorities are rapid seizure control and diagnosis. These patients should receive intravenous treatment with benzodiazepines and levetiracetam or valproate. If seizures are not rapidly controlled, intensive care management follows, the details of which are beyond the scope of this chapter.

FOLLOW-UP VISITS

The patient's report of seizures should be reviewed. It is important to analyse the history of further events. The importance of avoiding misdiagnosis of seizure mimics persists even after diagnosis. If seizures continue, adherence should be checked with therapeutic drug monitoring (TDM) if needed. If adherence is an issue, the reasons should be addressed. The ASM dose should be gradually titrated according to tolerance to achieve seizure control using TDM to ensure therapeutic serum levels are achieved as individuals vary in how the ASM is metabolized. The presence of lifestyle factors preventing complete control should also be reviewed (sleep, alcohol, stress). The common side effects should be sought out and TDM can be helpful in confirming the ASM as the cause (Table 25.2). Persistent failure of seizure control should lead to a review of the diagnosis. If the diagnosis remains secure, rational polytherapy or a switch to an alternative monotherapy can be tried.

Table 25.2 Antiseizure medication side effects and interactions

Drug	Important interactions	Important side effects and cautions
Valproate	An enzyme inhibitor. Increases serum levels of lamotrigine and phenobarbital. Increases the free fraction of phenytoin by displacing it from plasma protein. May cause side effects with carbamazepine due to increased carbamazepine epoxide. Avoid the combination of meropenem and valproate as valproate levels drop severely. Valproate may potentiate side effects of psychotropic medications	Severely teratogenic. Must not be used in women of child-bearing age without specialist advice and strict adherence to a valproate pregnancy prevention programme

Gastrointestinal complaints, tremor, weight gain, hair loss and changes to blood count (low white count and platelets)

Rarely severe liver dysfunction, mainly in children under age 2 years

May affect fertility by causing polycystic ovarian syndrome |
| Lamotrigine | Lamotrigine levels lowered by all enzyme inducers. Valproate increases lamotrigine levels. Follow *British National Formulary* advice when introducing lamotrigine in someone taking valproate | Rash: this must be sought out and lamotrigine stopped to avoid the rare complication of Stevens–Johnson syndrome. Slow titration reduces risk

Insomnia, anxiety and headache |
| Carbamazepine | An enzyme inducer with many interactions. It reduces serum levels of several ASMs and oral contraceptives (rendering them ineffective) and anticoagulants. Undergoes autoinduction requiring increased dose during titration. Carbamazepine toxicity occurs when clarithromycin or erythromycin are co-prescribed | Sedation, dizziness and double vision. Side-effects reduced when using a slow-release preparation

Generally benign drop in white cell count and serum sodium

Rash (requires discontinuation)

Very rare: Stevens–Johnson syndrome (a multisystem and rash disorder that is potentially fatal and more common in Asians. HLA-B*1502 can help predict risk in Asians |
| Oxcarbazepine | A weaker enzyme inducer than carbamazepine but reduces the effectiveness of oral contraceptives. Increases phenytoin concentrations | Like carbamazepine

Hyponatremia is more common |

(Continued)

Table 25.2 (Continued)

Drug	Important interactions	Important side effects and cautions
Eslicarbazepine	Prodrug of S(+)-licarbazepine, which is renally excreted. Minimal interaction with common ASMs except that phenytoin levels may increase. Oral contraceptives may be less effective	Like carbamazepine Hyponatremia is more common
Lacosamide	Minimal interactions	Like carbamazepine, but rash and blood parameter changes are rare
Phenytoin	Major enzyme inducer with many interactions. Reduces levels of many ASMs, oral contraceptives and warfarin. Unpredictable interaction with carbamazepine. Phenytoin levels increased by clobazam, oxcarbazepine, eslicarbazepine and topiramate. Absorption depends on formulation and is reduced by enteral feeding. Complex pharmacokinetics, which vary between individuals and half-life increases markedly at high serum levels with the potential for toxicity. Serum levels essential to guide dosing	Dizziness, double vision, unsteadiness Rash Long-term use: gum thickening, skin coarsening, osteomalacia, peripheral neuropathy
Levetiracetam	Minimal interactions	Mood disturbance and insomnia
Brivaracetam	Enzyme inducers may reduce brivaracetam levels. Co-administration with carbamazepine may lead to increased carbamazepine epoxide and side effects	Mood disturbance and insomnia (may be less in some patients than levetiracetam)
Topiramate	Oral contraceptives are less effective when topiramate exceeds 200 mg. Phenytoin levels may increase. Enzyme inducers lower topiramate levels	Sedation, weight loss (due to anorexia), cognitive slowing, including reduced verbal fluency, kidney stones, paraesthesia Teratogenic
Zonisamide	Enzyme inducers lower zonisamide levels otherwise no interactions. Caution when co-administering topiramate or acetazolamide	Sedation, weight loss (due to anorexia), cognitive slowing, including reduced verbal fluency, kidney stones, paraesthesia
Rufinamide	Enzyme inducers lower rufinamide levels. Valproate increases rufinamide levels	Sedation, mood change, vomiting
Cenobamate	Increases clobazam and phenytoin levels. Other interactions unknown as it is a new ASM	Sedation, dizziness, unsteadiness, drug reaction with eosinophilia and systemic symptoms
Ethosuximide	Levels reduced by enzyme inducing drugs and variable effects with valproate	Gastrointestinal symptoms, mood change, sedation
Benzodiazepines (clobazam, diazepam, clonazepam, lorazepam, midazolam)	Few interactions. Clobazam can increase phenytoin levels Levels of clobazam and its metabolites increased by cannabidiol and cenobamate	Sedation

Table 25.2   (Continued)

Drug	Important interactions	Important side effects and cautions
Phenobarbital	Potent enzyme inducer that reduces serum levels of many drugs and ASMs. Important ones: oral contraceptives (rendering them ineffective) and anticoagulants. Valproate increases phenobarbital levels significantly	Sedation, dizziness, unsteadiness, slowed thinking
Primidone	Like Phenobarbitone	Sedation, dizziness, unsteadiness, slowed thinking
Tiagabine	Minimal interactions except enzyme inducers reduce tiagabine levels	Sedation, dizziness, tremor, depression, psychosis, non-convulsive status
Vigabatrin	Minimal interactions	Sedation, depression, psychosis, irreversible peripheral field loss, weight gain
Stiripentol	Enzyme inhibitor. Increases clobazam, phenytoin, carbamazepine and valproate levels	Sedation, unsteadiness
Perampanel	Enzyme inducers reduce perampanel levels, especially carbamazepine	Mood change, aggression, sedation, unsteadiness
Gabapentin	No pharmacokinetic interactions. Caution with dosing opioids and gabapentin (respiratory depression)	Sedation, weight gain
Pregabalin	No pharmacokinetic interactions. Caution with dosing opioids and gabapentin (respiratory depression)	Sedation, weight gain
Cannabidiol	Enzyme inhibitor potentially affecting several ASMs. Elevates clobazam metabolite (N-desmethylclobazam) levels causing somnolence. Bioavailability increased after high fat meals. Recommended that it is taken with meals	Sedation, diarrhoea, requires liver enzymes monitoring during titration

ASM, antiseizure medication. The important interactions, side effects and cautions for antiseizure drugs. Only the most essential facts are covered. The prescriber is urged to read the *British National Formulary* and/or the Summary of Product Characteristics for each drug at www.medicines.org.uk, particularly for enzyme inducers and inhibitors.

In inadequately controlled focal epilepsy in both men and women, and in generalised epilepsy in women of childbearing potential, lamotrigine may typically be combined with levetiracetam. In poorly controlled generalised epilepsy in men, valproate should be combined with lamotrigine levetiracetam or zonisamide or topiramate or perampanel. More specifically, in problematic myoclonus, valproate may be combined with either levetiracetam or clonazepam. In problematic absence epilepsy, valproate and ethosuximide may be combined. In generalised epilepsy in women of childbearing potential under the age of 55, if seizures remain uncontrolled, zonisamide or clobazam may be added to a lamotrigine and levetiracetam combination. In any woman, including those of childbearing potential, with poorly controlled generalised tonic-clonic seizures, one must consider the use of sodium valproate to minimise seizure related harms (including SUDEP) if alternative ASMs are ineffective. In this instance, in women of childbearing potential, the valproate pregnancy prevention program must be rigorously applied with the use of highly effective contraception.

Beyond these combinations, neurologists will often look to use ASM combinations that combine different mechanisms of action, with choice dictated mainly by expert opinion due to a lack of clinical trial evidence. Combining ASMs with a similar mechanism (e.g., sodium channel) runs the risk of increasing the side effects of that type of ASM. When combining ASMs, careful attention should be paid to the many potential pharmacokinetic interactions (Chapter 9) using online resources and references (Table 25.2) (Patsalos 2013a,b, 2022). Many older ASMs are cytochrome P450 inducers, which cause serum levels of co-medicated ASMs and other medications to fall (usually gradually), with potential loss of therapeutic effect. Other ASMs (valproate, cannabidiol, stiripentol) are enzyme inhibitors and can cause serum levels of co-medicated ASMs to rise, often quickly.

TDM is an important tool in avoiding toxicity, particularly with drugs such as phenytoin, which has a narrow therapeutic window and complex pharmacokinetics. Similarly, interactions with important non-ASMs such as oral contraceptives, anticoagulants and some antibiotics must be borne in mind. Whenever focal seizures remain intractable, a careful review of the MRI should be done to ensure a subtle structural lesion has not been overlooked. These lesions may be amenable to epilepsy surgery after comprehensive assessment.

EMERGENCY HOSPITAL ADMISSIONS

When reviewing a patient admitted with a relapse in seizures, the assessment should start by confirming that epileptic seizures did occur. Common causes of relapse include non-adherence, intercurrent illness (febrile illness or diarrhoea and vomiting), inadequate dosing and alcohol excess. If a patient has experienced prolonged (more than 4 or 5 minutes) tonic-clonic seizures, they, and their carer, should be instructed in the use of home rescue treatment.

For prolonged tonic-clonic seizures in an adult, or serial brief tonic-clonic seizures, over approximately an hour, midazolam should be administered into the buccal cavity. On first use, it is wise to seek medical support until it is known the regimen works. For clusters of focal seizures with recovery or for tonic-clonic seizures spaced apart by hours, clobazam can be offered. The aim of all home rescue plans is to minimise hospitalization.

Antiseizure medications are critical drugs. Extra care should be taken to ensure that during any hospital admission, patients with epilepsy are prescribed their regular medications at the correct dosage and time intervals without interruption. When oral access is not an option, specialist advice should be sought to switch to an alternative administration route or alternative medicine (Bank et al. 2017).

SPECIAL GROUPS

WOMEN WITH EPILEPSY

The treatment of epilepsy in women must consider contraception, conception, pregnancy and lactation as well as menstruation-exacerbated seizures (known as catamenial epilepsy) (Stephen et al. 2019). Several ASMs interact with hormonal contraception, and both epilepsy and ASMs affect reproductive hormones. The most important interactions are:

1. the lowering of lamotrigine levels by oestrogen-containing oral contraceptives

2. the reduced efficacy of all oral contraceptives when taking enzyme-inducing ASMs (carbamazepine and related ASMs, phenytoin, topiramate, perampanel, primidone and phenobarbital).

Individualised advice on the interactions and contraceptive options should be sought from the guidelines produced by the Faculty of Sexual and Reproductive Healthcare (https://www.fsrh.org/standards-and-guidance/). Women with epilepsy may experience seizure exacerbations in the premenstrual or ovulatory phase. Short courses of clobazam at the appropriate time or use of progesterone may help (Feely and Gibson 1984; Maguire and Nevitt 2021).

Epilepsy and ASMs have been reported to affect fertility and sexual function in complex ways in women and men, with some evidence that older enzyme-inducing ASMs and valproate cause more problems (Rathore et al. 2019). Women taking valproate may present with polycystic ovarian syndrome (Isojärvi et al. 1993).

The treatment of epilepsy in pregnancy should be in a multidisciplinary clinic. The risks to mother and unborn child from uncontrolled seizures and the risks to the foetus from the ASM need to be considered (Craig et al. 2021). Confidential inquiries into maternal deaths reveal that pregnancy is a time of elevated risk of SUDEP. Causes include poor adherence to ASM regimes and low levels of ASM due to the pharmacokinetic effects of pregnancy. The risk factors for SUDEP include poorly controlled convulsive seizures, sleep seizures and absence of good preconception advice. These risks should be evaluated with the prospective mother before conception to allow for an individualised plan for pregnancy. A serum ASM level should be taken pre-conception as a guide to monitoring during the pregnancy.

The teratogenic potential of several ASMs, in particular the serious harm caused by valproate, must be assessed (Battino et al. 2024). Recent guidance from the UK MHRA suggests that lamotrigine and levetiracetam show a good safety profile in pregnancy (MHRA 2021). The choices if these two drugs are ineffective are complex and require specialist advice that is beyond the scope of this chapter. Folic acid should be prescribed pre-conception at 5 mg for 3 months during the pregnancy (UK Teratology Information Service 2023).

Serum monitoring of ASMs that undergo a major reduction in serum levels (lamotrigine, levetiracetam, oxcarbazepine) is recommended every 4–8 weeks during the pregnancy by many specialists, even though the only randomised trial on this issue was not clear on the benefits (Thangaratinam et al. 2018). The option of proactive adjustment to lamotrigine and levetiracetam doses from the end of the first trimester with serum monitoring should be discussed with women, especially if a drop of >25% in serum level occurs. After the delivery, the lamotrigine and levetiracetam doses will need reducing over 2–4 weeks if the dose has been increased (Arfman et al. 2020). Generally, breast feeding is encouraged with most ASMs, but close observation of the baby is recommended for those that are sedative and pass extensively in breast milk (clobazam, phenobarbital and ethosuximide).

EPILEPSY IN THE OLDER PERSON

Epilepsy may persist from youth into old age or may start in older life. The incidence of new epilepsy increases with advancing age, is nearly always focal epilepsy and may be particularly prevalent in nursing home residents (Sen et al. 2020). Cerebrovascular disease and dementia are the most common causes. Genetic generalised epilepsies rarely start at this age. Acute asymptomatic seizures are commonly caused by metabolic derangements and alcohol. Diagnosing epilepsy may be particularly difficult in older people who live alone, have cognitive impairments that make taking a seizure history more difficult and have multiple comorbidities to consider before establishing a diagnosis. Excluding cardiac presentations of collapse is vital. The investigation is as in younger adults but focuses on detecting structural brain pathology and less often requires EEG.

Treatment in the older person requires slower drug titrations and lower initial target doses to avoid side effects, with careful consideration of comorbidities (e.g., cardiac, renal) and concomitant medication. Lamotrigine and levetiracetam offer the fewest side effects and are the best drugs to start with (Sen et al. 2020). Frailty, seizures and ASM side effects (bone thinning and impaired balance) all increase the risk of fractures and falls. Risks can be reduced in all age groups by avoiding enzyme-inducing ASMs, monitoring for low mineral bone density and vitamin D deficiency, and treating both as needed (Andersen and Jørgensen 2020).

PEOPLE WITH INTELLECTUAL DISABILITY

A fifth of people with intellectual disability (ID) are diagnosed with epilepsy, with a greater incidence in those with severe intellectual disability. People with ID often present with complex and intractable seizures in the context of other cognitive and neurological impairments (sensory, motor and autism). These difficulties mean that special efforts need to be made to obtain accurate seizure histories, with video evidence being particularly valuable. The occurrence of subtle seizures and non-epileptic behavioural events needs careful evaluation and distinction. Regular attention should be paid to monitoring for side effects of ASMs, which often present as a change in behaviour, mood, appetite or weight. Side effects may be more common in this population because of the use of polytherapy for epilepsy and psychiatric comorbidity.

People with ID may have other health problems that directly affect epilepsy control, for example disordered sleep initiation and obesity. These problems should be regularly discussed, as communication difficulties means people may not directly raise these with the prescriber. None of this should prevent a pro-active approach to treatment in people with ID as it can be just as effective as in those without ID (Kerr et al. 2009). Working together with the community learning disability team is important for holistic management. Reinvestigating patients whose diagnosis was often made before the availability of MRI and genetic technologies can be helpful (Nashef et al. 2019). There is an increased incidence of psychiatric comorbidity that may need multidisciplinary management with psychiatrists with expertise in ID (van Ool et al. 2016; Watkins et al. 2019).

YOUNG PEOPLE IN TRANSITION FROM PAEDIATRICS

When young people with epilepsy aged 16–18 years are referred for transition to an adult service, this is an opportunity to review the diagnosis and consider the individualised prognosis for the epilepsy into adulthood. Cases broadly divide into young people with well-controlled epilepsy and few other impairments, and those with complex needs. For the former, important topics for discussion will include whether life-long treatment is needed, promoting healthy lifestyle with epilepsy, giving advice on adherence, alcohol and drugs, risk taking, contraception, conception, employment, driving and safety. It is important also to detect potentially hidden problems of anxiety, depression, confidence, stigma, bone health and cognitive effects of ASMs.

For those with complex needs, and potentially a lifetime with epilepsy, it is important to develop a therapeutic relationship with the individual and their family. A thorough review of investigations and previously attempted treatments is needed before a plan can be drawn up. In the coming years it is likely that further genomic testing will reveal more personalised approaches for those with severe epilepsy from early life. Current examples are everolimus for tuberous sclerosis (French et al. 2016), ketogenic diet for those with glucose transporter deficiency (Pong et al. 2012) and avoidance of sodium channel drugs and use of rare drugs (stiripentol, cannabidiol and fenfluramine) in those with Dravet syndrome (Andrade et al. 2021).

HOLISTIC CARE

Epilepsy can be a complex and life-long disorder with many facets to its management. The prescriber must become expert in the use and monitoring of common ASMs, and know when to call for help with rarer or novel drugs, or when non-pharmacological treatment (vagal nerve stimulation, epilepsy surgery or ketogenic diet) might be the way forward. At times, a difficult decision must be made that further changes to treatment are meddlesome and will not improve the patient's quality of life. The prescriber should also provide a supportive role, helping to manage comorbidities, mood disorder, anxiety, confidence and morale. Efforts should be made to promote independence, and some patients will need support accessing appropriate government benefits. All of this should be seen within the context of improving the quality of life of people with epilepsy.

STOP AND THINK

In females, how do contraception and childbearing age affect the choice of antiseizure drugs?

SUMMARY

- Epilepsy is a clinical diagnosis made after careful history taking from the patient and witnesses, supported, if possible and safe, by video of seizures made on mobile phones. Magnetic resonance imaging and electroencephalography provide more information, which allows classification of the epilepsy syndrome and aetiology.

- Antiseizure medication (ASM) choice is governed by seizure type, side-effect profile and patient-specific factors such as gender, co-medication and comorbidity.

- The choice of ASM is informed by the results of large, randomised trials. Lamotrigine is the first-line ASM for focal epilepsy in all adults, with levetiracetam as an alternative. Lamotrigine and/or levetiracetam is the first choice for women with generalised epilepsy

- The first-line ASM choice for men aged <55 with generalised epilepsy as of 2024 is contentious, especially in the UK. Sodium valproate has a higher likelihood of seizure freedom, but carries risks of infertility and a potentially greater risk of neurodevelopmental delay in offspring (as of 2024 not yet fully established). The prescriber is urged to be aware of the most up-to-date evidence when counselling patients about treatment choice. In the UK as of February 2024, valproate must not be used in men and women under 55 of childbearing age without specialist advice, and it requires two specialist signatures on a consent form and for women it requires participation in the Valproate Pregnancy Prevention Program. Patients with seizure clusters or prolonged seizures should have access to home rescue treatment with buccal midazolam and/or clobazam.

- The cornerstones of good management are multidisciplinary team working (neurologist and specialist nurse), slow upward titration of the dose of the most appropriate ASM monotherapy, treatment concordance and management of lifestyle factors. Rational polytherapy is used in patients who do not achieve seizure freedom. Referral to a specialist centre should be made in patients who are not seizure-free after trials of two ASMs.

ACTIVITY

1. Which one of the following drugs is a powerful enzyme inducer, associated with a number of key drug interactions?

    (a) Carbamazepine

    (b) Clobazam

    (c) Lamotrigine

    (d) Levetiracetam

    (e) Sodium valproate

2. What pharmacokinetic effect is the combined oral contraceptive likely to have on lamotrigine?

   (a) Decrease in elimination

   (b) Decrease in plasma clearance

   (c) Decrease in volume of distribution

   (d) Increase in plasma half-life

   (e) Increase in plasma clearance

3. Which one of the following is the site of action of carbamazepine?

   (a) AMPA (glutamate) receptor

   (b) Calcium channels

   (c) GABA

   (d) Sodium channels

   (e) SV2a

4. In assessing a patient's complaint of dizziness and unsteadiness during therapy with lamotrigine or carbamazepine, which one of the following tests is most helpful?

   (a) Serum glucose

   (b) Full blood count

   (c) Liver function tests

   (d) Serum drug level

   (e) Urea and electrolytes

5. Which one of the following is an appropriate treatment for the termination of status epilepticus?

   (a) A benzodiazepine (such a midazolam)

   (b) A Z-drug (such as intravenous zoplicone)

   (c) An antipsychotic (such as intramuscular haloperidol)

   (d) An opioid (such as intravenous diamorphine)

   (e) Ketamine

6. In discussing withdrawal of antiseizure treatment, which one of the following is a key consideration?

   (a) During withdrawal, driving should be continued.

   (b) Withdrawal is not possible as therapy is lifelong.

   (c) Withdrawal is usually possible in genetic generalized epilepsy.

   (d) Consideration of the consequences of seizure relapse is as important as estimating the risk of a relapse.

   (e) Withdrawal should be carried out under the cover of a benzodiazepine.

USEFUL WEBSITES

Epilepsy Action. www.epilepsy.org.uk

The Epilepsy Society. www.epilepsysociety.org.uk

REFERENCES

Andersen, N.B. and Jørgensen, N.R. (2022) Impaired bone health as a co-morbidity of epilepsy. *Best Pract Res Clin Rheumatol* 36:Article 101755.

Andrade, D.M. et al. (2021) Dravet syndrome: A quick transition guide for the adult neurologist. *Epilepsy Res* 177:106743.

Arfman, I.J. et al. (2020) Therapeutic drug monitoring of antiepileptic drugs in women with epilepsy before, during, and after pregnancy. *Clin Pharmacokinet* 59:427–445.

Bank, A.M. et al. (2017) What to do when patients with epilepsy cannot take their usual oral medications. *Pract Neurol* 17:66–70.

Battino, D. et al. (2024) Risk of congenital malformations and exposure to antiseizure medication monotherapy. *JAMA Neurol* e240258.

Berg, A.T. (2008) Risk of recurrence after a first unprovoked seizure. *Epilepsia* 49(Suppl 1):13–18.

Berkovic, S.F. and Perucca, E. (2024) Restricting valproate prescribing in men: wisdom or folly? *Pract Neurol* 2024 Epub ahead of print: doi:1136/pn-2024-004097.

Bonnett, L.J. et al. (2022) Risk of seizure recurrence in people with single seizures and early epilepsy: model development and external validation. *Seizure* 94:26–32.

Chaves, J. and Sander, J.W. (2005) Seizure aggravation in idiopathic generalized epilepsies. *Epilepsia* 46 (Suppl 9):133–139.

Craig, J.J., Scott, S. and Leach, J.P. (2021) Epilepsy and pregnancy: identifying risks. *Pract Neurol* 22(2):98–106.

Feely, M. and Gibson, J. (1984). Intermittent clobazam for catamenial epilepsy: tolerance avoided. *J Neurol Neurosurg Psychiatry* 47:1279–1282.

Fisher, R.S. et al. (2005) Epileptic seizures and epilepsy: definitions proposed by the International League Against Epilepsy (ILAE) and the International Bureau for Epilepsy (IBE). *Epilepsia* 46:470–472.

Fisher, R.S. et al. (2014) ILAE official report: a practical clinical definition of epilepsy. *Epilepsia* 55:475–482.

Fisher, R.S. et al. (2017) Operational classification of seizure types by the International League Against Epilepsy: Position Paper of the ILAE Commission for Classification and Terminology. *Epilepsia* 58:522–530.

French, J.A. et al. (2016) Adjunctive everolimus therapy for treatment-resistant focal-onset seizures associated with tuberous sclerosis (EXIST-3): a phase 3, randomised, double-blind, placebo-controlled study. *Lancet* 388:2153–2163.

Gayatri, N.A. and Livingston, J.H. (2006) Aggravation of epilepsy by anti-seizure drugs. *Dev Med Child Neurol* 48:394–398.

Giussani, G. et al. (2023) Sudden unexpected death in epilepsy: a critical review of the literature. Epilepsia Open (2023) 8:728–757.

Isojärvi, J.I. et al. (1993) Polycystic ovaries and hyperandrogenism in women taking valproate for epilepsy. *N Engl J Med* 329:1383–1388.

Kerr, M. et al. (2009) Consensus guidelines into the management of epilepsy in adults with an intellectual disability. *J Intellect Disabil Res* 53:687–694.

Kim, L.G. et al. (2006) Prediction of risk of seizure recurrence after a single seizure and early epilepsy: further results from the MESS trial. *Lancet Neurol* 5:317–322.

Löscher, W. and Klein, P. (2021) The pharmacology and clinical efficacy of antiseizure medications: from bromide salts to cenobamate and beyond. *CNS Drugs* 35:935–963.

Maguire, M.J. and Nevitt, S.J. (2021) Treatments for seizures in catamenial (menstrual-related) epilepsy. *Cochrane Database Syst Rev* 9:CD013225.

Marson, A. et al. (2005) Immediate versus deferred antiepileptic drug treatment for early epilepsy and single seizures: a randomised controlled trial. *Lancet* 365:2007–2013.

Marson, A.G. et al. (2007a) The SANAD study of effectiveness of carbamazepine, gabapentin, lamotrigine, oxcarbazepine, or topiramate for treatment of partial epilepsy: an unblinded randomised controlled trial. *Lancet* 369:1000–1015.

Marson, A.G. et al. (2007b) The SANAD study of effectiveness of valproate, lamotrigine, or topiramate for generalised and unclassifiable epilepsy: an unblinded randomised controlled trial. *Lancet* 369:1016–1026.

Marson, A. et al. (2021a) The SANAD II study of the effectiveness and cost-effectiveness of levetiracetam, zonisamide, or lamotrigine for newly diagnosed focal epilepsy: an open-label, non-inferiority, multi-centre, phase 4, randomised controlled trial. *Lancet* 397:1363–1374.

Marson, A. et al. (2021b) The SANAD II study of the effectiveness and cost-effectiveness of valproate versus levetiracetam for newly diagnosed gener-alised and unclassifiable epilepsy: an open-label, non-inferiority, multicentre, phase 4, randomised controlled trial. *Lancet* 397:1375–1386.

MHRA (2021) Anti-seizure drugs: review of safety of use during pregnancy. Medicines and Healthcare Products Agency (accessed 21 April 2024). https://www.gov.uk/government/publications/public-assessment-report-of-antiepileptic-drugs-review-of-safety-of-use-during-pregnancy/antiepileptic-drugs-review-of-safety-of-use-during-pregnancy

MHRA (2023) Update on new study on risk in chil-dren born to men taking valproate. Medicines and Healthcare Products Agency (accessed 10 April 2024). https://www.gov.uk/government/news/mhra-update-on-new-study-on-risk-in-children-born-to-men-taking-valproate

Nashef, L. et al. (2019) Investigating adults with early-onset epilepsy and intellectual or physical disability. *Pract Neurol* 19:115–130.

NICE Guideline (2022) Epilepsies in children, young people and adults. NICE guidance 217.

Patsalos, P. (2022) *Antiseizure Medication Interactions*, 4th edn. Springer.

Patsalos, P.N. (2013a) Drug interactions with the newer antiepileptic drugs (AEDs). Part 1: Pharmacokinetic and pharmacodynamic interactions between AEDs. *Clin Pharmacokinet* 52:927–966.

Patsalos, P.N. (2013b) Drug interactions with the newer antiepileptic drugs (AEDs). Part 2: Pharmacokinetic and pharmacodynamic interactions between AEDs and drugs used to treat non-epilepsy disorders. *Clin Pharmacokinet* 52:1045–1061.

Pong, A.W. et al. (2012) Glucose transporter type I deficiency syndrome: epilepsy phenotypes and out-comes. *Epilepsia* 53:1503–1510.

Rathore, C. et al. (2019) Sexual dysfunction in people with epilepsy. *Epilepsy Behav* 100(Pt A):106495.

Scheffer, I.E. et al. (2017) ILAE classification of the epi-lepsies: Position Paper of the ILAE Commission for Classification and Terminology. *Epilepsia* 58:512–521.

Sen, A. et al. (2020) Epilepsy in older people. *Lancet* 395:735–748.

Shorvon, S., Perucca, E. and Engel, J. (eds) (2015) *The Treatment of Epilepsy*, 4th edn. Wiley-Blackwell.

Sills, G.J. and Rogawski, M.A. (2020) Mechanisms of action of currently used antiseizure drugs. *Neuropharmacology* 168:107966.

Smith, P.E. (2012) Epilepsy: mimics, borderland and chameleons. *Pract Neurol* 12:299–307.

Stephen, L.J. et al. (2019) Management of epilepsy in women. *Lancet Neurol* 18:481–491.

Thijs, R.D. et al. (2019) Epilepsy in adults. *Lancet* 393:689–701.

Thangaratinam, S. et al. (2018) AntiEpileptic drug Monitoring in PREgnancy (EMPiRE): a double-blind randomised trial on effectiveness and accept-ability of monitoring strategies. *Health Technol Assess* 22:1–152.

UK Teratology Information Service. Uktis.org/official-position-statement-high-dose-folic acid-wwe-cancer. (accessed April 2024). https://uktis.org/monographs/use-of-folic-acid-in-pregnancy/.

van Ool, J.S. et al. (2016) A systematic review of neu-ropsychiatric comorbidities in patients with both epilepsy and intellectual disability. *Epilepsy Behav* 60:130–137.

Watkins, L.V., Pickrell, W.O. and Kerr, M.P. (2019) Treatment of psychiatric comorbidities in patients with epilepsy and intellectual disabilities: Is there a role for the neurologist? *Epilepsy Behav* 98 (Pt B):322–327.

CLINICAL GUIDELINES

NICE Guideline (2022) Epilepsies in children, young people and adults. NICE Guidance 217.

Pain and Analgesia

Roger Knaggs

CHAPTER 26

LEARNING OUTCOMES

By the end of this chapter the reader should be able to:

- define pain and distinguish between different types of pain

- briefly describe the processes involved in pain transmission

- outline the major steps in prostaglandin biosynthesis

- describe the gate control theory of pain and discuss its significance

- describe the basic and clinical pharmacology of simple analgesics, non-steroidal anti-inflammatory drugs and opioids

- explain and apply the principles of the World Health Organization ladder for pain.

Pain, more than many other topics in this book, is something that most, if not all, of us have all experienced. Acute and persistent pain are massive issues throughout the world. A Europe-wide telephone survey suggested that between 12% and 30% of people had persistent pain, defined as pain lasting for longer than 6 months (Breivik et al. 2006) and this causes a great deal of suffering, which in turn affects quality of life. In a more recent systematic review of studies in the UK, Fayaz et al. (2016) reported that between one-third and one-half of the population of the UK experience chronic pain. Before considering the drugs used to control pain in more detail, it is important to think about what pain actually is and how pain signals are transmitted in the body.

WHAT IS PAIN?

Put most simply, pain is what the patient says it is. Unlike many illnesses, there is no biochemical or physiological test that tells us how much pain someone is experiencing. The International Association for the Study of Pain (2020) defines pain as 'An unpleasant sensory and emotional experience associated with, or resembling that associated with, actual or potential tissue damage'. This helpful definition reminds us that pain is usually associated with some form of tissue damage and that although pain is predominantly a sensory phenomenon, emotions contribute to the degree of pain that someone is experiencing. The definition is expanded on by the addition of six key notes to provide valuable context.

- 'Pain is always a personal experience that is influenced to varying degrees by biological, psychological, and social factors.

- Pain and nociception are different phenomena. Pain cannot be inferred solely from activity in sensory neurons.

- Through their life experiences, individuals learn the concept of pain.

- A person's report of an experience as pain should be respected.

The New Prescriber: An Integrated Approach to Medical and Non-medical Prescribing, Second Edition. Edited by Joanne Lymn, Alison Mostyn, Roger Knaggs, Michael Randall, and Dianne Bowskill. © 2024 John Wiley & Sons Ltd. Published 2024 by John Wiley & Sons Ltd.

- Although pain usually serves an adaptive role, it may have adverse effects on function and social and psychological well-being.

- Verbal description is only one of several behaviours to express pain; inability to communicate does not negate the possibility that a human or a nonhuman animal experiences pain.' (International Association for the Study of Pain 2020)

Acute pain is something that we have all experienced and usually signals impending or actual tissue damage, allowing the individual to avoid further injury or to allow tissue healing. Persistent (chronic or long-term) pain is much harder to define. Previously it was defined as pain that lasts for longer than 6 months. More recently, it has been thought of as pain that persists longer than normal healing; usually this is considered to be 3 months.

PAIN PHYSIOLOGY

The processes by which the body understands that someone is in pain can be thought of in a series of steps (Figure 26.1).

PAIN DETECTION

Initially, tissue damage is detected by special pain receptors in nerves (nociceptors). There are different receptor types according to what has caused the injury. This may be because of temperature changes (too hot or cold), mechanical damage (pressure) and chemical changes (as occur in inflammation). The intensity of the pain is influenced by the relative number of nociceptors (some areas of the body, such as the head and neck, have many more than others, the limbs for example) and by the frequency with which nerve impulses are generated by them. Damaged tissue releases many chemicals, including prostaglandins, histamine, bradykinin and serotonin, that increase the sensitivity of the nociceptors and act as mediators of inflammation.

Inflammatory mediators

Prostaglandins are a family of chemicals that are produced by phospholipids, found in the cell membrane of all human cells (Figure 26.2). Initially, arachidonic acid is formed from phospholipids found in cell membranes using the enzyme phospholipase A_2. Arachidonic acid is metabolised

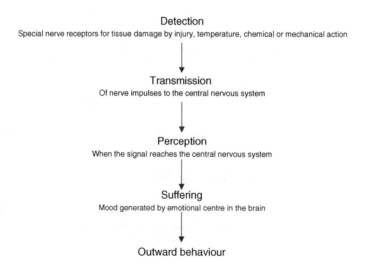

FIGURE 26.1   Physiology of pain.

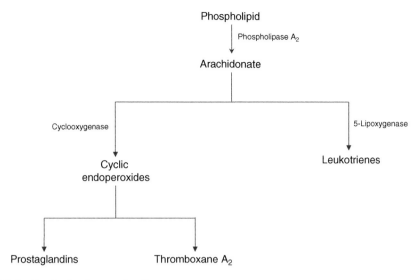

FIGURE 26.2   Synthesis of prostaglandins.

by two enzymes, lipoxygenase and cyclooxygenase (COX), to produce leukotrienes and endoperoxides, respectively. Leukotrienes are inflammatory chemicals causing narrowing of the airways and blood vessels, and increased capillary permeability but have little effect on pain. Prostaglandins and thromboxane A_2 are produced from the very unstable endoperoxides.

Prostaglandins, along with other hormones and chemicals, control many normal physiological functions, including secretion of gastric acid, renal blood flow, salt and water excretion by the kidney, and temperature regulation (Table 26.1). In addition, prostaglandins have been

Table 26.1   Physiological functions of prostaglandins

Prostaglandin	Physiological function
Prostaglandin D_2	Inhibit platelet aggregation
	Vasodilator
	Relaxation of gastrointestinal and uterine smooth muscle
Prostaglandin E_2	Vasodilator
	Increase gastric acid secretion
	Decrease mucus production in stomach
	Control renal blood blow
	Alter Na^+ and water excretion from kidney
	Bronchoconstrictor
Prostaglandin $F_2\alpha$	Bronchoconstrictor
	Myometrial contractions
Prostaglandin I_2	Vasodilator
	Inhibition of gastric acid secretion
	Decrease mucus production in stomach
	Inhibit platelet aggregation
	Control renal blood blow
	Alter Na^+ and water excretion from kidney

Table 26.2   Functions of different forms of COX enzyme

COX-1	COX-2	COX-3
Always present in most cells (constitutive)	Only induced in inflammatory cells	Normally present in the brains of some animals
Required for normal homeostasis	Important in pain and inflammatory states	Involved in sensing pain
• gastrointestinal tract		Little involvement in inflammation
• kidney		Role in humans unclear
• platelet		

found to play an important role in local sensitisation of tissues to inflammatory mediators and pain perception.

In 1991, scientists discovered that two forms of the cyclooxygenase enzyme, named COX-1 and COX-2. COX-1 is present in most tissues and is responsible for maintaining normal homeostasis and tissue function in many organs, such as the gastrointestinal (GI) tract, kidney, lung and platelet. On the other hand, COX-2 is largely associated with inflammatory states (Table 26.2). More recently, another form of the COX enzyme (COX-3) has been found in some animal models. However, the relevance of COX-3 to humans remains unclear (Pickering et al. 2008).

PAIN TRANSMISSION

Once a painful stimulus has been generated, the signals are passed from the area of tissue damage to the spinal cord and ultimately to the brain. Individual nerve fibres covering the same area of skin join to make a single spinal nerve that enters the spinal cord. In the spinal cord these signals are processed before being sent to the brainstem. There is another synapse in the brainstem and a third neuron sends the signal to the cortex, where the brain is able to determine where the pain is coming from (Figure 26.3).

There are relatively few places where drugs may modify transmission of pain signals:

• site of tissue damage or inflammation

• peripheral nerves carrying pain signals

• spinal cord

• brain.

Gate control theory

The gate control theory of pain suggests that the spinal cord has a key role in determining why some people develop persistent pain, and takes into account both the physiological and psychological components of pain. The key principle of gate control theory is that impulses flow from the periphery to the brain through a 'gate' in the spinal cord, which may be opened or closed by other nerve circuits (Figure 26.4).

Put simply, the amount of stimulation passing through the gate is dependent on the relative activities in large-diameter myelinated A-β nerve fibres, smaller diameter A-delta nerve fibres and unmyelinated C nerve fibres. When the amount of information passing through the gate reaches a critical level (i.e., C-fibre activity is greater than A-β fibre and A-delta fibre), there is increased activity in areas of the brain associated with pain and increases in the level of pain that a patient is

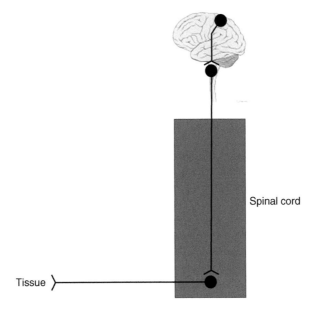

FIGURE 26.3   Pain transmission.

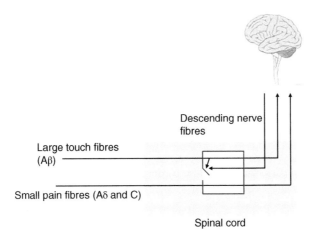

FIGURE 26.4   Gate control theory.

experiencing. The gate is closed by increased stimulation of ascending A-β nerves and descending signals from several brainstem areas.

PAIN PERCEPTION

In the brain there are many nerve pathways that are activated when a painful stimulus is detected. These activate memories of previous painful experiences, interact with the emotional centres in the brain and are modified by cultural influences. The brainstem also probably helps initiate the response of the autonomic nervous system to pain, including the initiation of nervous impulses resulting in muscular contraction so that you move away from the source of the pain.

ANALGESIC PHARMACOLOGY

PARACETAMOL

Paracetamol is regarded as the mainstay analgesic for almost all types of acute and musculoskeletal pain, although there have recent questions raised regarding efficacy and safety for conditions such as low back pain and osteoarthritis (Saragiotto et al. 2019).

Mechanism of action

Despite being used in clinical practice for over 50 years, it is still unclear how paracetamol exerts its pharmacological effect, although it is thought that its mechanism of action is within the central nervous system as it has antipyretic effects (fever reducing) as well as being a painkiller.

Pharmacokinetics

Following oral administration, the bioavailability of paracetamol is around 60%. If given by the rectal route, bioavailability is much lower and much more variable. Therapeutic plasma levels are reached within 30 minutes of oral administration. The elimination half-life of paracetamol is relatively short ($t_{1/2}$ = 2–4 hours), so frequent dosing is required to maintain its analgesic effect.

Paracetamol metabolism and toxicity

With normal doses the majority of paracetamol is metabolised and inactivated in the liver, undergoing a phase II conjugation reaction with glucuronic acid (Figure 26.5). A small proportion of a dose is metabolised using a CYP450-mediated reaction that forms a reactive intermediate, *N*-acetyl-*p*-benzoquinimine (NAPQI). Usually NAPQI can be deactivated by conjugation with glutathione in the liver. However, following ingestion of a large amount of paracetamol, the hepatic stores of both glucuronic acid and glutathione become depleted, leaving free NAPQI to cause liver damage. Toxicity may occur following ingestion of approximately twice the normal daily dose (14–16 paracetamol 500-mg tablets).

STOP AND THINK

Liver damage following paracetamol overdose occurs because the liver's supplies of glutathione are depleted. How is paracetamol overdose treated?

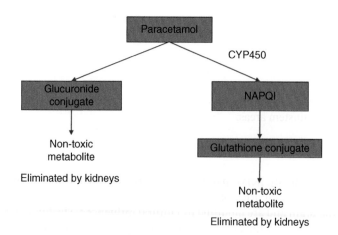

FIGURE 26.5 Paracetamol metabolism in liver. CYP450, cytochrome P450; NAPQI, *N*-acetyl-*p*-aminobenzoquinoimine.

Side effects

Thankfully, given the availability of paracetamol, side effects are uncommon. Occasionally rash, jaundice, blood disorders (such as thrombocyopaenia) or anaphylactic type reactions may occur.

Combination products

There are many over-the-counter preparations and several prescription products that contain paracetamol in addition to other drugs. These must always be considered prior to recommending and/or prescribing a paracetamol product.

PRACTICE APPLICATION

Combination analgesic preparations (e.g., co-codamol and co-dydramol) containing varying amounts of paracetamol and a weak opioid are not recommended for routine prescribing as the opioid content is generally too low to be effective as an analgesic but is sufficient to cause opioid side effects. It is not possible to titrate the doses of the individual component drugs either. Co-proxamol was withdrawn from the UK market in 2007 because it was implicated in a significant number of suicides.

NON-STEROIDAL ANTI-INFLAMMATORY DRUGS

Non-steroidal anti-inflammatory drugs (NSAIDs) are particularly effective in acute pain, such as tension headache and postoperative pain, and where a disease process produces significant inflammation (e.g., rheumatoid arthritis). Commonly prescribed NSAIDs include aspirin (see Chapter 18 for its use as an antiplatelet), ibuprofen and naproxen.

Mechanism of action

NSAIDs are effective painkillers as they inhibit the cyclooxygenase enzyme, responsible for arachidonate metabolism to cyclic endoperoxides (Figure 26.2). By doing this, the production of prostaglandins and thromboxane A_2 is reduced.

STOP AND THINK

Given the normal physiological roles of prostaglandins, what potential side effects of NSAIDs can you predict?

Pharmacokinetics

All NSAIDs are almost completely absorbed after oral absorption, but the rate of absorption may be altered by changes in GI blood flow or motility or if taken with food. Some NSAIDs have been formulated with an enteric coating that is only broken down in the small intestine to reduce the direct irritant effect on the GI mucosa. Most NSAIDs are weak organic acid compounds, so although absorption does begin in the stomach, the majority occurs in the small intestine due to a much-increased surface area.

Following absorption, there is significant binding of NSAIDs to plasma proteins, including albumin (>95% in most cases). Reduction in the amount of serum albumin will result in more unbound drug in the systemic circulation, with potential additional harm. Because there is only a limited amount of plasma proteins, other drugs (e.g., oral anticoagulants such as warfarin) that are also highly bound to plasma proteins may compete for the albumin-binding sites and hence cause drug interactions.

Side effects

The side effects of NSAIDs are produced as a result of decreasing prostaglandin production required for normal body function, particularly in the GI and respiratory systems, kidneys and platelets, and are responsible for a third of hospital admissions for adverse drug reactions. Most of these adverse drug reactions are avoidable as it is possible to predict vulnerable groups and drug interactions (Davis and Robson 2016).

Although effective in conditions in which there is an inflammatory contribution to pain, NSAIDs have serious, potentially fatal, side effects that may be remembered by the acronym GRAB:

G – gastrointestinal: Gastrointestinal side effects are the most common unwanted effects of NSAIDs. These may be non-specific and less serious (e.g., dyspepsia, diarrhoea, nausea and vomiting) or more serious (e.g., ulceration, bleeding, intestinal obstruction).

R – renal: In susceptible individuals, especially the elderly, NSAIDs may cause acute renal failure. Also, NSAIDs alter salt and water homeostasis, which may worsen heart failure and produce a small increase in blood pressure.

A – asthma: NSAIDs, particularly aspirin, may worsen asthma in some patients.

B – blood disorders: All NSAIDs reduce platelet aggregation and increase the risk of bleeding, not just from the GI tract.

Probably the safest NSAID as an analgesic is ibuprofen (200–400 mg three times daily). At higher doses (up to 800 mg three times daily) the incidence of side effects increases to levels similar to other NSAIDs.

STOP AND THINK

What is the underlying mechanism for NSAIDs to worsen control of asthma symptoms?

Cautions and contraindications

NSAIDs should be used with caution in patients with many other conditions.

- Cardiac disease: Patients with hypertension, congestive heart failure, ischaemic heart disease, peripheral arterial disease or cerebrovascular disease need careful assessment before considering NSAID therapy due to an increased risk of thromboembolic events with some NSAIDs. Similar consideration should be made before initiating longer-term treatment of patients with risk factors for cardiovascular events.

- Impaired cardiac or renal function, including patients being treated with diuretics: NSAIDs have the opposite effect to diuretics on salt and water elimination in the kidney, hence acting as physiological antagonists.

- Haematological disorders: Increased risk of bleeding.

- Older people: Increased incidence of GI, renal and cardiac side effects.

- Children under the age of 16 years: Increased chance of developing Reye's syndrome if aspirin is given to children.

- Other contraindications: Due to the potential for side effects, NSAIDs are contraindicated in:

  - active, or history of, GI ulcers, bleeding or perforation

  - previous hypersensitivity reactions (e.g., asthma, angio-oedema, urticaria or acute rhinitis) to ibuprofen, aspirin or other NSAIDs

  - severe hepatic, renal or heart failure

  - pregnancy (especially third trimester).

Routes of administration

NSAIDs have been formulated for administration by a variety of routes. The oral route is the most common and is the preferred route for both acute and long-term administration. If the area of inflammation is relatively localised, a topical NSAID may be considered (NICE 2022). A smaller number of NSAIDs (e.g., diclofenac, ketorolac, parecoxib) have been marketed as injections for parenteral administration, but serious side effects (e.g., abscess formation) have limited their routine use.

COX-2 SELECTIVE DRUGS

COX-2 selective inhibitors, or coxibs, were developed to reduce the GI side effects of NSAIDs. Clinical experience has demonstrated that coxibs are as effective as full NSAID comparators but are no better. GI side effects are reduced but not eliminated completely and hence these drugs are best reserved for patients who have more significant risk factors for a GI bleed.

It now apparent that COX-2 is important in normal physiology as well as pain and that a balance between COX-1 and COX-2 is necessary for optimum NSAID activity. Concern has been expressed about the cardiovascular safety of coxibs, and an increased incidence of myocardial infarction and stroke led to the withdrawal of rofecoxib in September 2004.

Those coxibs still available (celecoxib, etoricoxib) should not be given to patients with established ischaemic heart disease, cerebrovascular disease or symptomatic heart failure. Caution should be exercised if patients have risk factors for developing ischaemic heart disease (hypertension, hyperlipidaemia, diabetes mellitus and smoking).

PRACTICE APPLICATION

- MHRA guidance on NSAID use suggests that the lowest effective dose of NSAID or COX-2 selective inhibitor should be prescribed for the shortest time necessary. The need for long-term treatment should be reviewed periodically.

- Prescribing should be based on the safety profiles of individual NSAIDs or COX-2 selective inhibitors, and on individual patient risk profiles (e.g., GI and cardiovascular).

- Prescribers should not switch between NSAIDs without careful consideration of the overall safety profile of the products and the patient's individual risk factors, as well as the patient's preferences.

- Concomitant aspirin (and possibly other antiplatelet drugs) greatly increases the GI risks of NSAIDs and severely reduces any GI safety advantages of COX-2 selective inhibitors. Aspirin should only be co-prescribed if absolutely necessary.

- Patients at risk of gastric bleed or peptic ulceration should be considered for gastric protection using a proton-pump inhibitor.

OPIOIDS

Opioids have been used for thousands of years although morphine and other active constituents of the opium poppy were only extracted in the early 19th century. An opioid is any substance that produces morphine-like effects.

Opioids traditionally have been classified as either weak or strong (Table 26.3). Weak opioids have a lower analgesic potency, but are capable of producing the same side effects, including constipation and respiratory depression, as more potent opioids.

MECHANISM OF ACTION

The human body has specific protein receptors for naturally occurring opioid compounds (the enkephalins and endorphins) throughout the body. Opioid drugs act by augmenting, or increasing, the effects of the enkephalins and endorphins in the spinal cord and brain. In the spinal cord, opioids prevent the transmission of pain signals through the 'gate' mechanism in the dorsal horn and spinal reflexes. Descending signals from the brainstem back to the spinal cord are also modified.

Three types of opioid receptor have been identified, each contributing to the overall pharmacological effects observed (Table 26.4). Although predominantly found within areas of the central nervous system (CNS) associated with processing of pain signals, opioid receptors are also found in other CNS areas (e.g., those associated with control of breathing and the cough and vomiting reflexes) and other tissues, such as the GI tract.

Table 26.3   Opioid classification

Weak opioids	Strong opioids
Codeine	Morphine
Dihydrocodeine	Oxycodone
Dextropropoxyphene	Fentanyl
Tramadol	Buprenorphine
	Methadone

Table 26.4   Opioid receptor subtypes

Receptor	Site of action	Physiological effects
Mu (OP_3) (u)	Brainstem	Analgesia at spinal level
	Spinal cord	Analgesia at supraspinal level
		Respiratory depression
		Sedation
		Euphoria
		Constipation
Kappa (OP_2) (κ)	Cortex	Analgesia at spinal level
	Brainstem	Sedation
	Spinal cord	
Delta (OP_1) (δ)	Spinal cord	Analgesia
		Alteration of mood

Pharmacokinetics

The physical and chemical properties, and hence pharmacokinetics, of opioids vary considerably. A comprehensive description of the pharmacokinetics of individual opioids is beyond the scope of this book. If information is required, specialist data should be consulted.

Side effects

There are numerous side effects associated with opioids.

- Nausea and vomiting: Brain areas associated with the regulation of vomiting (chemoreceptor trigger zone) can be stimulated when an opioid is given.
- Constipation: Opioids increase smooth muscle tone and reduce motility in the GI tract, leading to constipation. Unlike other side effects, constipation tends to persist with prolonged opioid therapy. Prophylactic treatment with a stimulant laxative (e.g., senna) and stool softener (e.g., docusate sodium) should be considered.
- Sedation: Sedation and drowsiness are common on initiation of opioid therapy and on dose escalation. Most patients develop tolerance to these effects within days to weeks.
- Respiratory depression: Breathing is controlled by several areas in the brainstem. These areas contain opioid receptors and are stimulated when a patient is given an opioid, leading to decreased frequency (i.e., respiratory rate) and depth (i.e., tidal volume) of breathing.
- Hypotension: Opioids cause vasodilatation by reducing the tone of vascular smooth muscle and through local histamine release at the site of administration.
- Urinary retention: Opioids cause urinary retention because of loss of the natural voiding reflex.
- Other problems: Concerns regarding tolerance, dependence and addiction with long-term opioid use continue to trouble public and healthcare professionals alike and sometimes are barriers to effective pain relief.

Cautions and contraindications

Thankfully, there are relatively few cautions and contraindications when using opioids. In the treatment of pain, morphine should be used with caution in the following situations.

- Hypotension: As opioids produce vasodilatation, blood pressure may be lowered further.
- Asthma/COPD, although a relative and not an absolute contraindication. Opioids cause central respiratory depression and may compromise breathing. For patients with existing respiratory disease, this may be problematic.
- Ileus: If large quantities of oral opioid are given in the early postoperative period, significant amounts of morphine may be absorbed from the small intestine when GI transit returns to normal. This has been implicated in deaths in the United Kingdom and other countries.
- Hepatic and/or renal impairment: Empirical dose reduction or conversion to an alternative opioid may be necessary.
- Pregnancy/breastfeeding: Lipophilic opioids may be transferred to the foetus and neonate in substantial quantities.

Routes of administration

Almost all routes of drug delivery have been used at some point with opioids. Patients who experience inadequate pain relief or intolerable side effects with one opioid often may be successfully treated with another opioid or with the same opioid delivered by a different route.

PRACTICE APPLICATION

Common routes of opioid administration include:

- oral (liquid, tablet, capsule)
- rectal
- parenteral (intramuscular, subcutaneous, intravenous)
- transdermal
- buccal
- spinal (epidural, intrathecal).

OTHER ANALGESICS

A wide variety of other drugs (e.g., antidepressants, antiepileptics and muscle relaxants) may have a role in the management of specific types of persistent pain, but this is beyond the scope of this discussion.

PRACTICE APPLICATION

Other drugs used for pain:

- antidepressants (e.g., amitriptyline, nortriptyline)
- antiepileptics (e.g., carbamazepine, gabapentin, pregabalin)
- corticosteroids
- nefopam
- local anaesthetics
- 5-hydroxytryptamine agonists (e.g., sumatriptan)
- capsaicin.

Local anaesthetics, such as lidocaine and bupivacaine, are used most commonly for acute pain management during and after surgery, although there is a lidocaine 5% medicated plaster for postherpetic neuralgia, a type of neuropathic (nerve) pain. They work in excitable tissues by reducing the generation of action potentials blocking voltage-gated sodium channels. In doing so, they inhibit action potentials in nociceptive nerve fibres and so block the transmission of pain impulses. As the binding site on the sodium channel is intracellular, the local anaesthetic must enter the cell to have its effects.

Side effects may occur when there is inadvertent significant systematic absorption. The major tissues affected are the CNS and the cardiovascular system. In the CNS the initial excitatory symptoms include numbness of the tongue, slurred speech and light headedness. If left unnoticed this may progress to drowsiness, tremor and facial twitches before more generalised CNS depression causes coma and respiratory arrest. Blockade of sodium channels in the heart causes depression in myocardial contractility and heart arrythmias.

WORLD HEALTH ORGANIZATION PAIN LADDER

In 1986 the World Health Organization proposed an analgesic ladder for use in cancer pain (Figure 26.6). One of the intentions of developing this ladder was to increase the availability and appropriate use of opioid analgesics in low- and middle-income countries. Although not intended

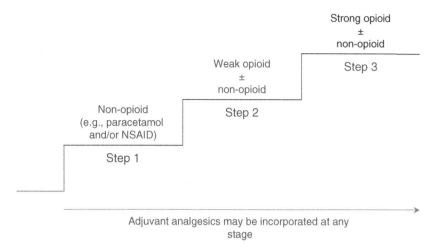

FIGURE 26.6 World Health Organization analgesic ladder. NSAID, non-steroidal anti-inflammatory drug.

for use in other pain conditions, it provides a good basis for safe prescribing in some other types of pain, such as in acute severe postoperative pain, where it may be more appropriate to consider the ladder in reverse.

GUIDANCE

The National Institute for Health and Care Excellence (NICE) has developed guidance on the diagnosis and management of a range of painful conditions, including neuropathic pain, osteoarthritis and low back pain. The guidance emphasises the need for holistic care, the importance of non-pharmacological strategies and the limited role for medicines in managing many types of persistent pain.

SUMMARY

- To feel a painful stimulus requires:
  - detection using specific receptors
  - transmission of the signals to the spinal cord and brain, and
  - interpretation and perception of those signals once they have reached the brain.
- The gate control theory recognises the importance of the spinal cord in interpreting painful stimuli and how physiological and psychological factors contribute to pain.
- Paracetamol is the mainstay of analgesia, although its mechanism of action is not fully understood. To prevent liver and kidney damage, it is important that the maximum recommended dose is followed.
- Non-steroidal anti-inflammatory drugs are effective analgesics, inhibiting the production of the inflammatory prostaglandins. Despite their efficacy, side effects are relatively common and must be monitored.
- Opioids interact with specific opioid receptors.
- The World Health Organization pain ladder provides a step-wise approach to analgesic use.

ACTIVITY

For each of the statements 1–10 choose the most appropriate option from A to L. Each option may be used once, more than once or not at all.

Options

A	Morphine	B	Dihydrocodeine
C	Ibuprofen	D	Amitriptyline
E	Gabapentin	F	Paracetamol
G	Glyceryl trinitrate	H	Aspirin
I	Buprenorphine	J	Tramadol
K	Diamorphine	L	Oxycodone

1. A drug that should not be given to children under the age of 16 due to the risk of Reye's syndrome.

2. A drug that treats the pain associated with angina pectoris.

3. A drug that would be appropriate to reduce fever in a 10-year-old boy.

4. A drug that would be appropriate to prevent further ischaemic events in a 65-year-old woman who has recently suffered a myocardial infarction.

5. An opioid drug used in the immediate treatment of a myocardial infarction.

6. A drug that would be appropriate to treat a 36-year-old man suffering from tennis elbow.

7. An opioid that is formulated for transdermal administration.

8. An opioid drug that is contraindicated in epilepsy.

9. An antiepileptic drug used in the management of neuropathic pain.

10. An opioid used almost exclusively in palliative care because of high water solubility that allows smaller volumes to be infused by the subcutaneous route.

REFERENCES

Breivik, H., Collett, B., Ventafridda, V., et al. (2006) Survey of chronic pain in Europe: prevalence, impact on daily life, and treatment. *Eur J Pain* 10:287–333.

Davis, A. and Robson J. (2016) The dangers of NSAIDs: look both ways. *Br J Gen Prac* 66:172–173.

Fayaz, A., Croft, P., Langford, R.M., et al. (2016) Prevalence of chronic pain in the UK: a systematic review and metaanalysis of population studies. *BMJ Open* 6:e010364. doi: 10.1136/bmjopen-2015-010364

NICE (2022) Osteoarthritis in over 16s: diagnosis and management. NICE guideline [NG226]. https://www.nice.org.uk/guidance/ng226.

Pickering, G., Estève, V., Loriot, M.A., Eschalier, A. and Dubray, C. (2008) Acetaminophen reinforces descending inhibitory pain pathways. *Clin Pharmacol Ther* 84:47–51.

Raja, S.N., Carr, D.B., Cohen, M., et al. (2020). The revised International Association for the Study of Pain definition of pain: concepts, challenges, and compromises. *Pain* 161:1976–1982.

Saragiotto, B.T., Abdel Shaheed, C. and Maher, C.G. (2019) Paracetamol for pain in adults. *BMJ* 367:l6693. doi: 10.1136/bmj.l6693

USEFUL WEBSITES

British National Formulary (online). BMJ Group and Pharmaceutical Press, London. https://bnf.nice.org.uk/.

NICE. Scenario: NSAIDs – prescribing issues. https://cks.nice.org.uk/topics/nsaids-prescribing-issues/management/nsaids-prescribing-issues/.

Medicines & Healthcare products Regulatory Agency guidance on the use of coxibs and NSAIDs. www.mhra.gov.uk/Safetyinformation/General safetyinformationandadvice/Product-specificinformationandadvice/CardiovascularsafetyofCOX-2inhibitorsandnon-selectiveNSAIDs/CON019582.

CLINICAL GUIDANCE

NICE (2020) Low back pain and sciatica in over 16s: assessment and management. NICE guideline [NG59]. https://www.nice.org.uk/guidance/ng59.

NICE (2020) Neuropathic pain in adults. Pharmacological management in non-specialist settings. Clinical guideline [CG173]. https://www.nice.org.uk/guidance/cg173.

NICE (2022) Osteoarthritis in over 16s: diagnosis and management. NICE guideline [NG226]. https://www.nice.org.uk/guidance/ng226.

NICE (2021) Perioperative care in adults. NICE guideline [NG180]. https://www.nice.org.uk/guidance/ng180.

NICE (2021) Chronic pain (primary and secondary) in over 16s: assessment of all chronic pain and management of chronic primary pain. NICE guideline [NG193]. https://www.nice.org.uk/guidance/ng193

NICE (2021) Headaches in over 12s: diagnosis and management. NICE guideline [CG150]. https://www.nice.org.uk/guidance/cg150.

NICE (2022) Medicines associated with dependence or withdrawal symptoms: safe prescribing and withdrawal management for adults. NICE guideline [NG215]. https://www.nice.org.uk/guidance/ng215.

FURTHER READING

Dickenson, A.H. (2002) Gate control theory stands the test of time. *Br J Anaesth* 88:755–777.

Melzack, R. and Wall, P.D. (1965) Pain mechanisms: a new theory. *Science* 150:971–979.

Ritter, J.M., Flower, R., Henderson, G., et al. (2023) *Rang and Dale's Pharmacology*, 10th edn. Elsevier, Amsterdam.

Royal College of Surgeons of England and the College of Anaesthetists. (1990) *The Commission on the Provision of Surgical Services. Report of the Working Party*. Royal College of Surgeons, London.

Schug, S.A., Scott, D.A., Mott, J.F., et al. (2020) *Acute Pain Management: Scientific Evidence*, 5th edn. ANZCA & FPM, Melbourne.

Twycross, R., Wilcock, A. and Stark Toller, C. (2021) *Introducing Palliative Care*, 6th edn. Royal Pharmaceutical Society, London.

Wilcock, A., Howard, P. and Charlesworth, S. (2022) *Palliative Care Formulary*, 8th edn. Royal Pharmaceutical Society, London.

CHAPTER 27

Drugs of Misuse

Michael Randall

LEARNING OUTCOMES

By the end of this chapter the reader should be able to:

- describe types of commonly misused drugs, including cannabinoids, cocaine, ketamine and opioids
- describe non-therapeutic drugs of misuse, for example alcohol and nicotine
- describe the mechanisms of drug addiction, including tolerance and dependence
- understand the health risks of drug addiction
- describe the principles of treatment for addiction.

Whilst drugs have many medicinal uses, some medicinal and non-medicinal drugs are also subject to misuse. Drug abuse (or substance misuse disorder) has far-reaching consequences for the individual, their family and friends, and also societal impacts. In most countries there are laws and categories of drugs of misuse, designed to reduce the access and limit the impact of drugs of misuse, with criminal penalties associated with the use or supply of drugs.

There are a number of psychoactive drugs, such as cannabinoids, cocaine and opioids, that are well recognised as drugs of misuse. However, the recreational use of alcohol and nicotine is probably far more widespread and associated with significant harm to health. Indeed, Nutt et al. (2010) carried out an analysis of harm due to drugs and identified alcohol as being associated with the greatest harm. One could also argue that nicotine through smoking-related cancers and respiratory and cardiovascular diseases is associated with the highest level of mortality; 50% of smokers die from smoking-related disease.

PRACTICE APPLICATION

Always ask patients about their consumption of alcohol and nicotine. Patients should be asked their smoking history, whether they are current smokers, ex-smokers or never smoked. Patients who are current smokers should be offered advice and support around smoking cessation (NICE 2018).

CLASSIFICATION OF DRUGS OF MISUSE

In the UK, there are currently several legal categories of controlled drugs:

Class A: includes opioids (e.g., morphine, diamorphine), cocaine, Ecstasy (3,4-methylenedioxy methamphetamine, MDMA), methamphetamine, lysergic acid diethylamide (LSD)

Class B: includes weak opioids (e.g., codeine), cannabis, amphetamine, ketamine

Class C: includes benzodiazepines (e.g., diazepam), gabapentin, pregabalin, the opioid buprenorphine.

The New Prescriber: An Integrated Approach to Medical and Non-medical Prescribing, Second Edition.
Edited by Joanne Lymn, Alison Mostyn, Roger Knaggs, Michael Randall, and Dianne Bowskill.
© 2024 John Wiley & Sons Ltd. Published 2024 by John Wiley & Sons Ltd.

The legal class signifies the control and legal consequences of their use, with Class A being the highest and Class C the lowest category. Chapter 3 considers the law and prescribing of controlled drugs.

ADDICTION, DEPENDENCE AND TOLERANCE

Many drugs of misuse are abused because of their initial euphoric effects. This is often via the stimulation of the nervous system and is often associated with the 'dopamine reward' pathway. Rapid administration via inhalation or the intravenous route leads to a more rapid effect associated with drug misuse. The euphoric effects and the body's response to the drug are associated with addiction. Addiction is a state where the person no longer has control over their drug use and it is harmful.

Drug use, to varying degrees, can show dependence, where the individual develops the need or craving to repeat the consumption and for some drugs (e.g., opioids) this is due to profound and unpleasant withdrawal reactions.

Tolerance means that higher doses are required to exert the same pharmacological effect as that seen in naïve individuals as they start to abuse. Tolerance can be pharmacodynamic, where the drug receptors become downregulated by regular stimulation and/or reduced coupling to second messenger systems. In the case of alcohol, tolerance can also be pharmacokinetic, with induction of the metabolic enzymes for alcohol metabolism, leading to increased clearance.

CANNABINOIDS

Cannabis, derived from *Cannabis sativa*, has been used for millennia. It contains over 60 cannabinoids, of which $\Delta 9$-tetrahydrocannabinol (THC) is the main psychoactive ingredient. The main effect of cannabis is to lead to mild euphoria and is thought to be mediated via cannabinoid receptors (such as the CB_1 receptor). Cannabinoids have been widely researched over the past three decades, with the identification of endogenous lipids such as anandamide. The medicinal potential of cannabinoids has been widely explored and cannabis extract is licenced in the UK for spasticity associated with multiple sclerosis and cannabidiol for seizures associated with Lennox–Gastaut and Davet syndromes.

In recent years, synthetic cannabinoids such as 'Spice' have been commonly abused, leading to severe effects including catatonia, paranoia and psychosis. There is also concern that cannabinoid use in younger subjects and those with a history of psychosis may uncover schizophrenia.

OPIOIDS

Opioids were originally derived from the opium poppy and have a long history of misuse. Morphine is the archetypal opioid and heroin (or diamorphine) is a more water-soluble synthetic derivative. Opioids have major roles in pain management (Chapter 26) and palliative care, but are common drugs of misuse. Heroin is commonly smoked or injected intravenously to give a rapid 'rush' or euphoria. The pharmacological effects of opioids are mediated via opioid receptors (μ, δ, κ), which are responsible for their medicinal properties in analgesia but also their euphoric (μ) and hallucinogenic (κ) effects.

Opioids are highly addictive, with profound withdrawal reactions (cravings, diarrhoea, goose bumps) on stopping and this reinforces or maintains their misuse. Opioid use also leads to tolerance, where repeated use results in high doses being needed for the same pharmacological and euphoric effect. Opioid overdose can occur and is associated with respiratory depression, which can be managed by administration of the opioid receptor antagonist naloxone. Intravenous administration of opioids carries the risk of blood-borne viruses, including the human immunodeficiency virus (HIV) and hepatitis C.

COCAINE

Cocaine is derived from coca leaves and has a long history of use as a local anaesthetic and misuse. Cocaine is often 'snorted' or injected and when used as the free base is referred to as 'crack'. Cocaine blocks the reuptake of noradrenaline, dopamine and 5-hydroyxtryptamine in the peripheral and central nervous systems, leading to euphoria and a range of peripheral effects, including raised blood pressure, tachycardia and dilated pupils.

KETAMINE

Ketamine is a dissociative anaesthetic, which leads to analgesia with amnesia. Ketamine is now a drug of misuse leading to dissociative euphoria or 'out of body' experiences. Ketamine is an *N*-methyl-D-aspartate receptor (NMDA) antagonist.

LYSERGIC ACID DIETHYLAMIDE

LSD is a hallucinogenic drug that changes sensory perception and emotions. LSD has a complex action, acting as an agonist at dopamine D_2 receptors and a range of 5-hydroxytryptamine receptors and is thought to lead to excitation via glutamate release.

AMPHETAMINES

Amphetamines are central nervous system stimulants by causing the release of noradrenaline and dopamine.

'ECSTASY', 3,4-METHYLENEDIOXY METHAMPHETAMINE

MDMA has both psychedelic and stimulatory effects via the release of neurotransmitters, noradrenaline, dopamine and 5-hydroxytryptamine. Hyperthermia is a rare but potentially fatal unpredictable adverse effect of MDMA.

SOME OTHER THERAPEUTIC DRUGS SUBJECT TO POTENTIAL ABUSE

In addition to opioids, other prescribed medicines are subject to potential misuse. Benzodiazepines were widely used long-term for anxiety until the 1980s, when their addiction potential and withdrawal reactions were first more widely recognised. Their use is now limited to short-term therapy for 2–4 weeks. The action of benzodiazepines is to enhance the actions of the inhibitor neurotransmitter γ-aminobutyric acid (GABA).

The anticonvulsant drugs gabapentin and pregabalin (gabapentinoids) (Chapters 25 and 26) also have abuse potential, with highs and euphoric states, and their misuse appears to have significantly increased.

ALCOHOL

Alcohol has been widely used and misused over millennia. It is a social and cultural norm in some societies and illegal in other communities. Alcohol has depressant effects via reduced release of GABA and disinhibition, which initially leads to excitatory effects prior to depressant effects. Alcohol is widely used and in the UK the recommendation is not to consume more than 14 units of alcohol a week (where one unit is a small glass of wine, a single measure of spirits or half a pint of weak beer), that individuals should have two or three alcohol-free days and to avoid binges. Alcohol should not be consumed at all during pregnancy due to its harmful effects on the foetus (foetal alcohol syndrome). In addition to societal impact, long-term alcohol misuse is associated with alcoholic liver disease, including cirrhosis of the liver and an increase in some cancers (including oesophageal). Suicide is also more prevalent in individuals who misuse alcohol.

Alcohol is associated with tolerance and dependence. In alcohol dependence, there can be withdrawal reactions, including 'the shakes' (delirium tremens) through to convulsions.

NICOTINE

Tobacco is commonly smoked in cigarettes, cigars or pipes, taken as snuff or inhaled in vapours via electronic cigarettes. Nicotine is a highly addictive drug that reinforces the need to maintain the habit. Smoking tobacco is extremely harmful, with the carcinogenic tars being linked to lung cancer but also a range of cancers including mouth, oesophagus, and bladder. Added to this, more than 90% of cases of chronic obstructive pulmonary disease are smoking-related and smoking is the largest modifiable risk factor for cardiovascular disease.

PERFORMANCE-ENHANCING DRUGS

A number of therapeutic and non-therapeutic drugs are misused with the intention of enhancing physical performance. Certain anabolic steroids, such as stanozolol and nandrolone, are taken with the aim of their catabolic effects enhancing muscle build up. The use of these anabolic steroids is associated with a range of significant side effects, including behavioural changes such as aggression.

Erythropoietin (EPO), the endogenous hormone which stimulates the production of red blood cells, has been widely used for a number of years, with the intention that an increase in red cell count will enhance oxygen delivery to muscle.

Stimulants, such as sympathomimetics found in common cold remedies, are banned in sports due to their ability to enhance performance. In other sports where fine control is required, β-blockers have been used to control tremor. UK Anti-Doping (www.ukad.uk) provides clear guidance on the prohibition and use of drugs in sport.

TREATMENT OF DRUG ADDICTION

Given the health and societal consequences of drug misuse and addiction, there are a range of therapeutic approaches that can be helpful in helping overcoming addiction. Some pharmacological approaches help to overcome cravings and withdrawal reactions.

SUPPORT FOR OPIOID ABUSE

The use of synthetic oral opioids (such as methadone) is a common approach to help support withdrawal. These oral opioids are commonly prescribed to help support patients with opioid addiction and are provided in pharmacies for supervised dosing. In addition, the oral opioid means that the patient is no longer at risk of blood-borne infections associated with needle sharing and intravenous drug use.

Other approaches involve using the opioid receptor antagonist naltrexone once the person is detoxified from opioid use, otherwise there is a risk of precipitating a withdrawal reaction if the patient is still taking opioids. This opposes the actions of the opioid and so the person no longer experiences euphoria and the misuse potential is reduced.

STOP AND THINK

Buprenorphine is a partial opioid agonist that is increasingly used in opioid substitution treatment. What effects would you expect it to have in a person who was taking other opioids?

NICOTINE THERAPY

Nicotine is highly addictive and support for nicotine addiction can be found through giving nicotine via patches, gum, lozenges or inhalers to reduce the craving and to prevent the damage due to smoking. In the last decade, electronic cigarettes that deliver nicotine in a vapour have been advocated as supporting nicotine addiction. However, this is controversial as there is no long-term evidence of the effects of the vapours on the lungs and there is some evidence of lung damage.

Bupropion is an atypical antidepressant that has also been found to be beneficial in nicotine addiction.

STOP AND THINK

Should you or should you not recommend e-cigarettes to promote smoking cessation?

ALCOHOL DEPENDENCE

There are several approaches to support patients who abuse alcohol. Chronic alcohol consumption is associated with vitamin deficiencies and patients are routinely given vitamin B_6 and thiamine to prevent this. To help support alcohol dependence, benzodiazepines such as chlordiazepoxide are often used to help minimise the withdrawal reactions. Benzodiazepines are also associated with dependency and so their use is restricted over a number of days, with a reducing regimen forming the basis of many protocols.

To prevent patients from actually drinking alcohol, the drug disulfiram is sometimes used. Disulfiram is an inhibitor of aldehyde dehydrogenase, and so the metabolism of alcohol is incomplete, leading to the accumulation of the toxic aldehyde metabolite. If alcohol is consumed whilst taking disulfiram, the patient has a severe reaction of nausea, flushing, hypotension and weakness, resulting in the patient avoiding alcohol. Other measures include using acamprosate antagonist (an NMDA receptor antagonist) and oral naltrexone (an opioid receptor antagonist). Naltrexone acts by reducing the effects of endogenous opioids released in response to alcohol.

SUMMARY

- Drug misuse disorder is associated with significant harm to the individual and society.
- There are several drugs that are open to misuse because of their ability to exert powerful central nervous system effects, which, depending on the drug, may include euphoria and altered perception.
- Nicotine and opioids are associated with the greatest addiction potential.
- The dopamine reward system is one mechanistic theory to explain the pleasurable effects of drug misuse disorders.
- Repeated drug use may be associated with tolerance and dependence.
- Many pharmacological approaches to help support drug use disorder are available.

ACTIVITY

1. The cannabis or the cannabinoid system has which one of the following features?

    (a) Anandamide is the endogenous ligand.

    (b) Cannabinoids are all highly addictive.

(c) Cannabinoids do not have therapeutic uses.

(d) Cannabis is used injected intravenously.

(e) Δ9-tetrahydrocannabinol is a cannabinoid receptor antagonist.

2. Which ONE of the following opposes the actions of opioids?

(a) Codeine

(b) Loperamide

(c) Naloxone

(d) Nandrolone

(e) Nicotine

3. Which ONE of the following describes the pharmacology of ketamine?

(a) It is a selective μ-opioid receptor agonist.

(b) It is a serotonin selective reuptake inhibitor.

(c) It is a sympathomimetic.

(d) It is a GABA modulator.

(e) It is an NMDA receptor antagonist.

4. Which ONE of the following is helpful in mitigating the adverse effects of alcohol withdrawal?

(a) Benzodiazepines

(b) Carbamazepine

(c) Disulfiram

(d) Neuromuscular blockers

(e) Opioids

REFERENCES

NICE (2018) Stop smoking interventions and services. NICE guideline NG92.

Nutt, D.J., King, L.A. and Phillips, L.D. (2010) Drug harms in the UK: a multicriteria decision analysis. *Lancet* 376:1558–1565.

FURTHER READING

Brunton, L. and Knollmann, B. (2022) *Goodman and Gilman's The Pharmacological Basis of Therapeutics*, 14th edn. McGraw Hill, New York.

Ritter, J.M., Flower, R., Henderson, G., et al. (2023) *Rang and Dale's Pharmacology*, 10th edn. Elsevier, Amsterdam.

Tracy, D.K., Wood, D.M. and Baumeister, D. (2017) Novel psychoactive substances: types, mechanisms of action, and effects. *BMJ* 356:i6848.

CLINICAL GUIDELINES

NICE (2012) Drug use disorders in adults. NICE Quality Standard QS23.

NICE (2018) Stop smoking interventions and services. NICE guideline NG92.

USEFUL WEBSITES

UK Anti-Doping. http://www.ukad.uk.

Antibacterial Chemotherapy

Tim Hills

LEARNING OUTCOMES

By the end of this chapter the reader should be able to:

- understand the difference between Gram-positive and Gram-negative bacteria

- understand the difference between anaerobic and aerobic bacteria

- understand the difference between bactericidal and bacteriostatic action

- understand what is meant by broad- and narrow-spectrum antimicrobials

- describe the four principal mechanisms of action of antibacterial agents and suggest examples of classes of drugs that utilise these mechanisms

- describe the principal clinical uses of major classes of antibiotics.

GENERAL PRINCIPLES OF ANTIMICROBIAL CHEMOTHERAPY

Antimicrobials act by exploiting the differences between how microorganisms and mammalian cells function to either kill or inactivate the microorganism without harming us. This is called selective toxicity.

BACTERIAL CLASSIFICATION

Bacteria are prokaryotes or single-celled organisms that contain proteins and genetic information (in the form of RNA and DNA). The DNA is generally confined to a central region, known as the nucleoid, but is not contained within a membrane. Bacteria are surrounded by a cell wall and sometimes a capsule. Bacteria can be described in terms of their cell wall structure, shape and oxygen requirements. Classification is important as some antibiotics affect only certain types of bacteria.

Gram stain

Gram staining is a basic laboratory staining process performed on most grown cultures. It separates bacteria into two groups (Gram positive and Gram negative) depending on their cell wall structure (Figure 28.1). Gram-positive bacteria have cell walls which contain more peptidoglycan than Gram-negative bacteria and it is this additional peptidoglycan that allows these bacteria to take up the crystal violet stain so the cells appear deep purple. Gram-negative cell walls have less peptidoglycan so stain poorly; they are viewed by the addition of a counterstain to give a red colour.

The New Prescriber: An Integrated Approach to Medical and Non-medical Prescribing, Second Edition.
Edited by Joanne Lymn, Alison Mostyn, Roger Knaggs, Michael Randall, and Dianne Bowskill.
© 2024 John Wiley & Sons Ltd. Published 2024 by John Wiley & Sons Ltd.

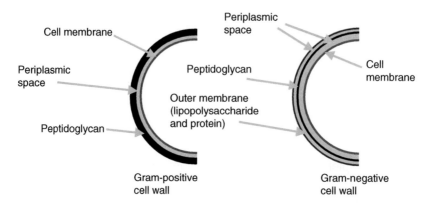

FIGURE 28.1   The differences in cell wall structure between a Gram-positive and a Gram-negative bacterium. Note the thicker peptidoglycan layer in the Gram-positive cell and the additional outer membrane in Gram-negative cells.

Cell shape and arrangement

The shape of a bacterium can give you a hint of what it might be. The majority of bacterial cells are shaped like a grape (cocci) or are more cylindrical (rods or bacilli). Cocci can be arranged in pairs (e.g., *Neisseria* species), chains (e.g., *Streptococcus* species) or clusters, like a bunch of grapes (e.g., *Stapylococcus* species).

Aerobic/anaerobic

Cultures are grown in the presence and absence of oxygen. Some bacteria prefer, or only grow in, conditions either containing oxygen (aerobic) or that are oxygen free (anaerobic).

These initial tests give the microbiologist an idea of what the bacteria involved might be (Table 28.1). They allow an informed decision about the appropriateness of empirical therapy before a definitive identification is made.

Further tests

The bacteria are grown on various selective media and/or are subjected to various tests that can further differentiate them into species (e.g., *Streptococcus*) and make a formal identification (e.g., *Streptococcus pyogenes*). They are also cultured with antibiotic discs to see if they inhibit bacterial growth and identify which antibiotics can be used to treat the infection (sensitivities) and to determine the lowest concentration of an antibiotic that will inhibit the bacteria's growth (minimum inhibitory concentration [MIC]).

Choosing empirical antibiotic therapy

There are a number of factors which should be considered when deciding which antibiotics to use and these can be remembered using the acronym CLEFS:

- *Cost*: Whilst it may be less important, if the differences between antibiotics are small, cost should be considered.

- *Local resistance patterns*: Different hospitals will have different problems, particularly in units that use many antibiotics (e.g., haematology units, intensive care units), and hospital policies will vary.

- *Environment*: What are the likely bugs in this environment? Is this a hospital- or community-acquired infection? What is the risk of methicillin-resistant *Staphylococcus aureus* (MRSA)? How severe is the disease?

Table 28.1 Bacterial classification by Gram stain, shape and aerobic/anaerobic nature

Gram positive				Gram negative			
Cocci		Bacilli		Cocci		Bacilli	
Aerobic	**Anaerobic**	**Aerobic**	**Anaerobic**	**Aerobic**	**Anaerobic**	**Aerobic**	**Anaerobic**
Staphylococcus spp.	Peptostreptococcus	Listeria	Clostridioides spp.	Neisseria	Rare	Pseudomonas spp.	Bacteroides
Streptococcus Pneumoniae						Escherichia coli.	
						'coliforms'	
						Legionella	

- *Patient factors*: These are comorbidity (e.g., myasthenia gravis, epilepsy) and other medication/interactions (erythromycin/rifampicin). What routes of administration are available? Is the patient pregnant or breastfeeding?

- *Site*: The antibiotics chosen must be able to penetrate the area where the infection occurs.

Most of the hard work will be done for you. Microbiologists and local experts will consider the factors above when producing your local acute/primary care trust guidelines. If you plan to prescribe antibiotics, it is essential that you obtain your trust's antibiotic guidelines.

STOP AND THINK

What route of administration would be most appropriate for a deep-seated infection (e.g., bone and joint infection, endocarditis) that requires high blood levels for effective antibiotic penetration and treatment?

ANTIBIOTICS: KEY DESCRIPTIONS

Before moving on to the mechanism of action of antibiotics, it is necessary to describe a few key terms that are important in antimicrobial chemotherapy.

Does the antibiotic kill bacteria or stop their growth?

Bactericidal antibiotics kill the bacteria while *bacteriostatic* antibiotics stop bacterial growth, thus allowing host defences to kill them. Generally, these differences do not matter. There are situations where bactericidal antibiotics may potentially be superior, however, and these include where the host defences are compromised (e.g., neutropenia) and when the host defences struggle to get to the site of the infection (e.g., central nervous system, endocarditis).

How does drug concentration affect efficacy? (Figure 28.2)

- *Time-dependent killing (time > MIC)*: The time for which the antibiotic concentration is above the MIC is the most important. How high above the MIC does not make a lot of difference (e.g., penicillins).

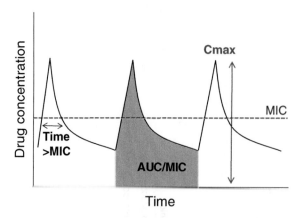

FIGURE 28.2 An example of a drug concentration against time graph for three drug doses. AUC, area under the curve; C_{max}, maximum drug serum concentration; MIC, minimum inhibitory concentration.

- Concentration-dependent killing (C_{max}): C_{max} is the maximum serum drug concentration gained during the dosing interval. The greater the concentration above the MIC, the more effective the bactericidal effect, but the duration for which the concentration remains high is less important (e.g., aminoglycosides).

- *Area under the curve divided by the MIC (AUC/MIC)*: Most antibiotic classes fit into this group the best. Here a mixture of concentration- and time-dependent aspects is important for efficacy.

Spectrum of activity

You may have heard of 'broad-spectrum' and 'narrow-spectrum' antibiotics. What this means exactly is not strictly defined but the broader the spectrum, the more species of bacteria the antibiotic can treat. Usually a broad-spectrum antibiotic would be able to treat a range of Gram-positive and Gram-negative organisms.

PRACTICE APPLICATION

The use of empirical broad-spectrum antibiotics is essential when the patient is septic and the range of possible pathogens is wide (e.g., ventilator-associated pneumonia). It is usually possible to change to more targeted narrow-spectrum therapy once the culture results are available.

MECHANISM OF ACTION OF ANTIBACTERIAL DRUGS

There are four key mechanisms of action employed by antibacterial drugs, all of which are based around the concept of selective toxicity. The main pharmacodynamic properties of the major classes of antibiotics are summarised in Table 28.2.

INHIBITION OF CELL WALL SYNTHESIS

Bacterial cells all have a cell wall while mammalian cells do not, making this an ideal target for antibacterial therapy. Peptidoglycan is a major constituent of many bacterial cell walls. It consists of polysaccharide chains with peptide cross-links and provides structure and strength to the cell (Figure 28.3). As mammalian cells do not contain peptidoglycan, antibiotics that target its formation will have selective toxicity.

Peptidoglycan synthesis is inhibited by β-lactam antibiotics (penicillins and cephalosporins) and glycopeptides (vancomycin).

β-lactam antibiotics

The β-lactam ring is the core active component for a number of antibiotics with various properties and spectra, including penicillins, cephalosporins, monobactams and carbapenems.

The mechanism of action of these antibiotics is related to the β-lactam ring itself. This acts as a false substrate for a bacterial transpeptidase enzyme (penicillin-binding protein [PBP]), which is involved in the final peptide cross-links of the peptidoglycan in the bacterial cell wall. The β-lactam ring mimics the structure of the natural substrate of PBP. While the bond between PBP and its natural substrate is temporary, β-lactam antibiotics form an irreversible bond, neutralising the transpeptidase enzyme and interrupting peptidoglycan synthesis, leading to cell lysis.

Penicillins

No other antibiotic class has been more important than penicillins, which were discovered by Sir Alexander Fleming in 1928. Benzylpenicillin (penicillin G) and the orally active

Table 28.2 A summary of the major antibiotic classes with example drugs and main pharmacodynamic features

Class	Examples	Action	Effect	Notes
Aminoglycosides	Gentamicin Tobramycin	Inhibit ribosomal protein synthesis.	Bactericidal	Synergy with antibiotics that act on cell walls, antagonised by bacteriostatic agents (e.g., tetracycline, chloramphenicol)
Carbapenems	Imipenem Meropenem	Inhibit peptidoglycan formation in cell wall	Bactericidal	8% cross-over allergy risk with penicillin-allergic patients
Cephalosporins	Cefuroxime Ceftriaxone	Inhibit peptidoglycan formation in cell wall	Bactericidal	2-16% cross-over allergy risk (often quoted as 10%) with penicillin-allergic patients
Glycopeptides	Vancomycin Teicoplanin	Inhibit peptidoglycan formation in cell wall	Bactericidal (bacteriostatic at low concentration)	
Macrolides	Clarithromycin Erythromycin	Inhibit ribosomal protein synthesis.	Bacteriostatic except at high concentration	Competes in binding on the ribosome with chloramphenicol, streptogamins and lincosamides, antagonistic and cross-resistance
Nitrofurantoin and nitroimidazoles	Nitrofurantoin Metronidazole	Free-radical damage to DNA, RNA and proteins	Probably bactericidal	Only useful for urinary tract infections (excluding pyelonephritis)
Quinolones	Ciprofloxacin Levofloxacin	Inhibit topoisomerases and DNA replication	Bactericidal	
Penicillins	Benzylpenicillin Amoxicillin	Inhibit peptidoglycan formation in cell wall	Bactericidal	
Rifamycins	Rifampicin	Interfere with DNA transcription to mRNA and thus protein synthesis	Bactericidal	Resistance occurs quickly: NOT to be used as monotherapy
Sulphonamides and diaminopyrimidines	Sulfamethoxazole Trimethoprim	Interfere with folate synthesis	Bacteriostatic combination treatment can be bactericidal	There is synergy between trimethoprim and sulphonamides which leads the combination to be bactericidal
Tetracyclines	Doxycycline Oxytetracycline	Inhibit ribosomal protein synthesis	Bacteriostatic	Stop iron tablets with most

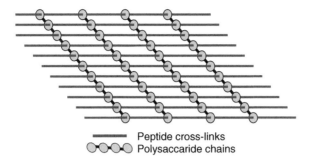

Peptide cross-links
Polysaccharide chains

FIGURE 28.3   Structure of peptidoglycan.

phenoxymethylpenicillin (penicillin V) are the original penicillins. Both are rapidly cleared by the kidneys, resulting in a short half-life and frequent dosing regimens (every 6 hours). They were originally active primarily against Gram-positive organisms, including staphylococci and streptococci, and are therefore useful in treating skin and soft tissue infection. However, resistance in staphylococci has emerged so these drugs can only be relied on now to cover streptococci. Over time, the structure of penicillin has been changed to develop semisynthetic penicillins such as amoxicillin and flucloxacillin with a broader spectrum of activity but with a similar short half-life (Table 28.3).

Penicillins are well known for causing 'allergies'. What this means varies greatly, ranging from mild skin reactions through to life-threatening anaphylaxis. Nausea, vomiting and diarrhoea are adverse drug reactions that can occur with any antibiotic and would not contraindicate its use. Patients describing minor non-confluent, non-pruritic rash of delayed onset, emerging over 72 hours after starting the drug, are probably not allergic. Penicillins can be used with caution in serious infections where alternatives are inferior or have other disadvantages. Patients describing severe reactions such as anaphylaxis, angioedema and systemic rashes, including urticaria, should not receive penicillin as these reactions are life-threatening.

Cephalosporins

Another group of β-lactam antibiotics, cephalosporins, is subdivided into different generations. Drugs within the same generation tend to have similar spectra of activity (Table 28.4).

Most cephalosporins, with the notable exception of ceftriaxone, have short half-lives and thus require frequent dosing regimens.

Up to 6.5% of patients allergic to a penicillin will also have a reaction with a cephalosporin. Cross-reactivity is thought to be due to the side chains rather than the β-lactam ring and is much more likely with first-generation cephalosporins. Patients who are severely allergic to penicillins (immediate-onset rash, urticaria, angioedema, anaphylaxis, etc.) should not generally receive a cephalosporin. However, in the case of life-threatening infections, where alternatives are inferior and where resuscitation/anaphylaxis management facilities are available (e.g., inpatient treatment of meningitis), third- (and more rarely second-) generation cephalosporins are sometimes used.

Cephalosporins have fallen out of favour in recent years due to their capacity for inducing *Clostridioides difficile* diarrhoea (Department of Health 2007). The clinical use of selected cephalosporins is shown in Table 28.5.

Glycopeptides

Glycopeptides also inhibit peptidoglycan synthesis. They bind to the growing peptide chain and prevent cross-link formation. The key glycopeptides in clinical use are vancomycin and teicoplanin. Both have very good Gram-positive cover (including MRSA) but are inactive against Gram-negative bacteria. Resistance to these antibiotics in *Staphylococcus aureus* is still quite rare, especially considering that vancomycin has been in use since the 1950s (Hiramatsu et al. 1997).

Table 28.3 Clinical uses of semisynthetic penicillins

Drug	Amoxicillin	Flucloxacillin
	An aminopenicillin that is better absorbed orally than phenoxy-methylpenicillin but is still broken down by all β-lactamases	A β-lactamase-resistant penicillin
Oral dose	500 mg three times a day (sometimes increased to 1 g three times a day)	500 mg four times a day (sometimes increased to 1 g four times a day)
Oral bioavailability	75–89% and unaffected by concurrent food	50–70% and reduced by concurrent food (advise taking on an empty stomach)
Main uses	• Otitis media • Bacterial sinusitis • Infective exacerbations of chronic bronchitis (although see above re *Haemophilus influenzae* resistance) • Non-severe community-acquired pneumonia • Sensitive urinary and biliary infections (not blind therapy)	• Skin and soft tissue infections (e.g., impetigo, cellulitis) • Bone and joint infections (under a specialist) • Most sensitive *Staphylococcus aureus* infections
Other notes	Clavulanic acid (a β-lactamase inhibitor) used in conjunction with a penicillin such as amoxicillin in co-amoxiclav • Irreversibly inactivates β-lactamase 'protecting' the penicillin • Extends spectrum of activity of amoxicillin leading to increased activity versus beta lactamase, producing *Staphylococcus aureus*/Gram-negative enteric organisms (e.g., *Escherichia coli*/anaerobes to give a 'similar' spectrum to using cefuroxime (see cephalosporins below) and metronidazole • Risk of cholestatic jaundice if use exceeds 14 days and in elderly patients	Risk of cholestatic jaundice, especially with use for more than 14 days or in elderly patients

Table 28.4   Cephalosporins in current UK practice

Generation	First	Second	Third	Fourth	Fifth
Oral	Cefalexin	Cefaclor	Cefixime	Cefepime	Ceftaroline
	Cefradine	Cefuroxime	Cefpodoxoime	Cefiderocol	Ceftolozane
	Cefadroxil				Ceftobiprole
Parenteral	Cefradine	Cefuroxime	Cefotaxime		
			Ceftriaxone		
			Ceftazidime		
Spectrum of activity	Good Gram-positive activity	Good Gram-positive activity	Reduced Gram-positive activity	Good Gram-positive activity	Broad-spectrum Gram-positive activity
	Unreliable Gram-negative activity	Improved Gram-negative activity (more resistant to β-lactamase)	Broad-spectrum Gram-negative activity	Broad-spectrum Gram-negative activity	Broad-spectrum Gram- negative activity

Table 28.5   Clinical uses of common cephalosporins

	Cefradine (first generation)	Cefaclor (second generation)
Oral dose	500 mg four times a day	500 mg three times a day
Oral bioavailability	90% and unaffected by concurrent food	93% and unaffected by concurrent food
Main uses	Generally not used as first-line treatment • Alternative for urinary tract infection • Soft tissue infections • Sometimes used in surgical prophylaxis • NOT suitable for respiratory infections (doesn't cover *Haemophilus influenzae*)	• Alternative for urinary tract infection • Alternative for respiratory infection (e.g., allergy)
Other notes	• Higher risk of *Clostridioides difficile* diarrhoea than penicilllins	• Higher risk of *Clostridioides difficile* diarrhoea than penicilllins • Limited clinical advantages over first-generation cephalosporins within the context of urinary tract infection

Vancomycin has a narrow therapeutic window so, when given intravenously, requires close monitoring to ensure efficacy and prevent toxicity.

Glycopeptides are not significantly absorbed orally. Systemic infections require parenteral treatment. Oral therapy is used for treating *C. difficile* (Chapter 29) as the infection is within the gastrointestinal tract lumen.

INHIBITION OF BACTERIAL PROTEIN SYNTHESIS

Bacterial cells, like mammalian cells, synthesise proteins by transcribing genes into messenger RNA, which is translated by ribosomes into an amino acid chain and then folded into a protein.

There are many antibiotic classes that act by inhibiting protein synthesis, so why do they not harm us? Fortunately, the structure and size of the bacterial ribosomes are sufficiently different from those of mammalian ribosomes. Antibiotics preferentially bind to the bacterial version whilst not affecting ours, thus allowing selective toxicity. Many antibiotics interfere with protein synthesis, including aminoglycosides, macrolides, tetracyclines and chloramphenicol (Figure 28.4).

Macrolides

The key macrolides in clinical use are erythromycin, clarithromycin and azithromycin. All can be given orally whilst erythromycin and clarithromycin are also available in intravenous form.

Macrolides are especially useful for their activity against atypical pathogens such as *Chlamydia*, *Mycoplasma* and *Legionella*. They are also active against most streptococci and *Staphylococcus aureus*, and are often used either as an alternative to penicillin, in allergic patients, for mild respiratory tract infection or skin/soft tissue infection or when atypical cover is required, for example in combination with a penicillin/cephalosporin in community-acquired pneumonia. Resistance does occur, so it is important that culture results are reviewed and patients are followed up.

All the macrolides inhibit enzymes in the cytochrome P450 system (see Chapter 9). Erythromycin and clarithromycin are potent inhibitors and have more clinically significant drug interactions than azithromycin. Clinical uses of erythromycin are shown in Table 28.6.

PRACTICE APPLICATION

It is always important to check the *British National Formulary* for interactions when prescribing erythromycin and clarithromycin, as many are clinically significant and contraindicate concurrent use.

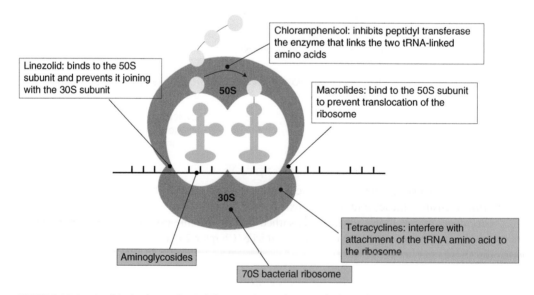

Chloramphenicol: inhibits peptidyl transferase the enzyme that links the two tRNA-linked amino acids

Linezolid: binds to the 50S subunit and prevents it joining with the 30S subunit

50S

Macrolides: bind to the 50S subunit to prevent translocation of the ribosome

30S

Tetracyclines: interfere with attachment of the tRNA amino acid to the ribosome

Aminoglycosides

70S bacterial ribosome

FIGURE 28.4 Antibiotic classes that inhibit protein synthesis and where they act. tRNA, transfer RNA.

Table 28.6   Clinical uses of erythromycin and doxycycline, both of which act by inhibiting bacterial protein synthesis

Drug	Erythromycin	Doxycycline
Oral dose	500 mg four times a day	200 mg loading dose then 100 mg once a day
		100 mg twice a day for sexually transmitted infections and more serious infections
Oral bioavailability	18-45%, varies on the salt form	93%
Main uses	• First choice for some STDs, e.g. *Chlamydia*	• Used to treat some sexually transmitted infections, e.g. *Chlamydia*
	• First choice for legionnaire's disease, usually in combination	• Respiratory infections
	• Used in combination with aminopenicillins for respiratory infection	• As an oral alternative in sensitive methicillin-resistant *Staphylococcus aureus* infections
	• As an alternative in skin/soft tissue infections	
Other notes	• Nausea and vomiting are sometimes troublesome; in these patients clarithromycin may be used	• Stop iron tablets whilst treating with doxycycline and restart after course
		• Sensitises the skin to sunlight

Tetracyclines

The key tetracyclines in clinical use are tetracycline, oxytetracycline, doxycycline and minocycline. All are only available orally in the UK and have quite a broad spectrum of activity.

Most tetracyclines bind with divalent ions (e.g., Ca^{2+} and Mg^{2+}) in the gut. These complexes cannot be absorbed by the body and so the antibiotic is rendered ineffective. For this reason, tetracyclines should not be taken at the same time as indigestion remedies or taken at all by patients taking iron supplements; some tetracyclines should not be taken at the same time as dairy products because of the calcium ions they contain. The affinity of tetracyclines for calcium is the reason why these drugs should not be used at all in children under 12 as they can lead to discoloured teeth. Apart from minocycline and doxycycline, tetracyclines should not be used in patients with kidney disease as they can cause renal impairment. The clinical uses of doxycycline are shown in Table 28.6.

STOP AND THINK

The interaction between tetracyclines and indigestion remedies is an example of which type of drug antagonism?

Aminoglycosides

The key aminoglycosides in clinical use are gentamicin, amikacin and tobramycin. None are absorbed orally so must be given intravenously for treating systemic infection. All aminoglycosides require close monitoring to ensure efficacy (from high enough peak levels) and avoid nephrotoxicity and ototoxicity (by ensuring low enough trough levels).

Aminoglycosides can exhibit synergy when used with β-lactams (lower doses/peak levels required for efficacy).

Over the last decade there has been a move towards giving the total dose of aminoglycoside as a single daily infusion in an attempt to maximise efficacy and minimise toxicity. A number of meta-analyses have shown reduced nephrotoxicity, with trends towards improved efficacy and similar ototoxicity (Barza et al. 1996).

INHIBITION OF BACTERIAL DNA SYNTHESIS

DNA synthesis is fundamental to growing life and hence antibiotics that interfere with DNA synthesis tend to be bactericidal. Obviously, mammalian cells also need to synthesise DNA and so these drugs have to be designed carefully to achieve selective toxicity. Key antibiotics that act by inhibiting bacterial DNA synthesis are the quinolones, metronidazole, nitrofurantoin and rifampicin.

Quinolones

The key quinolones in clinical use are ciprofloxacin (Table 28.7), levofloxacin, ofloxacin and moxifloxacin. Quinolones are very well absorbed orally and distribute extensively throughout the body so intravenous preparations are rarely necessary. Although the half-life varies, most quinolones can be given as once- or twice-daily regimens.

Resistance seems to occur rapidly and resistance to one fluoroquinolone generally means resistance to all.

Quinolone antibiotics inhibit DNA gyrase and topoisomerase IV, enzymes involved in the coiling of bacterial DNA and which are essential for DNA replication in bacteria. Mammalian cells do not contain DNA gyrase and so selective toxicity is assured.

PRACTICE APPLICATION

Although very effective, quinolones have fallen out of favour in recent years due to being highlighted as a risk factor for MRSA colonisation, extended-spectrum β-lactamase infections and *C. difficile* infection.

Table 28.7 Clinical uses of ciprofloxacin and metronidazole, both of which act by inhibiting bacterial DNA synthesis

Drug	Ciprofloxacin	Metronidazole
Oral dose	250-750 mg twice a day	400 mg three times a day
Oral bioavailability		100%
Main uses	• Alternative for urinary tract infections • Sometimes used for *Pseudomonal* infection	• Anaerobes (including *Clostridioides difficile*) • Some protozoa • Often used as part of a combination to cover anaerobes (gastrointestinal, gynae etc.)
Other notes	• Oral gives as good a level as IV: 400 mg IV = 500 mg oral, leading to 80% bioavailability (IV gives high levels more rapidly) • Usually give 750 mg twice a day as equivalent to 400 mg twice a day IV	• Avoid alcohol whilst taking and for 72 hours after

IV, intravenous

Metronidazole and nitrofurantoin

Metronidazole (Table 28.7) and nitrofurantoin are reduced intracellularly to reactive metabolites that interact with and cause direct damage to DNA, with bactericidal effect.

INHIBITION OF FOLATE SYNTHESIS

Folate is essential for DNA synthesis. Mammals obtain folate from their food while bacterial cells synthesise their own. Both mammals and bacteria have to reduce folate into its active form, tetrahydrofolate, before it can be used for DNA synthesis. Key antibiotics that act by inhibiting folate synthesis are trimethoprim and the sulphonamides.

Figure 28.5 highlights the two enzymes in folate metabolism inhibited by sulphonamides and trimethoprim.

For the sulphonamides, achieving selective toxicity is obvious as their target is not found in mammalian cells. For trimethoprim, it is more complicated. Dihydrofolate reductase (DHFR) is an enzyme common to both bacteria and mammals so why doesn't trimethoprim harm us? The reason is that whilst trimethoprim could inhibit mammalian DHFR, it is much less active against this than it is against the bacterial version (Table 28.8). The IC_{50} is the concentration necessary to inhibit 50% of the enzyme; the lower the IC_{50}, the more active the drug. Hence trimethoprim is about 50,000 times more active against bacteria than humans. Methotrexate is most active against the human DHFR and hence is a useful cytotoxic. Pyrimethamine is an antiprotozoal drug.

Sulphonamides

Sulphonamides are now rarely used as monotherapy due to growing resistance. However, they are still used in combination with DHFR inhibitors. Separately, sulphonamides and trimethoprim are bacteriostatic. Combined as co-trimoxazole, they work synergistically and are usually bactericidal, with enhanced activity against rarer organisms such as *Pneumocystis jiroveci* (formerly *Pneumocystis carinii*), which is an important opportunistic pathogen in the immunosuppressed. Sulphonamides (and co-trimoxazole) have an extensive side-effect profile, including serious blood dyscrasias and frequent rashes, so co-trimoxazole is usually restricted to infections where other options are not suitable.

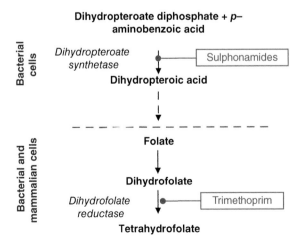

FIGURE 28.5   Action of antibiotics on bacterial folate synthesis.

Table 28.8 The relative potency of dihydrofolate reductase (DHFR) inhibitors

	IC_{50} for DHFR		
	Human	Protozoal	Bacterial
Trimethoprim	260	0.07	0.005
Pyrimethamine	0.7	0.0005	2.5
Methotrexate	0.001	~0.1	Inactive

Table 28.9 Clinical uses of trimethoprim

Spectrum	Generally active	Escherichia coli
		Most other urinary pathogens
		Some strains of *Staphylococcus aureus* (including some methicillin-resistant *Staphylococcus aureus*)
	Generally not active	Anaerobic bacteria
Oral dose	200 mg twice a day	
Oral bioavailability	90-100%	
Main uses	First line for urinary tract infections	
Other notes	Resistance is growing	

Trimethoprim

The clinical uses of trimethoprim are shown in Table 28.9.

SUMMARY

- Antimicrobials exploit differences between humans and microorganisms to cause selective toxicity.

- Bacteria are divided into Gram positives and Gram negatives based on their cell wall structure.

- Bacteria are divided into cocci or bacilli based on their shape under a microscope and into anaerobic and aerobic depending on whether they can grow in the presence or absence of oxygen.

- Broad-spectrum antibiotics treat many types of bacteria; narrow-spectrum agents are more targeted to specific species.

- Antibiotics either kill the bacteria (bactericidal) or prevent them from multiplying (bacteriostatic), allowing the host defences to kill them.

- Use your local antibiotic guidelines when deciding on empirical (blind) therapy.

- Review antibiotic choice with the results of microbiology cultures.

- Antibiotics within the same class have the same mechanism of action and, generally, a similar spectrum of activity.

- There are four principal mechanisms of antibacterial action: damaging the bacterial cell wall, inhibiting bacterial protein synthesis, inhibiting bacterial DNA synthesis and inhibiting bacterial metabolic pathways.

- β-lactam antibiotics and glycopeptides inhibit bacterial cell wall synthesis.
- Aminoglycosides, macrolides and tetracyclines all inhibit bacterial protein synthesis.
- Quinolones, metronidazole, nitrofurantoin and rifampicin all inhibit bacterial DNA synthesis.
- Trimethoprim and sulphonamides inhibit bacterial metabolic pathways.

ACTIVITY

1. Which of the following statements regarding bacteria and antibiotics are correct?

    (a) Ciprofloxacin is the first-line antibiotic to treat uncomplicated urinary tract infection.

    (b) Augmentin® can be used in patients allergic to a penicillin.

    (c) Trimethoprim and sulphonamides act on the same metabolic pathway and have synergy when used in combination.

    (d) *Staphylococcus aureus* is a Gram-positive organism.

    (e) Gentamicin's efficacy is linked to the amount of time its concentration is above the bacteria's MIC.

2. Which two of the following antibiotics would be effective against respiratory atypicals?

    (a) Co-amoxiclav

    (b) Cefuroxime

    (c) Clarithromycin

    (d) Doxycycline

    (e) Vancomycin

3. Which three of the following antibiotics act by inhibiting peptidoglycan synthesis?

    (a) Co-amoxiclav

    (b) Cefuroxime

    (c) Clarithromycin

    (d) Doxycycline

    (e) Vancomycin

4. Which two of the following organisms commonly cause skin and soft tissue infections (e.g., cellulitis)?

    (a) *Staphylococcus aureus*

    (b) *Haemophilus influenzae*

    (c) *Moraxella catarrhalis*

    (d) *Streptococcus pyogenes* (group A β-haemolytic Strep.)

    (e) *Bacteroides* spp.

5. Which of the following bacteria can be treated by metronidazole?

   (a) *Staphylococcus aureus*

   (b) *Haemophilus influenzae*

   (c) *Moraxella catarrhalis*

   (d) *Streptococcus pyogenes* (group A β-haemolytic Strep.)

   (e) *Bacteroides* spp.

REFERENCES

Barza, M., Ioannidis, J.P., Cappelleri, J.C. and Lau, J. (1996) Single or multiple daily doses of aminoglycosides: a meta-analysis. *BMJ* 312:338–345.

Department of Health (2007) *Saving Lives: Antimicrobial Prescribing, A Summary of Best Practice*. Department of Health, London.

Hiramatsu, K., Hanaki, H., Ino, T., Yabuta, K., Oguri, T., Tenover, F.C. (1997) Methicillin-resistant *Staphylococcus aureus* clinical strain with reduced vancomycin susceptibility. *J Antimicrob Chemother* 40(1):135–136.

FURTHER READING

Abbanat, D., Morrow, B. and Bush, K. (2008) New drugs in development for the treatment of bacterial infections. *Curr Opin Pharmacol* 8:582–592.

British National Formulary (online). BMJ Group and Pharmaceutical Press, London. https://bnf.nice.org.uk/

Drugs and Therapeutics Bulletin (2017) Penicillin allergy—getting the label right. *BMJ* 358:j3402.

Page, C.P., Curtis, M.J., Sutter, M.C., et al. (2006) *Integrated Pharmacology*, 3rd edn. Mosby, London.

Pai, M.P., Momarry, K.M. and Rodvold, K.A. (2006) Antibiotic drug interactions. *Med Clin North Am* 90:1223–1255.

Ranji, S.R., Steinman, M.A., Shojania, K.G. and Gonzales, R. (2008) Interventions to reduce unnecessary antibiotic prescribing: a systematic review and quantitative analysis. *Med Care* 46:847–862.

Ritter, J.M., Flower, R.J., Henderson, G., et al. (2023) *Rang and Dale's Pharmacology*, 10th edn. Elsevier, Amsterdam.

Thethi, A.K. and van Dellen, R.G. (2004) Dilemmas and controversies in penicillin allergy. *Immunol Allergy Clin North Am* 24:445–461.

USEFUL WEBSITES

NICE clinical knowledge summaries. https://cks.nice.org.uk/

REUSABLE LEARNING OBJECTS

Pharmacokinetic and pharmacodynamic influences of aminoglycoside dosing. www.nottingham.ac.uk/nursing/sonet/rlos/bioproc/aminoglycosides/

Antibiotic Resistance and Clostridioides Difficile

CHAPTER 29

Tim Hills

LEARNING OUTCOMES

By the end of this chapter the reader should be able to:

- demonstrate an understanding of how antibiotic resistance emerges and spreads

- discuss the main mechanisms of antibiotic resistance that bacteria employ

- describe how *Clostridioides difficile* infection (CDI) occurs

- outline the main risk factors associated with contracting CDI

- describe the treatment of CDI infection and know when to refer patients for specialist care.

BACTERIA AND THE HUMAN BODY

The human body is a bacterial ecosystem. There are 10 times more bacterial cells on, or in, our body than human cells (most live within the bowel). Whilst some of these are pathogenic and cause infection, most do no harm and many live alongside us performing useful functions such as synthesising vitamins (such as vitamin K) or aiding digestion. Moreover, our natural flora helps prevent overgrowth of pathogenic microorganisms by providing competitive pressure for space and nutrients. The use of antibiotics alters this natural human flora by killing off the sensitive bacteria, allowing the resistant species that are left to multiply with less competition. The broader the spectrum of antibiotic, the more species of bacteria affected and the more chance of a resistant colonisation occurring.

For example, if a patient has cellulitis in their right leg, most likely to be either haemolytic streptococci or *Staphylococcus aureus* (Figure 29.1a), one could treat with a narrow-spectrum antibiotic such as flucloxacillin. This will treat the infection; it will also kill the other haemolytic streptococci or *Staph. aureus* (and other sensitive bacteria) on the body that are not causing the infection (so-called 'innocent bystanders') but this is unavoidable (Figure 29.1b). Alternatively, one could choose to treat the infection with the broader-spectrum antibiotic cefuroxime. It would still treat haemolytic streptococci or *Staph. aureus* but also covers a range of Gram-negative enteric bacteria. Hence, it would select for resistance in more species of bacteria and have a greater impact on the natural flora, leaving only the resistant microorganisms (Figure 29.1c). With less competition for space and nutrients, these resistant microorganisms grow, colonise the patient (Figure 29.1d) and pass to another person. For this reason, it is generally best to use the most narrow-spectrum antibiotic available that will treat the infection effectively.

It is also important to use the antibiotics for the shortest duration that will effectively treat the infection (Haider et al. 2008; El Moussaoui et al., 2008; Lee et al. 2021). Longer durations of antibiotic therapy will suppress the natural flora for longer and increase the risk of acquiring a multiresistant colonisation.

The New Prescriber: An Integrated Approach to Medical and Non-medical Prescribing, Second Edition.
Edited by Joanne Lymn, Alison Mostyn, Roger Knaggs, Michael Randall, and Dianne Bowskill.
© 2024 John Wiley & Sons Ltd. Published 2024 by John Wiley & Sons Ltd.

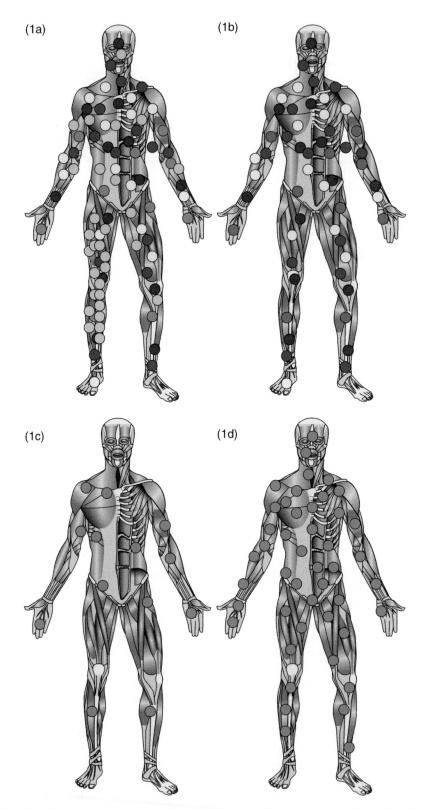

FIGURE 29.1 The effect of using narrow- and broad-spectrum antibiotics to treat a patient with cellulitis of the right leg on their natural flora. Different coloured spots represent different populations of bacteria. (1a) Patient has cellulitis in their right leg, most likely to be either haemolytic streptococci or *Staphylococcus aureus*. (1b) Infection treated with a narrow-spectrum antibiotic such as flucloxacillin. (1c) Infection treated with the broader spectrum antibiotic. (1d) Impact on natural flora of broader spectrum antibiotics. Nutrients resistant micro-organisms grow and colonise the patient.

STOP AND THINK

Can you think of examples of broad-spectrum antibiotics that have been used unnecessarily?

PRACTICE APPLICATION

If initial broad-spectrum antibiotic therapy is necessary (e.g., for neutropenic sepsis) it is important that microbiology cultures are taken and therapy reviewed in light of the results.

ANTIBIOTIC RESISTANCE

Antibiotic resistance is a well-documented problem both within secondary care and, increasingly, in the community. Resistance to an antibiotic varies between species and strains, being either native or following a mutation in the antibiotic's target.

NATIVE RESISTANCE

Some bacteria or strains were always resistant to the antibiotic even before it was introduced, these are called natively resistant. They either naturally contain an enzyme conferring resistance (e.g., some strains of *Escherichia coli* and β-lactamase) or their structure is such that the antibiotic cannot reach its target or the target does not exist (e.g., *Mycoplasma* sp. does not have peptidoglycan in its cell wall and therefore β-lactam antibiotics would never work against it).

RESISTANCE ACQUIRED FOLLOWING MUTATION

Point mutations tend to occur within the genome of one in about every 10^7 bacterial cells (Figure 29.2). If the mutation is part of the gene that encodes for the antibiotic's target, it may lead to resistance.

Genes that code for resistance may be positioned on a bacterial chromosome or contained on a plasmid (a separate ring of DNA that can be transferred to other bacteria). Resistance genes on a chromosome are spread clonally (Figure 29.2). Dividing bacteria colonise and may spread from patient to patient where infection control precautions are not perfect. A good example of this is methicillin-resistant *Staph. aureus* (MRSA), where two very successful epidemic clones account for the vast majority of UK healthcare-associated infections (Johnson et al. 2001).

Resistance genes on a plasmid spread clonally but can also be easily shared between strains and even species. For example, vancomycin resistance in enterococci (VRE) has been transferred

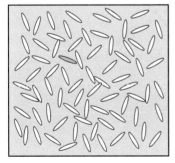
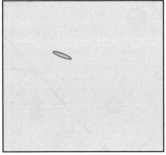
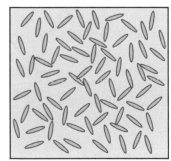

FIGURE 29.2   About every one in 10^7 bacteria will have a mutation (green). If this confers new resistance to an antibiotic that is used the sensitive population is killed, giving the resistant organism the chance to multiply and cause a resistant colonisation that may then be passed onto another patient.

in vitro to MRSA to produce a vancomycin-resistant MRSA (VRSA). The first report of a clinical infection with vancomycin-resistant MRSA was in a patient co-colonised with VRE and MRSA (Chang et al. 2003).

Potentially, resistance genes can also spread following cell lysis as some bacteria can scavenge DNA lying around the environment and incorporate it into their chromosome. Bacteriophages (viruses that infect bacteria) may also extract DNA from one bacterium and inject it into another one.

MECHANISMS OF RESISTANCE

The mechanisms of resistance that bacteria employ are varied, but most fit into one of six categories (Figure 29.3).

Efflux pumps

The antibiotic enters the cell but is actively pumped out by efflux pumps so that intracellular concentration does not become high enough to affect the target. Tetracycline resistance is often mediated through efflux pumping. Multidrug efflux pumps are sometimes expressed by *Pseudomonas aeruginosa* and are able to excrete a variety of antibiotics, including quinolones, β-lactams, trimethoprim, sulphonamides and aminoglycosides.

Enzymic degradation

The bacterial cell secretes an enzyme that is capable of inactivating the antibiotic before it is able to reach the target. The best-known example is β-lactamase, which can hydrolyse the β-lactam ring of some penicillins, cephalosporins and carbapenems. Aminoglycosides can also be degraded by specific secreted enzymes.

Bypass

The antibiotic inhibits an essential enzyme in a cell metabolic pathway. The bacteria manage to bypass this to produce the required metabolite using another pathway. This type of resistance can occur against sulphonamides.

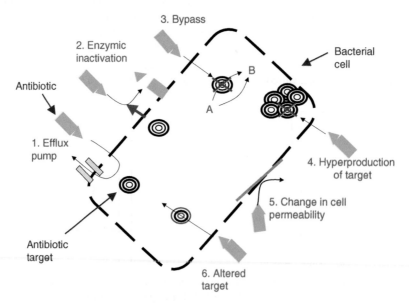

FIGURE 29.3 Mechanisms of resistance employed by bacteria.

Hyperproduction of target

The bacteria produce so much of the target enzyme that the antibiotic is unable to inhibit it all. Hyperproduction of dihydrofolate reductase can confer resistance to trimethoprim in some bacteria.

Change in cell permeability

Many antibiotics enter cells through porins in the cell wall. Alterations in these porins reduce the amount of antibiotic that enters the bacteria. Consequently, a higher concentration of antibiotic is necessary to obtain sufficient concentrations within the cell and leads to an increase in the minimum inhibitory concentration and resistance. Cephalosporins can sometimes be affected by porin alteration. Gentamicin resistance is sometimes conferred by alterations in the cell wall uptake mechanism.

Altered target

Direct mutations to the antibiotic target can led to decreased affinity and reduced antibiotic efficacy. Many antibiotics are potentially susceptible to mutation in their targets, including aminoglycosides, macrolides, clindamycin and quinolones.

MULTIRESISTANT BACTERIA

Methicillin-resistant Staph. aureus

The original 'superbug', MRSA is resistant to all current β-lactam antibiotics (penicillins, cephalosporins and carbapenems). Different strains have variable resistance to other antistaphylococcal antibiotics. All antibiotics that can treat *Staph. aureus* have the potential to select for MRSA, although quinolones have been highlighted as particularly high risk for MRSA colonisation. This is probably because they are excreted in sweat (MRSA colonises the groin, axillae and nose) and can induce the expression of *Staph. aureus* adhesion factors (Weber et al. 2003). Several new antibiotics have recently become available that are active against MRSA (and VRSA), including linezolid, daptomycin and tigecycline, and more are in development.

Extended-spectrum β-lactamase producers

A Gram-negative bacterium (e.g., *E. coli)* that produces an enzyme that inactivates a wider range of β-lactam antibiotics, including cephalosporins. Unfortunately, as well as cephalosporin resistance, these bacteria also tend to carry resistance to quinolones, gentamicin, trimethoprim, co-amoxiclav, piperacillin/tazobactam and in some cases nitrofurantoin. This can leave the carbapenems as the only option. With few antibiotics in the development pipeline that will treat extended-spectrum β-lactamase (ESBL) producers, and *E. coli* being such a successful pathogen, these are likely to be one of the major problem organisms in the near future.

Vancomycin-resistant enterococcus

Although a lower-grade pathogen than *E. coli* or *Staph. aureus*, enterococci still cause infections such as endocarditis in susceptible patients. Depending on the strain, VRE may be sensitive to amoxicillin, although nearly all are sensitive to the new anti-MRSA drugs linezolid, tigecycline and daptomycin.

Acinetobacter baumannii

Another low-grade pathogen that tends to affect immunocompromised patients or those who have had numerous antibiotics. Hospital strains tend only to be sensitive to colistin, tigecycline and sometimes the carbapenems.

ANTIBIOTIC-ASSOCIATED DIARRHOEA AND *CLOSTRIDIOIDES DIFFICILE*

Diarrhoea is one of the most common adverse effects with antibiotic use. It can occur with any antibiotic and is often attributed to *Clostridioides difficile.*

Clostridioides difficile is a Gram-positive spore-forming bacterium. Bacterial spores are like seeds: they can survive for months in the environment and are very hard to kill, even with disinfectants. If ingested, these spores move through the gastrointestinal tract to the lower bowel, where they germinate into vegetative bacteria. The patient's normal bowel flora is a useful defence but if it is disrupted by antibiotic, then the Clostridia are allowed to proliferate, colonise and, if the strain is able, produce toxin. Additionally, it appears that some antibiotics may actually encourage spore germination and/or toxin production and disease.

PRACTICE APPLICATION

Clostridioides difficile spores are not reliably killed by alcohol handrubs. When caring for patients with *Clostridioides difficile* infection or diarrhoea, it is important to use soap and water to clean hands.

Clostridioides difficile can produce three types of toxin, which together cause gut mucosal inflammation, epithelial cell apoptosis, and fluid and electrolyte leakage into the lumen, leading to offensive diarrhoea.

PRACTICE APPLICATION

The severity of disease that *Clostridioides difficile* infection causes varies from patient to patient. A few will be asymptomatic carriers, but may act as a reservoir for further spread. Some will only experience mild diarrhoea, while for others profuse diarrhoea may follow infection; these will require active treatment. In its severest form, *Clostridioides difficile* infection may cause life-threatening pseudomembraneous colitis. What determines the severity of disease is unclear but in part it may be due to the patient's ability to mount an immune response to the toxins and certainly the elderly and the immunosuppressed are at greatest risk of severe disease.

TREATMENT OF *CLOSTRIDIOIDES DIFFICILE* INFECTION

With confirmed or highly suspected *Clostridioides difficile* infection (CDI), the first job is to review and stop the causative antibiotic if at all possible, reviewing proton-pump inhibitors (PPIs) and ensuring adequate hydration and nutrition. Treatment of CDI usually involves specific antibiotics which target *Clostridioides difficile*, vancomycin, metronidazole or fidaxomicin.

STOP AND THINK

As *Clostridioides difficile* causes infection within the gut lumen, which route of administration would be most appropriate for treatment of this infection?

VANCOMYCIN

Vancomycin is the first-line antibiotic in UK guidelines (NICE 2021) due to its effectiveness and relatively low cost. Vancomycin does not cross the blood–gut barrier and therefore is usually given orally. The dose ranges from 125 to 500 mg four times a day depending on severity. In patients who cannot swallow, a nasogastric tube should be used. Rectal administration has been used, particularly in patients with ileus. Approximately 20–30% of patients who initially respond to therapy will experience recurrence, mostly within the first month. Half of these can be attributed to a different *Clostridioides difficile* strain and are therefore reinfections rather than relapses.

METRONIDAZOLE

This antibiotic was once first line for treatment but studies (Beinortas et al. 2018) have shown it to be inferior to other treatments. It is now restricted to combination therapy in refractory or life-threatening CDI where intravenous metronidazole (which can cross the blood–gut barrier) is added to oral vancomycin.

FIDAXOMICIN

Fidaxomicin is an oral antibiotic, as effective as vancomycin but with a narrower spectrum of activity that allows the re-establishment of a normal gut flora, leading to a reduced recurrence rate. It is, however, much more expensive and therefore restricted in the UK to patients who have experienced a recurrence of CDI as these patients are much more likely to experience subsequent recurrences.

Faecal microbiota transplants

Similar to an extremely high dose of probiotic (see below) faecal microbiota transplant (FMT) aims to fix the disrupted gut flora that allow *Clostridioides difficile* to establish colonisation and infection by administering a healthy donor's stool, usually via nasogastric tube to the infected patient. It has been effective in the treatment of acute infection, particularly in patients who have experienced recurrences (Baunwall et al. 2020; Dubberke et al. 2018). It is recommended by the National Institute for Health and Care Excellence (NICE) for patients with recurrent CDI and two or more previous episodes.

Bezlotoxumab

This is a neutralizing monoclonal antibody aimed at *Clostridioides difficile* toxin. It is used in addition to oral vancomycin to reduce recurrence by about 10%. Additional benefit with fidaxomycin is unclear due to limited use in the trials. It should be used in caution in patients with congestive heart failure. Currently it is not recommended in the recent NICE guidance due to its high cost.

MODULATION OF CDI RISK

Antibiotics

Many factors have been identified that increase the risk of contracting CDI, the most obvious being antibiotic usage. Antibiotics disrupt the normally protective gut bacteria flora and all are considered potential risk factors for CDI (including, paradoxically, oral vancomycin and metronidazole). Some groups have been shown to offer increased risk over others; these are generally the broad-spectrum agents (Table 29.1).

Using more than one antibiotic at once appears to increase the CDI risk, although it is difficult to say how much. What is clear is that extending the duration of the treatment course increases the risk of contracting CDI. With a more sustained disruption to bowel flora, the patient is without their natural defence for longer and there is more chance that if *Clostridioides difficile* spores are ingested, they will germinate (Pépin *et al.*, 2005).

Age and immune system

With the exception of the under-2s, the patient's CDI risk increases as their age increases, with those over 65 being especially at risk. The reason for this is probably multifactorial: older people often

Table 29.1 Examples of antibiotic classes and their risk of CDI

Risk of CDI	Antibiotic	Comment
High	Cephalosporins	Particularly third generation
		Also linked to promoting MRSA and VRE colonisation
	Quinolones	A recent study suggested that quinolones were the highest independent risk factor of all the antibiotic classes
		Also linked to encouraging MRSA colonisation
	Clindamycin	Implicated as the major causative antibiotic in many of the early CDI outbreaks
		Anecdotally some centres report seeing less CDI associated with higher (e.g., 600 mg qds) compared with lower doses
Moderate	Macrolides and aminopenicillins	Studies have linked macrolides, amoxicillin and co-amoxiclav to CDI, with co-amoxiclav expected to be higher risk due to its broader spectrum of activity and greater disruption of anaerobic bacteria
Low	Narrow-spectrum penicillins	Benzylpenicillin, flucloxacillin
	Tetracyclines	
	Metronidazole	
	Trimethoprim	
	Rifampicin	
	Glycopeptides (intravenous)	Glycopeptides do not distribute into the gut lumen and therefore do not disrupt gut flora when given intravenously
	Aminoglycosides (parenteral)	Aminoglycosides have broad-spectrum Gram-negative activity but do not partition across the gut mucosa and cause limited disruption of bowel flora when given parenterally
	Topical antibiotics (e.g., eye drops)	The risk of disrupting gut flora is low regardless of the class of antibiotic the eye drops contain

CDI, *Clostridioides difficile* infection; MRSA, methicillin-resistant *Staphylococcus aureus*; qds, four times a day; VRE, vancomycin resistance in enterococci.

have more comorbidities coupled with longer hospital stays and their immune systems also tend to be poorer. Patients who are unable to mount a significant immune response to *Clostridioides difficile* toxin are at much greater risk from recurrent CDI and are likely to experience more severe disease.

Characteristics of hospital stay

As a patient's stay in hospital continues, their risk from CDI increases. Some studies have also suggested that a stay on the intensive care unit increases risk. Patients who are sicker also tend to be more susceptible to CDI. Similarly, the presence of a nasogastric tube appears to increase the risk of contracting CDI, probably as this by-passes the protective stomach.

Proton-pump inhibitors

The theory is that increasing gastric pH reduces the protection that the stomach offers, allowing more spores through into the bowel, although current clinical evidence regarding PPI use is conflicting. Until subsequent evidence clarifies the situation, the prudent approach is to ensure that PPI use is in line with NICE guidance and ensure that patients are regularly reviewed to prevent CDI, with strong consideration to stopping PPI use in patients with recurrent disease.

Prebiotics and probiotics

Prebiotics are substances that are purported to promote an environment that encourages the growth of 'good bacteria' often being a source of their food. Probiotics are living microorganisms taken to promote a 'good' or 'friendly' large bowel flora, but doses are usually miniscule compared with the number of bacteria within the bowel. Although they have provoked much interest in the media in the prevention of CDI, most preparations have not been tested in controlled trials and those that have shown benefit have usually been used in a context of a higher CDI infection risk than is commonly seen today and so are not recommended.

SUMMARY

- Inappropriate use of antimicrobials does not just affect the patient (through side effects), but also impacts the community by encouraging resistance.

- Always use antibiotics in line with local guidelines and for the shortest duration that will treat the infection.

- If antibiotics are indicated, narrow down the spectrum in line with microbial sensitivities to reduce the impact on natural flora.

- Bacteria may have native resistance to antibiotics or acquire resistance following mutation.

- The mechanisms of resistance employed by bacteria fall into six categories: efflux pumps, enzymic degradation, bypass, hyperproduction of target, change in cell permeability and altered target.

- Most antibiotic-resistant bacteria are spread clonally; excellent infection control reduces their spread.

- Diarrhoea is one of the most common adverse effects seen with antibiotics and is often attributed to *Clostridioides difficile.*

- Risk factors for *Clostridioides difficile* infection (CDI) include antibiotic use, particularly broad-spectrum antibiotics and use of multiple antibiotics.

- Other risk factors for CDI include age, length of hospital stay, severe comorbidities, the presence of feeding tubes and possibly acid-suppressing agents.

- Oral vancomycin is the first-line agent for the treatment of CDI. It is combined with intravenous metronidazole in life-threatening disease.

- Oral fidaxomicin is as effective as oral vancomycin and has a lower rate of recurrence, but is currently much more expensive.

ACTIVITY

1. Using a broader-spectrum antibiotic reduces the risk of resistance as it can treat more infections.   True/False

2. *Clostridioides difficile* infection can be induced by the use of any antibiotic.   True/False

3. The risk of contracting *Clostridioides difficile* infection increases with age.   True/False

4. The risk of relapse following *Clostridioides difficile* infection is low (<5%).   True/False

5. An extended-spectrum β-lactamase producer (ESBL) is:

    (a) an antibiotic that kills most types of bacteria (e.g., meropenem)

    (b) a Gram-negative bacteria with resistance against all current cephalosporins and penicillins

(c) a strain of *Clostridioides difficile* that produces more toxin, causing more severe disease

(d) a form of MRSA that is particularly difficult to eradicate

6. Which of these antibiotics are considered higher risk for inducing *Clostridioides difficile* infection?

(a) Ciprofloxacin

(b) Doxycycline

(c) Piperacillin/tazobactam

(d) Gentamicin IV

7. Which of these is NOT a resistance mechanism employed by bacteria to evade antibiotic attack?

(a) Hyperproduction of the target

(b) Efflux pumps

(c) Ribosomal inhibition

(d) Changing the cell permeability

REFERENCES

Baunwall, S.M.D., Eriksen, M.K., Mullish, B.H., Marchesi, J.R. and Hvas, C.L. (2020) Faecal microbiota transplantation for recurrent *Clostridioides difficile* infection: An updated systematic review and meta-analysis. *EClinicalMedicine* 100642:29–30.

Beinortas, T., Burr, N.E., Wilcox, M.H. and Subramanian, V. (2018) Comparative efficacy of treatments for *Clostridium difficile* infection: a systematic review and network meta-analysis. *Lancet Infect Dis* 18(9):1035–1044.

Chang, S., Sievert, D.M., Hageman, J.C., et al. (2003) Vancomycin-resistant *Staphylococcus aureus* investigative team: infection with vancomycin-resistant *Staphylococcus aureus* containing the vanA resistance gene. *N Engl J Med* 348:1342–1347.

Dubberke, E.,R., Lee, C.H., Orenstein, R. et al. (2018) Results from a randomized, placebo-controlled clinical trial of a RBX2660—A microbiota-based drug for the prevention of recurrent *Clostridium difficile* infection. *Clin Infect Dis* 67(8):1198–1204.

El Moussaoui, R., Roede, B.M., Speelman, P., *et al.* (2008) Short-course antibiotic treatment in acute exacerbations of chronic bronchitis and COPD: a meta-analysis of double-blind studies. *Thorax* 63:415–422.

Haider, B.A., Saeed, M.A. and Bhutta, Z.A. (2008) Short-course versus long-course antibiotic therapy for non-severe community-acquired pneumonia in children aged 2 months to 59 months. *Cochrane Database Syst Rev* 2:CD005976.

Johnson, A.P., Aucken, H.M., Cavendish, S., et al., UK EARSS Participants (2001) Dominance of EMRSA-15 and -16 among MRSA causing nosocomial bacteraemia in the UK: analysis of isolates from the European Antimicrobial Resistance Surveillance System (EARSS). *J Antimicrob Chemother* 48:143–144.

Lee, R.A., Centor, R.M., Humphrey, L.L. et al. (2021) Appropriate use of short-course antibiotics in common infections: Best practice advice from the American College of Physicians. *Ann Intern Med.* https://doi.org/10.7326/M20-7355.

NICE (2021) *Clostridioides difficile* infection: antimicrobial prescribing NICE guideline [NG199]. https://www.nice.org.uk/guidance/ng199.

Pépin, J., Saheb, N., Coulombe, M.A., et al. (2005) Emergence of fluoroquinolones as the predominant risk factor for *Clostridium difficile*-associated diarrhea: a cohort study during an epidemic in Quebec. *Clin Infect Dis* 41:1254–1260.

Weber, S.G., Gold, H.S., Hooper, D.C., et al. (2003) Fluoroquinolones and the risk for methicillin-resistant *Staphylococcus aureus* in hospitalized patients. *Emerg Infect Dis* 9:1415–1422.

FURTHER READING

Cunningham, R. and Dial, S. (2008) Is over-use of proton pump inhibitors fuelling the current epidemic of *Clostridium difficile*-associated diarrhoea? *J Hosp Infect* 70:1–6.

NICE (2015) *Clostridium difficile* infection: risk with broad-spectrum antibiotics. Evidence Summary. https://www.nice.org.uk/guidance/esmpb1.

Van Prehen, J., Reigadas, E., Vogelzang, E.H. et al. (2021) European Society of Clinical Microbiology and Infectious Diseases: 2021 update on the treatment guidance document for *Clostridioides difficile* infection in adults. *Clin Microbiol Infect*, 27:S1–S21.

CHAPTER 30

Antifungal and Antiviral Drugs

Tim Hills

LEARNING OUTCOMES

By the end of this chapter the reader should be able to:

- understand the aetiology of fungal disease

- discuss the use, mechanism of action and problems associated with the following antifungal drugs:

  ○ nystatin

  ○ azole antifungals

  ○ terbinafine

- understand the nature of viruses and viral infections

- discuss the use, mechanism of action and problems associated with the following antiviral drugs:

  ○ acicolvir

  ○ zanamivir/oseltmivir

- discuss the use and mechanism of action of antiviral and neutralizing monoclonal antibodies directed at SARS-CoV 2.

MYCOLOGY AND CLASSIFICATION

Fungi are eukaryotes with a rigid cell wall, like plants but without the chlorophyll. Pathogenic fungi occur in two forms: unicellular yeasts (e.g., *Candida)* and filamentous moulds (e.g., *Aspergillus).* Some fungi are capable of growth in either form depending on the conditions and are called dimorphic. Fungi are able to reproduce independently of any host organism. Yeasts do so asexually through budding, whereas moulds produce airborne spores.

Fungi are generally seen as opportunistic pathogens. In normal hosts disease tends to be superficial, mostly occurring if the normal flora has been altered, for example by the use of broad-spectrum antibiotics (Chapter 28). In immunocompromised patients, however, fungi can cause difficult-to-treat deep and/or invasive infections that are often life-threatening (Lass-Flörl 2009).

PATHOGENIC MOULDS

Dermatophytes

These are a group of more than 30 species of fungi that live in the dead layers of nails and skin. Most are spore-forming moulds. Dermatophytes produce keratinase, an enzyme that digests keratin, the tough protein that provides structure. Keratin is the main component of nails and the top layer of the skin (stratum corneum). Dermatophytes cause a group of diseases known as ringworm. Ringworm, despite its name, has nothing to do with worms but derives its name from a moth (*Tinea)* whose worms produce similar-shaped holes when they grow in woollen blankets. Ringworm infections are also known as the 'tineas'.

The New Prescriber: An Integrated Approach to Medical and Non-medical Prescribing, Second Edition.
Edited by Joanne Lymn, Alison Mostyn, Roger Knaggs, Michael Randall, and Dianne Bowskill.
© 2024 John Wiley & Sons Ltd. Published 2024 by John Wiley & Sons Ltd.

Aspergillus spp.

Aspergillus is a naturally occurring spore-forming fungus. These spores are very common and can be found in decaying vegetation, soil, potted plants, pepper and spices. Whilst there are many species of *Aspergillus* (>250), only a few actually cause disease.

Aspergillus-related disease occurs in three forms:

- colonisation and allergic response, for example allergic bronchopulmonary aspergillosis
- colonisation of pre-existing cavities, for example an aspergilloma in the sinuses or in the lungs after tuberculosis infection
- invasive disease, generally only seen in the immunocompromised.

PATHOGENIC YEASTS

Candida spp.

This is the most common pathogenic yeast. It is found in small numbers in the normal skin flora and in the flora of the gastrointestinal and genitourinary tracts. Candidal overgrowth and mucocutaneous infection occur when the normal body microbial flora is altered (e.g., by broad-spectrum antibiotics). Infection develops as discrete small white patches on the mucosal surface that can join to form a pseudomembrane (e.g., oral thrush). Cutaneous infections present as spreading erythema, sometime with pustules or macerated skin. Cutaneous candidiasis only occurs in warm moist areas. In immunocompromised patients, invasive systemic infection involving any organ in the body may occur.

PRACTICE APPLICATION

Patients may be immunocompromised for a variety of reasons:

- cancer patients: cytotoxic chemotherapy leading to neutropenia
- transplant patients: immunosuppressive therapy to prevent organ rejection
- in the intensive care unit: many patients with multiple organ failure have a reduced immune response and have often received multiple courses of antibiotics and venous cannulae.

Cryptococcus Neoformans

Cryptococcus is a yeast-like fungus that is found naturally in bird faeces (especially pigeons). It is the most common cause of life-threatening fungal infection in people with HIV infection. Most common sites for infection are the lungs and the central nervous system, where *Cryptococcus* meningitis has been well studied.

ANTIFUNGAL DRUGS

Fungi, being eukaryotes, are fundamentally more similar to mammalian cells than bacteria. However, there are still plenty of targets for selective toxicity, particularly the fungal cell wall and the fungal cell membrane. There are fewer drugs available to treat fungal infections than bacterial ones and many of these seem to have quite toxic side effects.

CELL WALL ACTIVE DRUGS

Echinocandins

Echinocandins, such as caspofungin, prevent the synthesis of 1,3-β-glucan, an essential component of fungal cell walls. Remember, mammalian cells do not have a cell wall and hence antifungal drugs that target this structure will only act on the fungal cells and not on our cells. Preventing the synthesis of 1,3-β-glucan renders the fungal cell vulnerable to osmotic changes and is often fungicidal. Caspofungin is active against *Candida* spp. and *Aspergillus* spp., and is licensed in adult and paediatric patients for:

- treatment of invasive candidiasis

- treatment of invasive aspergillosis in patients who are refractory to or intolerant of amphotericin B, lipid formulations of amphotericin B and/or itraconazole. Refractoriness is defined as progression of infection or failure to improve after a minimum of 7 days of prior therapeutic doses of effective antifungal therapy

- empirical therapy for presumed fungal infections (such as *Candida* or *Aspergillus)* in febrile, neutropenic adult patients.

Anidulafungin and micafungin are similar echinocandins, although their indications are currently more limited than those of caspofungin.

Cell Membrane Active Drugs

Ergosterol is the main sterol in the fungal cell membrane; the mammalian equivalent sterol is cholesterol. Targeting ergosterol is therefore an ideal example of selective toxicity and as such it is a target for a variety of antifungal drug classes.

Interactions with Ergosterol

The polyenes are a class of fungicidal drugs that act by disrupting the fungal cell membrane, the best known of which are nystatin and amphotericin B. Eight polyene drug molecules combine with eight molecules of ergosterol to form a hydrophilic pore lined with hydroxyl groups (Figure 30.1). This pore allows the movement of intracellular ions and water across the membrane and leads to membrane depolarisation and cell death. While mammalian cell membranes do not contain ergosterol, polyenes have been shown to form pores with cholesterol. Fortunately, this is not a significant issue because polyenes complex preferentially with ergosterol rather than cholesterol, and the pores formed with cholesterol are less stable and are smaller and less effective carriers of cations (Baginski et al. 2005). The clinical uses of nystatin are outlined in Table 30.1.

Amphotericin B is a broad-spectrum antifungal that is given intravenously in the treatment of life-threatening infections. Its usefulness is limited by dose-related nephrotoxicity. Toxicity is reduced by combining amphotericin B in a lipid formulation (as AmBisome® and Abelcet®). Although these are more expensive, they are usually the only formulations available in UK practice to reduce the patient safety risk of overdose with the non-lipid amphotericin B formulation Fungizone©.

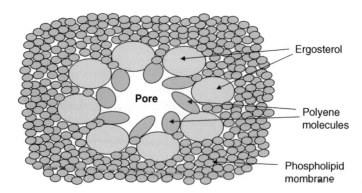

FIGURE 30.1 Polyene antifungal molecules combine with ergosterol to form a hydrophilic pore through the fungal cell membrane.

Table 30.1 Clinical uses of nystatin

Activity spectrum	Both moulds and yeasts, including *Candida* spp., *Aspergillus* spp. and *Cryptococcus neoformans*
Oral dose	For oral candida 100 000 units four times a day, usually for 7 days
Bioavailability	Insignificant absorption, currently only available in topical preparation
Excretion	Not applicable
Main uses	Cutaneous and mucocutaneous candidial infections
Other notes	An intravenous lipid-based preparation is likely to be available soon for systemic infection

PRACTICE APPLICATION

With all ampthotericin B preparations, it is important to give the patient an initial test dose and monitor them for 30 minutes for infusion-related reactions (fever, headache, chills, allergic reactions). These reactions are far less common with the lipid-associated preparations but if they do occur, symptoms can often be managed with paracetamol, antiemetics and antihistamines or by slowing the speed of the infusion. As well as renal function, patients should be closely monitored for changes in potassium, magnesium and calcium (initially daily).

Several of the enzymes involved in ergosterol synthesis are major targets for antifungal drug classes (Figure 30.2), including the azoles and terbinafine. The clinical uses of fluconazole and terbinafine are outlined in Table 30.2. Ergosterol is essential for maintaining the fluidity and permeability of the cell. Inhibition of these enzymes prevents the formation of ergosterol and compromises the cell. The azoles are the most numerous group of antifungal drugs (e.g., fluconazole). Most, when used systemically, are inhibitors of the cytochrome P450 group of metabolising enzymes, causing numerous drug interactions.

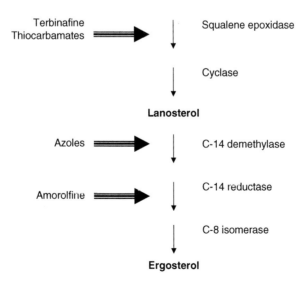

FIGURE 30.2 Many drugs interfere with ergosterol biosynthesis with actions at various enzymes within the biosynthetic pathway.

Table 30.2 Clinical uses of antifungal drugs that act by inhibiting ergosterol biosynthesis

Drug	Fluconazole	Terbinafine
Activity spectrum	*Candida albicans* and *Cryptococcus neoformans*	Active against most dermatophytes
		Also active vs *Candida* sp./ *Aspergillus* sp. but not used for systemic infections
Oral dose	Various depending on indication	Various depending on indication
Bioavailability	>90% absorbed	~40%
	Little need of IV unless 'nil by mouth'	
Excretion	Mostly renally excreted (60–90%)	Mixed excretion: requires dose reduction in renal impairment
		Avoid in liver impairment
Main uses	Cutaneous and mucocutaneous candidial infections that fail topical treatment	Drug of choice for treating fungal nail infections
	Deep infections caused by *Candida albicans* or other known sensitive *Candida* sp., especially as 'step-down' oral therapy following initial treatment with intravenous antifungals	Cutaneous fungal infection when oral therapy appropriate
Other notes	Hepatotoxic: not to be used in patients with liver impairment	Hepatotoxic: not to be used in patients with chronic or active liver impairment

STOP AND THINK

Have you checked your patient's current medication before prescribing an azole? Is the azole likely to inhibit metabolism of other prescribed medication?

PRACTICE APPLICATION

Resistance to one azole does not necessarily imply resistance to all. Voriconazole is a broad-spectrum azole antifungal that, although expensive, can still be used to treat fluconazole-resistant *Candida* strains.

VIRUSES

Viruses contain at least two types of macromolecules: proteins and genetic information contained in nucleic acid (either DNA or RNA but not both). They differ from the other major groups of microorganisms in that they require a living eukaryotic or prokaryotic host cell for replication, attaching and entering the cell with specific receptor-binding proteins. There are many types of virus, but this section will concentrate on three of the more common pathogens: herpes, influenza virus and SARS CoV 2.

ANTI-HERPES VIRUS DRUGS

Herpesviridae is a large family of viruses, many of which cause human disease. The most common are herpes simplex virus (HSV) which causes oral (HSV-1) and genital (HSV-2) herpes, varicella zoster virus (VZV), which causes chickenpox and shingles, Epstein–Barr virus (EBV), which

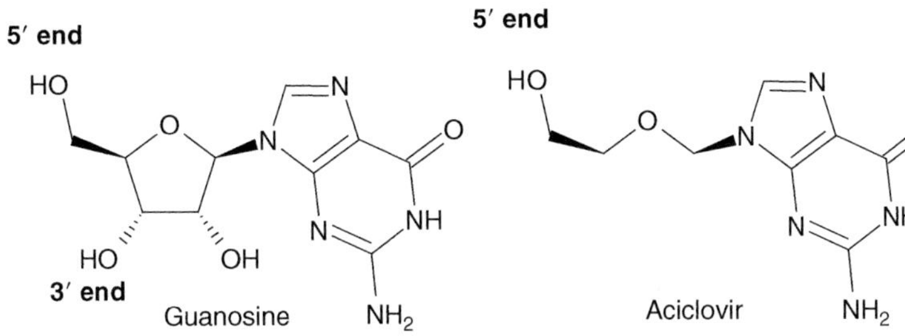

FIGURE 30.3   The structures of guanosine and acyclovir.

Table 30.3   Clinical uses of aciclovir

Activity spectrum	*Herpes viruses* family: most active vs herpes simplex, good activity vs varicella-zoster, slight activity vs Epstein-Barr virus, very slight activity vs cytomegalovirus
Oral dose	Varies with indication
Bioavailability	20%
Excretion	Mostly renally excreted
Main uses	Infections caused by herpes simplex and varicella-zoster viruses
	Prophylaxis of infection in immunocompromised
Other notes	Valaciclovir and famaciclovir are pro-drugs of aciclovir with better bioavailability, but they are more expensive

causes glandular fever, and cytomegalovirus (CMV). These viruses contain their genetic information in the form of DNA.

DNA is made up of a series of four 'bases', one of which is guanosine. Aciclovir is very similar in structure to guanosine (Figure 30.3) and, within cells infected with the herpes family of viruses, it actually acts as a guanosine analogue. After being activated by the addition of phosphate groups, aciclovir is incorporated into the viral DNA strands by the enzyme DNA polymerase. Once incorporated, it acts as a DNA chain terminator as there is nowhere to attach the next base.

Mammalian cells also use DNA polymerase in DNA synthesis but selective toxicity is assured because aciclovir is activated by viral enzymes and is much more effective at inhibiting viral DNA polymerase compared to the cellular version DNA polymerase (Elion 1983). The clinical uses of aciclovir are shown in Table 30.3.

ANTI-INFLUENZA VIRUS DRUGS

The influenza virus contains eight segments of single-stranded RNA, the genetic code for making new virus/enzymes contained in a capsid. On the virus surface are two protruding glycoproteins: haemagglutinin and neuraminidase.

Haemagglutinin aids the adhesion and phagocytosis of the virus into the host cell. Once inside, the viral RNA uses the host's organelles to manufacture further copies of the RNA viral code and the protein capsid, which together are packaged into new viral particles. These bud at the surface of the cell and, with the help of neuraminidase, are released to infect other host cells (Figure 30.4).

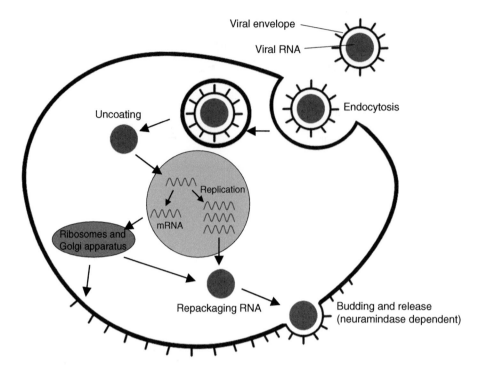

FIGURE 30.4 Reproduction cycle of the influenza virus.

Oseltamivir and zanamivir are neuraminidase inhibitors and prevent the release of the viral particles from the infected cell and hence the spread of infection within the body. As most of the spread occurs early in the infection, the drugs are more effective the sooner they can be started after symptoms appear. Both zanamivir and oseltamivir are licensed for the treatment of patients who present with flu-like illness when influenza A or B is circulating in the community, who can start taking the medicine within 48 hours of the onset of symptoms. Oseltamivir is additionally indicated for postexposure prevention in adults and adolescents 13 years of age or older following contact with a clinically diagnosed influenza case when influenza virus is circulating in the community.

The National Institute for Health and Care Excellence (NICE; www.nice.org.uk/) has evaluated both neuraminidase inhibitors and suggested that their use be restricted to the treatment of at-risk patients and post-exposure prophylaxis of at-risk patients or residents of care establishments (regardless of vaccination status). 'At-risk' individuals are those over 65 years or who have one of the following conditions:

- chronic respiratory disease, including asthma and COPD
- significant chronic heart disease (excluding hypertension)
- chronic renal disease
- chronic liver disease
- diabetes mellitus
- chronic neurological conditions
- immunosuppression.

SARS-COV-2/COVID-19

Many will remember early 2020 for the beginning of the pandemic caused by the coronavirus SARS-CoV-2. SARS-CoV-2 is a single-stranded RNA virus first isolated in December 2019 within the Wuhan province of China. The infection had high hospitalization and mortality rates, particularly in the older or higher risk groups, and overwhelmed many healthcare systems across the world. An international effort to develop, trial, manufacturer and distribute both vaccines and drugs led to a number of effective treatments, reducing the morbidity and mortality for those infected. At the time of writing supplies of many of these treatments were still limited within the NHS and therefore use was restricted to patients who met specific eligibility criteria.

PRACTICE APPLICATION

Before considering prescribing you should check your local trust guidance for more advice.

Neutralising Monoclonal Antibodies

Neutralising monoclonal antibodies (nMabs) are identical human antibodies engineered to specifically bind to antigens on the SARS-CoV-2 virus particles. At the time of writing, Ronapreve© (casirivimab with imdevimab) and sotrovimab were available within the UK. Both bind to the SARS-CoV-2 spike protein, preventing entry into the host cell. nMabs are intended to supplement an individual's endogenous antibodies and have uses in the prophylaxis and early treatment of infection. Sotrovimab has key advantages compared to casirivimab, with imdevimab being less complex to prepare for infusion and less susceptible to resistance from mutations of the spike protein such as those found in the Omicron variant.

SARS-CoV-2 Antiviral Drugs

At the time of writing three antiviral treatments were available within the UK for the treatment of SARS-CoV-2. These are involved in ongoing trials.

Remdesivir was the first antiviral licensed in the UK for the treatment of COVID-19 after originally being developed to treat ebola virus. It has shown benefit in the early treatment of patients at high risk of disease progression and is administered parenterally. After in vivo addition of phosphate groups, it acts as an adenosine triphosphate (ATP) analogue, being incorporated by RNA polymerase into RNA chains, delaying chain termination.

Molnupiravir was the first orally active antiviral licensed in the UK for the treatment of COVID-19. At this point it appears to be less effective at preventing disease progression in high-risk patients than nMabs, sotrovimab, Paxlovid© or remdesivir, although head-to-head studies have not occurred. Similar to remdesivir, it is metabolized to the active triphosphate form before incorporation into viral RNA by viral RNA polymerase, where it causes errors in the viral genome, preventing replication.

Paxlovid© is a combination of nirmatrelvir and ritonavir. Nirmatrelvir is active against the 3CL protease produced by SARS-CoV-2. It prevents the production of proteins required for replication. Nirmatrelvir is metabolized by the cytochrome P450 (CYP) 3A enzyme with an active half-life of 2 hours. Whilst ritonavir is also an antiviral protease inhibitor, it's not active against SARS-CoV-2. Ritonavir is a potent inhibitor of CYP3A that interacts to slow nirmatrelvir metabolism and increase its half-life to 6 hours, allowing a clinically effective twice-daily regimen. Ritonavir also inhibits CYP2D6 and the *p*-glyoprotein transport system, and it induces a number of other CYP enzymes. All in all, this leads to a large number of interactions, many of which are serious or potentially life-threatening. The University of Liverpool has developed a range of resources to check interactions with COVID treatments, including Paxlovid© (see www.covid19-druginteractions.org/). The clinical use of Paxlovid© is shown in Table 30.4.

Table 30.4 Clinical uses of Paxlovid© (nirmatrelvir with ritonavir)

Activity spectrum	SARS-CoV-2 virus
Oral dose	300 mg (2 × 150 mg tablets) of nirmatrelvir with 100 mg ritonavir twice a day for 5 days. The Paxlovid pack contains five blister strips each with one day's treatment. The dose is reduced in moderate renal impairment to 150 mg nirmatrelvir with 100 mg ritonavir twice a day for 5 days. Careful counselling is required to ensure the patient understands how to take the reduced dose.
Excretion	Faeces and renal
Main uses	Early treatment of COVID-19 in patients at high risk of disease progression to severe illness
Other notes	Numerous drug-drug interactions potentially leading to serious or life-threatening events. Take a full drug history and see www.covid19-druginteractions.org/ for more information.

SUMMARY

- Invasive fungal infections usually affect compromised patients. In normal hosts fungal infections tend to be superficial.

- The most common invasive fungal pathogens are *Candida* spp., *Aspergillius* spp. and *Cryptococcus neoformans*.

- The dermatophytes cause superficial skin and nail infections.

- Polyene antifungals (amphotericin B and nystatin) punch holes through the fungal cell membrane by forming a complex with ergosterol.

- Azole antifungals (e.g., fluconazole, voriconazole) and terbinafine inhibit the biosynthesis of ergosterol.

- Azole antifungals inhibit cytochrome P450 enzymes and have numerous drug–drug interactions.

- Terbinafine is particularly useful for the treatment of fungal nail infections. It can be hepatotoxic.

- Viruses need to enter a eukaryotic or prokaryotic cell to replicate.

- Aciclovir prevents viral DNA synthesis in cells infected by the herpes viruses, particularly herpes simplex and varicella zoster viruses.

- Oseltamivir and zanamivir inhibit neuraminidase to prevent the spread of influenza A and B virus.

- An international effort led to a range of treatments for COVID-19, including neutralizing monoclonal antibodies and antivirals.

- Paxlovid© an effective oral combination antiviral, active against SARS-CoV-2. It contains ritonavir, which is used to boost the levels of the active drug. It has numerous drug–drug interactions, potentially leading to severe or life-threatening adverse effects.

ACTIVITY

1. Invasive fungal infections only affect patients who have recently received chemotherapy.   True/False

2. The dermatophytes are a group of fungi that cause fungal lung infections.   True/False

3. Voriconazole is a broad-spectrum antifungal with good activity against *Candida* and *Aspergillus*.   True/False

4. Aciclovir has poor bioavailability, so the intravenous route should be used for treating life-threatening viral infections such as herpes simplex encephalitis.   True/False

5. Oseltamivir should be started as soon as possible after flu symptom onset but certainly within the first 48 hours.   True/False

6. Lipid-associated formulations of amphotericin B are more effective for treating fungal infections.   True/False

7. Fluconazole is the drug of choice for treating fungal nail infections.   True/False

8. Molnupiravir is first-line treatment for mild COVID-19 infection in high-risk patients.   True/False

REFERENCES

Baginski, M.J., Sternal, K., Czub, J. and Borowski, E. (2005) Molecular modelling of membrane activity of amphotericin B, a polyene macrolide antifungal antibiotic. *Acta Biochim Polon* 52:655–658.

Elion, G.B. (1983) The biochemistry and mechanism of action of acyclovir. *J Antimicrob Chemother* 12(Suppl B):9–17.

Lass-Flörl, C. (2009) The changing face of epidemiology of invasive fungal disease in Europe. *Mycoses* 52:197–205.

USEFUL WEBSITES

NICE technology appraisals for the prevention and treatment of influenza infection by zanamivir, amantadine and oseltamivir (TA168). www.nice.org.uk.

COVID-19 Drug interactions website. University of Liverpool. http://www.covid19-druginteractions.org

FURTHER READING

British National Formulary (online). BMJ Group and Pharmaceutical Press, London. https://bnf.nice.org.uk/

Cappelletty, D. and Eiselstein-Mckitrick, K. (2007) The echinocandins. *Pharmacotherapy* 27:369–388.

Chapman, S.W., Sullivan, D.C. and Cleary, J.D. (2008) In search of the holy grail of antifungal therapy. *Trans Am Clin Climatol Assoc* 119:197–215.

Pappas, P.G., Kauffman, C.A., Andes, D.R., et al. (2016) Clinical Practice Guideline for the Management of Candidiasis: 2016 Update by the Infectious Diseases Society of America. *Clin Infect Dis* 62:e1–e50.

Patterson, T.F., Thompson, G.R., Denning, D.W., et al. (2016) Practice Guidelines for the Diagnosis and Management of Aspergillosis: 2016 Update by the Infectious Diseases Society of America. *Clin Infect Dis* 63:e1–e60.

Reece, P.A. (2007) Neuraminidase inhibitor resistance in influenza virus. *J Med Virol* 79:1577–1586.

Wainberg, M.A. (2009) Perspectives on antiviral drug development. *Antiviral Res* 81:1–5.

CHAPTER 31

The Endocrine System

Alison Mostyn and Daniel Shipley

LEARNING OUTCOMES

By the end of this chapter the reader should be able to:

- describe how glucose homeostasis is maintained by the hormones insulin and glucagon

- describe the differences between type 1 and type 2 diabetes

- describe, using named examples, the pharmacodynamics, pharmacokinetics and therapeutics of drugs used to treat diabetes and their place in national guidelines

- understand the principles of prescribing insulin

- describe the hypothalamic–pituitary regulation and physiological function of thyroxine (T4) and triiodothyronine (T3), and relate this to the symptoms of hypo- and hyperthyroidism

- understand how to interpret blood tests for hypo- and hyperthyroidism

- describe, using named examples, the pharmacodynamics, pharmacokinetics and therapeutics of drugs used to treat hypo- and hyperthyroidism

THE ENDOCRINE SYSTEM

The endocrine system is composed of a diverse range of organs, tissues and cells that regulate most of our body systems (Figure 31.1). The signalling molecules released from endocrine organs are called hormones and they act on target cells which contain receptors specific for that hormone. Hormones may be classified as either circulating or local. A circulating hormone travels via the circulation to reach distant target cells (Figure 31.2), for example insulin is released from the pancreas and travels via the bloodstream to distant organs such as the liver and skeletal muscle. Local hormones can be either paracrine or autocrine. Paracrine hormones act on neighbouring cells, therefore negating the need to enter the bloodstream; the term *para* means 'beside'. Autocrine hormones, as the name suggests, act on the same endocrine cell from which they were released (Figure 31.2).

> **STOP AND THINK**
>
> Classify the following list of hormones as autocrine, paracrine or endocrine: adrenaline, oestrogen, gastrin, insulin, growth hormone.

MECHANISMS OF HORMONE ACTION

Hormones act on specific receptors on target cells, which can be classified by their location within the target cell as either membrane-bound or intracellular.

The New Prescriber: An Integrated Approach to Medical and Non-medical Prescribing, Second Edition.
Edited by Joanne Lymn, Alison Mostyn, Roger Knaggs, Michael Randall, and Dianne Bowskill.
© 2024 John Wiley & Sons Ltd. Published 2024 by John Wiley & Sons Ltd.

Major endocrine glands

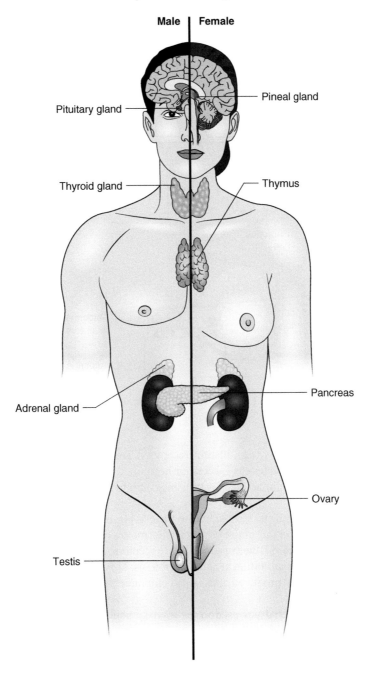

FIGURE 31.1   Location of the major glands and endocrine hormones (www.commons.wikimedia.org/wiki/Image:Illu endocrine system.jpg).

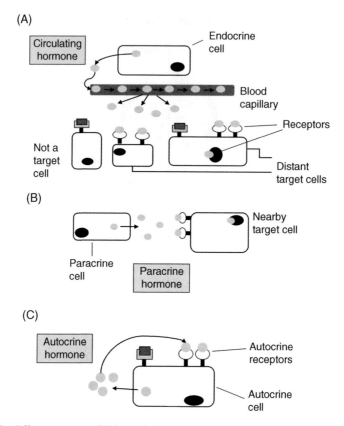

FIGURE 31.2 The differing actions of (A) circulating, (B) paracrine and (C) autocrine hormones.

Membrane-bound receptors (e.g., insulin receptors) are located within the plasma membrane of the target cell; this provides easy access for hormones within the interstitial fluid. Generally, these receptors initiate a cellular effect by utilising components which already exist within the cell, eliciting a fast response.

Intracellular receptors may be located within the cytoplasm (the glucocorticoid receptor) or nucleus (thyroid hormone receptor) of the target cell; hormones must cross the plasma membrane and enter the target cell to interact with intracellular receptors. Activated intracellular receptors then initiate the production or inhibition of cellular proteins. This effect takes several hours as new cellular components have to be produced or existing components degraded before cellular changes become apparent.

This chapter will focus on drugs used in the management of diabetes mellitus and thyroid disorders.

GLUCOSE HOMEOSTASIS AND DIABETES MELLITUS

THE ENDOCRINE PANCREAS

Plasma glucose concentrations are tightly regulated by the hormones insulin and glucagon. The organ responsible for the maintenance of normal plasma glucose is the pancreas. The pancreas consists of both non-endocrine cells, which are responsible for the production of digestive juices (the exocrine pancreas), and endocrine cells (the endocrine pancreas); the endocrine pancreas

Table 31.1 The function of each of the three cell types located in the endocrine pancreas

Cell type	Hormone	Function
Alpha (α) cells	Glucagon	Raises blood glucose concentrations
Beta (β) cells	Insulin	Lowers blood glucose concentrations
Delta (δ) cells	Somatostatin	Acts as a paracrine hormone to inhibit both insulin and glucagon

accounts for only 1–1.5% of the mass of the whole pancreas. Within the endocrine pancreas are 0.7–1 million clusters of cells named pancreatic islets or islets of Langerhans. There are three main cell types located within the endocrine pancreas (Table 31.1). These cells manufacture and secrete the hormones insulin, glucagon and somatostatin.

The most potent stimulator of insulin secretion is glucose. After ingestion of a meal, glucose stimulates insulin secretion from β-cells. Insulin circulates in the blood and acts on insulin receptors in target tissues to promote glucose uptake and reduce plasma glucose levels. The release of insulin from β-cells, just like the release of neurotransmitters from nerve cells (Chapters 14 and 21), occurs through the process of calcium-mediated exocytosis. Glucose has an inhibitory effect on glucagon secretion, therefore between meals, when plasma glucose concentrations are low, this inhibitory effect of glucose is removed. Glucagon is released from α-cells and promotes the breakdown of stored glycogen and stimulates gluconeogenesis. This increases the available energy for tissues (Figure 31.3). The effects of insulin in the body can be described as endocrine, paracrine and cellular effects, and these are described below.

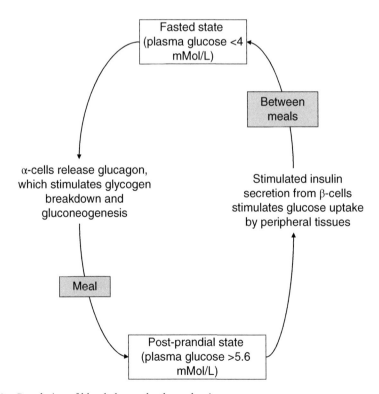

FIGURE 31.3 Regulation of blood glucose by the endocrine pancreas.

ENDOCRINE (PERIPHERAL) EFFECTS OF INSULIN

Insulin promotes the storage of nutrients in most of the organs and tissues of the body. However, there are three organs and tissues that are particularly specialised for the purpose of energy storage: skeletal muscle, adipose tissue and the liver.

The first organ insulin reaches via the bloodstream is the liver. Insulin acts on the liver in two ways: by promoting glycogen synthesis and storage, and by inhibiting both the production of new glucose (gluconeogenesis) and the breakdown of glycogen stores into glucose (glycogenolysis). In skeletal muscle, insulin promotes protein and glycogen synthesis and increases glucose transport into muscle cells. Adipose tissue responds to insulin signalling by promoting triglyceride storage, inhibiting lipolysis or breakdown of stored triglycerides and increasing glucose transport into adipocytes.

PARACRINE EFFECTS OF INSULIN

As well as regulating metabolism in distant organs, insulin has a paracrine role in the pancreas. Insulin has an inhibitory effect on the α-cells within the pancreatic islets, which reduces glucagon secretion.

CELLULAR ACTIONS OF INSULIN

The biological effects of insulin are mediated through the insulin receptor (Figure 31.4), which is located within the plasma membrane of the cell. Insulin binding activates the receptor and initiates biological changes, leading to a reduction of plasma glucose levels. One group of cellular proteins stimulated by the activated insulin receptor are the insulin receptor substrates (IRSs), which initiate a cascade of cellular events that culminate in the reduction of plasma glucose (Figure 31.5). The IRS-stimulated pathway is known to mediate many metabolic changes within the cell, including glycogenesis and decreased gluconeogenesis.

Insulin binding also stimulates the recruitment of glucose transporter 4 (GLUT4) to the cell membrane. When insulin is not bound to its receptor, GLUT4 remains in intracellular vesicles; on insulin receptor activation, these vesicles relocate to the membrane and fuse with it, allowing

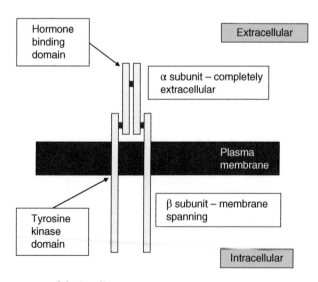

FIGURE 31.4 The structure of the insulin receptor.

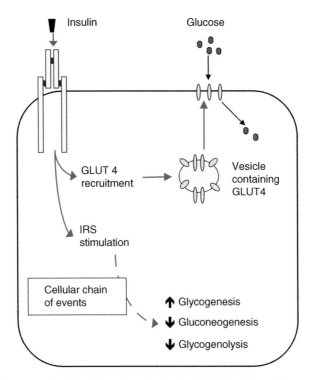

FIGURE 31.5   Mechanism of insulin action at a cellular level. GLUT4, glucose transporter 4; IRS, insulin receptor substrate.

glucose to flow into the cell (Figure 31.5). Not all tissue types require GLUT4 to take up glucose; the brain and liver utilise insulin-independent transporters.

Several other cellular pathways exist to facilitate insulin-stimulated protein synthesis, glycogenesis, antilipolysis and decreased glycolysis and gluconeogenesis. All these systems act together to reduce plasma glucose concentrations.

DIABETES MELLITUS

Diabetes mellitus is a disorder characterised by hyperglycaemia (elevated blood glucose). There are two types of diabetes: insulin-dependent (IDDM, type 1) and non-insulin-dependent (NIDDM, type 2).

Type 1 diabetes mellitus is often referred to as juvenile onset because a diagnosis is often made during childhood. One study in the UK gave the average age of diagnosis of type 1 diabetes as 20.6 years in 2005 (Sharp et al. 2008), but more recent evidence indicates that the most common age of diagnosis is between 10 and 14 years (Royal College of Paediatrics and Child Health 2022). An autoimmune reaction destroys pancreatic β-cells so no insulin is produced. This type of diabetes must be treated with insulin replacement therapy. The incidence of type 1 diabetes mellitus in the UK is increasing (Royal College of Paediatrics and Child Health 2022).

Type 2 diabetes mellitus used to be referred to as age-onset diabetes, but this terminology may now be outdated as more young people are being diagnosed. Indeed, the age of diagnosis of type 2 diabetes decreased between 1992 and 2005 from 57.1 to 54 (Sharp et al. 2008) and the first children with type 2 diabetes mellitus were diagnosed in 2000 (Whicher et al. 2020). Individuals with NIDDM typically produce insulin, sometimes at lower concentrations than normal, but their cells do not respond to insulin signalling. This means that insulin is not always required to treat NIDDM.

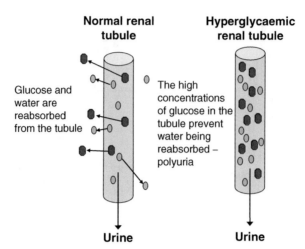

FIGURE 31.6 Demonstration of glycosuria.

The word 'diabetes' means 'a siphoning of water through the body', which refers to the frequent need to urinate experienced by diabetics. This polyuria is caused by osmotic diuresis. Under normal conditions, very little glucose reaches the proximal tubules of the kidney as it is taken up for storage in tissues. Any glucose that does reach the proximal tubule is normally reabsorbed into the bloodstream by a specific transporter, sodium-glucose co-transporter-2 (SGLT-2). If the blood glucose level exceeds the capacity of the transporters to reabsorb all the glucose present in the glomerular filtrate, the renal threshold is reached and glucose spills into the urine (glycosuria) (Figure 31.6). Osmotic diuresis occurs as the osmotic pressure of the glucose 'holds' water molecules in the tubule; this large volume of urine leads to polyuria.

Ketoacidosis results when cells in the body become deficient in glucose, which occurs when insulin is not stimulating the uptake of glucose into cells. As a result, the cells start to utilise other energy sources, including metabolising fatty acids. A byproduct of fatty acid metabolism is ketones, which are harmful to the body and therefore the kidney will attempt to remove them via the urine. The build-up of ketones in the blood is called ketoacidosis.

TREATMENT OF DIABETES

INSULIN

Insulin replacement therapy is always used to treat IDDM (type 1) and some cases of NIDDM (type 2). Almost all insulins used today are analogues of human insulin made by recombinant DNA technology, rather than being extracted and purified from the pancreas of animals.

STOP AND THINK

As insulin is a protein, it is destroyed by the juices of the gastrointestinal tract. This limits the possible routes of administration of insulin. Which of the following routes of administration would be suitable: oral, intravenous, subcutaneous injection?

Many different formulations of insulin exist, but they can be broadly classified as being rapid, short, intermediate or long acting (Table 31.2). A regimen using these preparations will be

Table 31.2 The different formulations of insulin available

Insulin type	Pharmacokinetics
Short-acting or soluble insulins	Rapid onset of action, 30–60 minutes Duration of action of up to 8 hours
Rapid-acting insulins (insulin lispro)	Designed to work in the same way as the insulin normally produced to cope with a meal
	Onset of action of ~15 minutes
	Duration of action of between 2 and 5 hours
Intermediate-acting insulins (isophane insulin, insulin zinc suspension)	Intermediate action
	Onset of action of approximately 1–2 hours
	Duration of action of 16–35 hours
Long-acting insulins (insulin glargine)	Normally used once a day
	Achieve a steady-state level after 2–4 days

devised to match an individual's requirements. NICE has type 1 diabetes guidelines which should be used when making clinical decisions.

Human insulin is crystalline zinc insulin dissolved in a clear solution at pH 3.5. However, insulin is more physiologically active at a neutral pH so is mixed with a buffer to achieve this. Regular insulin produces a rapid and short-lived effect. The chemical and pharmacokinetic properties of regular insulin can be altered by attaching other molecules to it or changing the amino acid sequence. This can alter the onset and/or duration of action, for example three amino acids are altered in the insulin molecule to produce the long-acting insulin glargine. Insulin glargine is soluble at pH 4 and becomes neutral when injected subcutaneously; this forms a precipitate that slowly releases insulin glargine into the plasma.

INSULIN PRESCRIBING PRINCIPLES

The prescribing of insulin can be challenging. For those conducting medicines reconciliation, identifying all the salient information is a challenge. Whilst insulin preparations can invariably be identified using both repeat records and discharge prescriptions, the precise details of the regimen are rarely recorded. Deciphering the number of units being injected along with times of administration requires conversation with patients, carers and relatives. The propensity for human error is high.

This is further complicated in secondary care, where arrangements for patient self-administration vary. Typically, a patient's capacity and suitability to self-administer insulin is assessed and recorded in the medical notes. To prevent duplication, the prescriber should enter the insulin regimen on the drug chart and instruct the nursing team to record self-administered doses. Any changes to the patient's health may necessitate reassessment. If the patient has an insulin infusion pump, this should also be noted on the drug chart.

Due to the frequency of errors, some hospital trusts mitigate the prescribing of insulin on separate stationery. These charts are designed not only to facilitate blood glucose monitoring but also eradicate abbreviation of the word 'units'. Deemed a "never event" by NHS England, using the letter 'u' instead of 'units' carries the risk of being mistaken for a zero, thereby leading to a 10-fold dose increase.

Insulin not only needs to be prescribed by brand, but also requires device designation. Generic insulin prescribing does not account for the lack of bioequivalence across preparations, with significant variation in release profile, onset of action etc. Furthermore, the patient's preferred delivery system is required to validate the prescription. Due to issues relating to supply, dexterity and adherence, insulin preparations are available in a range of devices.

Another prescribing peculiarity concerns biphasic insulin preparations. Brand names should be accompanied by a number that denotes the percentage of rapid or short-acting component contained in the insulin suspension. For example, in Novomix 30 (100 units/ml), there are 30 units of short-acting insulin in 1 ml. This means the remaining 70 units are intermediate acting.

PRACTICE APPLICATION

Examples of rapid, short, intermediate and long-acting insulins are provided in Table 31.3.

Table 31.3   Examples of rapid-, short-, intermediate- and long-acting insulins

Type	Examples
Rapid-acting	Insulin aspart, insulin lispro, insulin glulisine
Short-acting	Soluble insulin
Intermediate-acting	Isophane insulin
Long-acting	Insulin glargine, insulin detemir

TYPE 2 DIABETES MANAGEMENT

It is important to recognise that diabetes is major contributor towards both cardiovascular and chronic kidney disease. The optimisation of blood glucose is a component of prevention alongside the initiation of antihypertensives, statins and lifestyle intervention. The number of drugs available to manage type 2 diabetes can be overwhelming. National stratification of management is achieved by NICE guidelines, although patient factors are the main determinant affecting antiglycaemic prescribing.

If tolerated, metformin is typically started as monotherapy, with the dosage being upwardly titrated towards response. For those with chronic heart failure or established atherosclerotic cardiovascular disease, the addition of gliflozins is recommended.

Any further additions meanwhile are subject to an individual's clinical circumstances, such as comorbidities, contraindications, weight, risks from polypharmacy etc. Some drugs, for example, can cause weight gain (e.g., sulphonylureas), whilst other drugs are contraindicated in congestive heart failure (e.g., thiazolidinediones).

ORAL ANTIDIABETIC AGENTS

Oral antidiabetic agents are used to treat type 2 diabetes, sometimes in combination with insulin. Antidiabetic drugs included in the NICE guidance include sulphonylureas, biguanides, dipeptidyl peptidase-4 (DPP-4) inhibitors, SGLT-2 inhibitors and thiazolidinediones (Table 31.4).

Sulphonylureas

Sulphonylureas are the only group of oral antidiabetic agents which increase insulin secretion from the pancreas; in this respect, some β-cell functionality is required. As described previously, calcium ions are required to stimulate insulin release from β-cells. Under resting conditions, K^+ ions exit β-cells via a specific channel, maintaining cellular polarisation. The sulphonylurea drugs bind to a receptor on this K^+ channel, causing it to close and allowing the β-cell to become depolarised. This depolarisation allows the entry of Ca^{2+} into the β-cell and the Ca^{2+} ions stimulate the release of insulin by exocytosis (Figure 31.7).

Table 31.4   The main groups of antidiabetic drugs

Group	Drug examples	Physiological mechanism
Biguanides	Metformin	Reduce glucose production in the liver and increase peripheral glucose uptake
Sodium-glucose co-transporter-2 (SGLT-2) inhibitors (flozins)	Dapagliflozin Empagliflozin	Block the re-uptake of glucose into the bloodstream, resulting in excretion of glucose in the urine
Dipeptidyl peptidase-4 (DPP-4) inhibitors (gliptins)	Alogliptin Linagliptin	Potentiate the action of incretin hormones, creating a feeling of fullness
Thiazolidinediones	Pioglitazone	Sensitise peripheral tissues to insulin Stimulate glucose and fatty acids uptake into adipocytes Stimulate transcription of genes involved in insulin signalling
Sulphonylureas	Gliclazide Glibenclamide Tolbutamide	Increase insulin secretion from the β-cells of the pancreas
Glucagon-like peptide 1 (GLP-1) mimetics (incretin mimetics)	Semaglutide Liraglutide	Mimic incretin hormones Simulate insulin release, inhibit glucagon, slow digestion and create a feeling of fullness

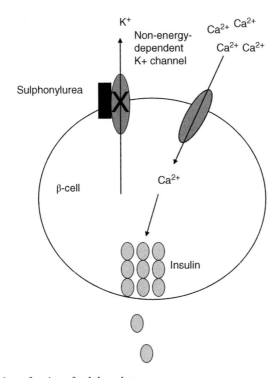

FIGURE 31.7   Mechanism of action of sulphonylureas.

Table 31.5 Potential molecular mechanisms of metformin action

Mechanism	Outcome
Enhanced muscle uptake of insulin	Improved signalling of insulin
Restoration of enzyme activity in the insulin-signalling cascade	Increased stimulation of insulin-dependent cellular events, e.g. increased glucose transporter 4 translocation to the membrane
Inhibition of enzymes in the gluconeogenic pathway in the liver	Reduction of gluconeogenesis
Reduction of the uptake of gluconeogenic substrates in the liver	Reduction of gluconeogenesis
Reduction of hepatic mitochondrial respiration	Reduced energy supply to the liver, resulting in reduced gluconeogenic ability
Stimulation of adenosine monophosphate-activated protein kinase	Inhibition of hepatic glucose production and increased glucose uptake in skeletal muscle

Biguanides

Metformin is the only biguanide drug available in the UK. It does not increase insulin secretion but decreases hepatic gluconeogenesis and increases peripheral glucose uptake. The molecular mechanisms behind these physiological changes are not well described, despite metformin being developed in the 1950s. The potential molecular mechanisms of metformin are listed in Table 31.5. This is not an exhaustive list and the mechanisms are not all conclusive.

Thiazolidinediones

The thiazolidinedione group of drugs (sometimes referred to as 'glitazones') are agonists of peroxisome proliferator activated receptor (PPAR) γ. PPARγ is a nuclear receptor found mainly in adipose tissue. The main physiological action of thiazolidinediones is to sensitise peripheral tissues to insulin. Despite PPARγ being found predominantly in adipose tissue, the improvement in insulin sensitivity observed with thiazolidinediones occurs mostly in the skeletal muscle. PPARγ is thought to modulate adipose tissue cytokines, which may communicate between adipose tissue and skeletal muscle.

As well as improving insulin sensitivity, thiazolidinediones also promote redistribution of lipid within the body. Extra-adipocyte lipid storage, for example in the liver and skeletal muscle, is thought to play a role in insulin resistance. By redistributing these stores of lipid to adipose tissue, insulin sensitivity can be improved.

DPP-4 inhibitors (gliptins)

Incretins are a family of hormones which are released following the ingestion of food. Their purpose is to maintain glucose homeostasis by simulating insulin release, inhibiting glucagon, slowing digestion and creating a feeling of fullness. Potentiating the action of incretin hormones is therefore a desirable mechanism in diabetes. This can be achieved using gliptins, which inhibit the DPP-4 enzyme. DPP-4 catalyses the inactivation of incretins like glucagon-like peptide 1 (GLP-1) and glucose-dependent insulinotropic polypeptide (GIP). By inhibiting DPP-4, incretin levels are increased.

SGLT-2 inhibitors (gliflozins)

SGLT-2 facilitates most glucose reabsorption from the proximal tubule back into the bloodstream. In diabetes this process is undesirable. Gliflozins inhibit this transporter and in doing so promote the excretion of glucose in the urine. As a result, even well-controlled diabetic patients will test positive for glucose in the urine.

GLP-1 MIMETICS (INCRETIN MIMETICS)

GLP-1 analogues, such as semaglutide and liraglutide, are agents that mimic the action of incretins. GLP-1 mimetics are considered if triple therapy with metformin and two other oral antidiabetic drugs is not effective, not tolerated or contraindicated.

Tirzepatide, a new dual GIP and GLP-1 analogue, was authorised in November 2023. Tirzepatide is a weekly injectable drug and is indicated for use when triple therapy with metformin and two other oral antidiabetic agents has been ineffective, not tolerated or contraindicated.

THE THYROID GLAND

THYROID FUNCTION

The thyroid gland is located in the neck in front of the larynx and trachea. The primary hormone secreted from the thyroid gland is thyroxine (T_4); tri-iodothyronine (T_3) is secreted in smaller concentrations. In the periphery, T_4 is transformed into T_3 by the enzyme 5'-deiodinase. As the name tri-*iodo*thyronine suggests, iodine is an essential component in these hormones.

Release of the thyroid hormones from the thyroid gland is regulated via the hypothalamic pituitary-thyroid axis. Stimuli, such as decreased plasma glucose or exercise, promote the hypothalamus to release thyrotrophin-releasing hormone (TRH). Once released, TRH acts on the anterior pituitary gland to stimulate the secretion of thyroid-stimulating hormone (TSH or thyrotrophin). TSH stimulates the release of T_4 and T_3 from the thyroid gland (Figure 31.8) as well as iodine metabolism and cell growth. Once secreted, T_3 and T_4 circulate widely in the body, affecting many different organ systems, for example adipose tissue. Thyroid hormones travel bound to a thyroid-binding globulin, which facilitates their transport. To maintain thyroid function homeostasis, T_3 can negatively feedback to the hypothalamus and pituitary to 'switch off' TRH and TSH secretion, respectively.

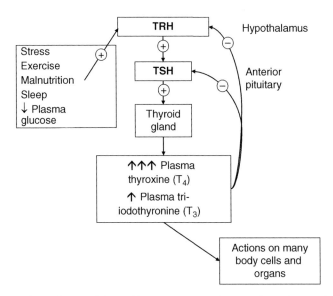

FIGURE 31.8 Feedback regulation of thyroid hormones. TRH, thyrotrophin-releasing hormone; TSH, thyroid-stimulating hormone.

Table 31.6 Summary of thyroid effects within the body

Metabolism	Growth	Development
↑ Basal metabolic rate	Necessary for growth in children	Essential for the growth and development of the foetal and neonatal brain
↑ Body heat production		
↑ Fat mobilization		
↑ Insulin-dependent entry of glucose into cells		
↑ Gluconeogenesis and glycogenolysis		
↑ Sympathetic activation in the heart, and skeletal and adipose tissue		

PRACTICE APPLICATION

Laboratory blood results contain information on 'free' and 'total' thyroid hormones. The free T_4 (FT_4) is the T_4 in the blood that is not bound to thyroid-binding globulins and is therefore freely available to bind to thyroid receptors. Total T_4, as the name suggests, is the total concentration of T_4 in the blood and includes free and bound T_4.

Thyroid hormones exert the majority of their biological effects via a nuclear receptor. Once T_4 reaches its target cell, it is converted into the more active T_3, which then interacts with the thyroid receptor. As described previously, biological effects exerted via nuclear receptors take some time to occur, up to days, due to the transcriptional and translational changes that must take place in the cell.

Thyroid hormones regulate a number of biological processes (Table 31.6), which can be grouped into metabolic effects and regulation of growth and development. Thyroid hormones have a key role in regulating growth and development in the foetus and neonate. The fetus begins to produce its own thyroid hormones after about 3 months, but in early gestation relies on the transfer of thyroid hormones across the placenta from the mother. A lack of dietary iodine during foetal and neonatal development or genetic impairment of the genes which produce thyroid hormones causes a disorder known as cretinism, which is associated with muscle weakness and mental impairment.

HYPOTHYROIDISM

Insufficient thyroid hormone secretion is known as hypothyroidism. There are many potential causes, including:

- autoimmune disease: causes a failure of the thyroid gland to produce thyroid hormones in sufficient quantities (most common cause)

- congenital lack of thyroid gland: born with no thyroid gland

- deficiency of TRH (hypothalamus) or TSH (pituitary) secretion

- surgical removal

- lack of iodine in the diet (rare in the UK).

STOP AND THINK

After reviewing the physiological effects of thyroid hormones (Table 31.6), what are the potential symptoms of hypothyroidism?

When there is a deficiency of thyroid hormones, the normal negative feedback of T_3 and T_4 to the hypothalamus and pituitary (Figure 31.8) is halted. With the 'brakes' removed from the pituitary, increased TSH is released and continues to stimulate the thyroid gland in an attempt to increase plasma T_3 and T_4. TSH promotes cell growth in the thyroid gland and this may produce goitre.

Hypothyroidism can be treated pharmacologically by replacing deficient hormones. Most commonly, T_4 is administered in the form of levothyroxine sodium. T_4 can be transformed into T_3 in the tissues by the enzyme 5′-deiodinase; the pharmacodynamics of levothyroxine are the same as those of the endogenous hormone. Liothyronine (T_3) can also be used but has a much shorter duration of action and is usually reserved for hypothyroid emergencies. Drugs for the treatment of hypothyroidism do not alter the synthesis or release of hormones from the thyroid gland, they simply provide an exogenous source of hormone.

HYPERTHYROIDISM

Overproduction of thyroid hormones is termed hyperthyroidism; the clinical result of a high plasma concentration of thyroid hormones is referred to as thyrotoxicosis. The most common cause of hyperthyroidism is an autoimmune disease (Graves' disease).

Again, considering the physiological effects of thyroid hormones (Table 31.6), the potential symptoms of hyperthyroidism can be determined. There is an increase in metabolism which leads to weight loss, excessive sweating and poor tolerance of warm temperatures, fatigue due to muscle weakness as muscle proteins are broken down, abnormally fast heart rate/palpitations and abnormally acute alertness making the individual irritable, tense or anxious.

When there is excessive secretion of thyroid hormones, the normal negative feedback of T_3 and T_4 to the hypothalamus and pituitary (Figure 31.8) is enhanced. This decreases TSH and TRH secretion from the hypothalamus and pituitary to decrease plasma T_3 and T_4. However, the thyroid does not respond to the reduced signals and continues to produce T_3 and T_4.

Hyperthyroidism may be treated pharmacologically with a group of drugs known as thioureylenes (carbimizole and propylthiouracil) which:

- prevent the incorporation of iodine into the structure of the thyroid hormone

- block the peripheral conversion of T_4 to (more active) T_3.

These drugs do not act on preformed thyroid hormones. The thyroid gland stores large amounts of preformed hormone so thioureylenes may take 2–3 weeks to be clinically effective. If the thyroid continues to overproduce thyroid hormones, alternative treatments such as radioiodine or surgical removal of the thyroid gland may be required.

Some of the symptoms of hyperthyroidism are caused by increased adrenoceptor stimulation, such as tachycardia and palpitations. Symptomatic relief from these symptoms can be provided with β-adrenergic receptor blockers (e.g., propranolol; Chapters 15 and 17).

SUMMARY

- The endocrine system regulates a diverse range of physiological and biochemical functions within the body.

- Glucose homeostasis is regulated by the hormones insulin and glucagon, which are secreted from the pancreas.

- Insulin acts on a membrane-bound receptor to facilitate the storage of glucose, thereby reducing plasma concentrations.

- Insulin is not secreted from the pancreas in individuals with insulin-dependent diabetes.

- Exogenous insulin treatments are used in type 1 diabetes; a range of short-, medium- and long-acting insulins are available.

- Non-insulin-dependent diabetes mellitus (type 2 diabetes) is characterised by insulin resistance.

- Several drugs, including sulphonylureas (which improve insulin secretion), biguanides (which improve peripheral responsiveness to insulin) and SGLT-2 inhibitors (which increase glucosuria) are used to treat type 2 diabetes.

- The thyroid gland regulates growth and metabolism via secretion of thyroxine (T_4) and tri-iodothyronine (T_3).

- T_4 is enzymatically transformed to T_3 (the active form of the hormone), which acts primarily on a nuclear receptor.

- Hypo- and hyperactive thyroid states can be treated pharmacologically with levothyroxine and carbimazole, respectively.

ACTIVITY

1. Pancreatic β-cells produce which hormone?

   (a) Cortisol

   (b) Glucagon

   (c) Insulin

   (d) Tri-iodothyronine

2. Insulin promotes the storage of glucose in body tissues.   True/False

3. Insulin is a protein.   True/False

4. Which group of oral antidiabetic drugs increases plasma insulin?

   (a) Biguanides

   (b) Sulphonylureas

   (c) Thiazolidinediones

   (d) SGLT-2 inhibitors

   (e) DPP-4 inhibitors

5. Skeletal muscle uptake of glucose occurs through which channel?

   (a) Calcium channel

   (b) GLUT4

   (c) Sodium pump

6. SGLT-2 inhibitors reduce glucosuria   True/False

7. Tri-iodothyronine (T_3) is more active than thyroxine (T_4).   True/False

8. Carbamizole takes a few weeks to exert a clinical effect. Why?

   (a) Patients forget to take it.

   (b) Preformed thyroid hormones are unaffected.

   (c) The drug is taken very slowly from the gut to the thyroid gland.

REFERENCES

Royal College of Paediatrics and Child Health (2022) National Paediatric Diabetes Audit (NPDA) annual reports.

Sharp, P.S., Brown, B. and Qureshi, A. (2008) Age at diagnosis of diabetes in a secondary care population: 1992–2005. *Br J Diabetes Vasc Dis* 8:92–95.

Whicher, C.A., O'Neill, S. and Holt, R.I.G. (2020) Diabetes in the UK: 2019. *Diabetic Med* 37:242–247.

FURTHER READING

Bassett, J.H., Harvey, C.B. and Williams, G.R. (2003) Mechanisms of thyroid hormone receptor-specific nuclear and extra nuclear actions. *Mol Cell Endocrinol* 213:1–11.

British Medical Association and Royal Pharmaceutical Society of Great Britain (2010) *British National Formulary*, 59th edn. BMJ Publishing, London.

Brunton, S.A. (2008) The changing shape of type 2 diabetes. *Medscape J Med* 10:143.

Delange, F. (2007) Iodine requirements during pregnancy, lactation and the neonatal period and indicators of optimal iodine nutrition. *Public Health Nutr* 10:1571–1580.

Devdhar, M., Ousman, Y.H. and Burman, K.D. (2007) Hypothyroidism. *Endocrinol Metab Clin North Am* 36:595–615.

Gardner, D.G., Shoback, D.M. and Greenspan, F.S. (2011) *Greenspan's Basic & Clinical Endocrinology*, 9th edn. McGraw-Hill, London.

Lepore, M., Pampanelli, S., Fanelli, C., et al. (2000) Pharmacokinetics and pharmacodynamics of subcutaneous injection of long-acting human insulin analog glargine, NPH insulin, and ultralente human insulin and continuous subcutaneous infusion of insulin lispro. *Diabetes* 49:2142–2148.

Page, C.P., Curtis, M.J., Sutter, M.C., et al. (2006) *Integrated Pharmacology*, 3rd edn. Mosby, London.

Ritter, J.M., Flower, R., Henderson, G., et al. (2023) *Rang and Dale's Pharmacology*, 10th edn. Elsevier, Amsterdam.

Rossetti, P., Porcellati, F., Fanelli, C.G., et al. (2008) Superiority of insulin analogues versus human insulin in the treatment of diabetes mellitus. *Arch Physiol Biochem* 114:3–10.

Whicher, C. A., O'Neill, S. and Holt, R.I.G. (2020) Diabetes in the UK: 2019. *Diabetic Med* 37:242–247.

USEFUL
WEBSITE

Thyroid Disease Manager. https://www.thyroid manager.org/.

Diabetes UK. www.diabetes.org.uk.

CLINICAL
GUIDANCE

NICE guideline [NG28]. Type 2 diabetes in adults: management. https://www.nice.org.uk/guidance/ng28.

NICE guideline [NG17]. Type 1 diabetes in adults: diagnosis and management. https://www.nice.org.uk/guidance/ng17.

NICE guideline [NG18]. Diabetes (type 1 and type 2) in children and young people: diagnosis and management. https://www.nice.org.uk/guidance/ng18.

NICE guideline [NG145]. Thyroid disease: assessment and management. https://www.nice.org.uk/guidance/ng145.

Contraception and Reproductive Health

CHAPTER 32

Alison Mostyn and Anna Soames

LEARNING OUTCOMES

By the end of this chapter the reader should be able to:

- describe the clinical uses, effectiveness, pharmacodynamics, pharmacokinetics, risks and non-contraceptive benefits of contraception containing oestrogen and progestogen

- describe the clinical uses, effectiveness, pharmacodynamics, pharmacokinetics, risks and non-contraceptive benefits of progestogen-only contraception

- describe the clinical uses, effectiveness, pharmacodynamics, pharmacokinetics and risks of emergency hormonal contraception

- understand the drug–drug interactions associated with the failure of contraception or other medication

- understand the clinical use of oestrogen and progesterone as hormone replacement therapy in the perimenopause and menopause.

ENDOCRINE REGULATION OF THE FEMALE REPRODUCTIVE SYSTEM

Like many body systems, female reproduction is tightly regulated by hormones. This regulation begins in the hypothalamus with the secretion of gonadotrophin-releasing hormone (GnRH). GnRH travels along the hypophyseal portal vessels to the anterior pituitary gland, where it stimulates the release of both follicle-stimulating hormone (FSH) and luteinising hormone (LH). FSH and LH travel to target organs to exert their biological effects, which include stimulating the ovaries (and testes in the male) to secrete oestrogen, progesterone and testosterone (Figure 32.1). Oestrogen, progesterone and testosterone exert several effects around the body and eventually plasma levels will reach a high enough concentration to cause negative feedback to the pituitary and hypothalamus.

FSH causes one oocyte (egg) in each ovarian cycle to mature and become the dominant follicle that will be released at ovulation. LH concentrations peak midcycle and promote ovulation.

Oestrogen and progesterone are the body's own sex hormones; they are steroid hormones that are derived from cholesterol (Figure 32.2). The main oestrogen found in the human body is oestradiol. Most oestrogens are secreted from the ovary and placenta. Oestrogens have a wide range of effects on the body (Table 32.1). As well as their reproductive, metabolic and somatic (affecting cells other than sperm and ova) effects, oestrogens also have neural effects, including feminisation of the brain.

Progesterone, the body's natural 'progestogen', is secreted by the corpus luteum and the placenta. Small amounts are also secreted by the testes and adrenal cortex. Synthetic steroids that mimic the actions of endogenous progesterone are called progestins. Progestogens have a role in several physiological functions (Table 32.2).

The New Prescriber: An Integrated Approach to Medical and Non-medical Prescribing, Second Edition.
Edited by Joanne Lymn, Alison Mostyn, Roger Knaggs, Michael Randall, and Dianne Bowskill.
© 2024 John Wiley & Sons Ltd. Published 2024 by John Wiley & Sons Ltd.

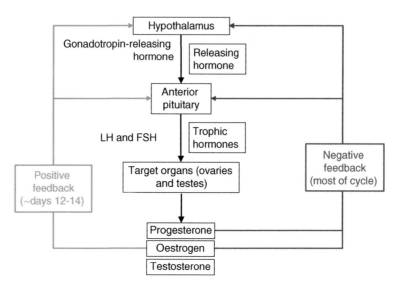

FIGURE 32.1 Endocrine regulation of the female reproductive system. FSH, follicle-stimulating hormone; LH, luteinising hormone.

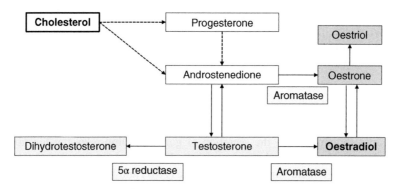

FIGURE 32.2 Production of oestrogens, progesterone and testosterone from cholesterol (adapted from Ritter et al. 2023).

Table 32.1 Summary of the main effects of oestrogens

Reproductive system	Metabolic effects	Somatic effects
Stimulates growth and maturation of the internal and external genitalia and breasts at puberty	Anabolic effects Stimulates Na⁺ reabsorption by the renal tubule (inhibits diuresis)	Stimulates lengthening of long bones and feminisation of the skeleton (pelvis)
Promotes the proliferative phase of the uterine cycle	Increases high-density lipoprotein (reduces low-density lipoprotein) blood levels	Inhibits bone resorption
Promotes oogenesis and ovulation	Enhanced coagulability of the blood	Promotes hydration of the skin
Stimulates capacitation of sperm		Stimulates the female pattern of fat deposition
		Appearance of axillary and pubic hair

Table 32.2 Physiological functions of progestogens

Reproductive system	Other effects
Glandular development of the breasts	Increased insulin levels
Cyclic glandular development of the endometrium	Competes with aldosterone at the renal tubule, causing decreased Na^+ reabsorption
Critical for successful reproduction	
	Increases body temperature

MECHANISM OF ACTION OF OESTROGEN AND PROGESTERONE

Oestrogen and progesterone, like most steroid hormones, act primarily on intracellular receptors. The mechanism of action (Figure 32.3) is very similar to that of tri-iodothyronine (Chapter 31). Oestrogen (ER) and progesterone receptors (PR) act as transcription regulators involved in diverse physiological functions, including regulation of the female reproductive system, mammary gland development, metabolism and bone density. ERs and PRs can interact directly with specific target sequences of DNA known as oestrogen or progesterone response elements.

ERs and PRs are not restricted to the reproductive system and are located throughout the body. Oestrogen binding to receptors outside the reproductive system, for example in the gastrointestinal tract, is responsible for some side effects associated with contraceptive drugs.

Once activated, response elements modulate transcription of a target gene. This modulation can be to either increase protein production or repress transcription, which will decrease the production of the associated protein. It is important to remember that increasing or decreasing proteins takes time (hours), so the clinical effect is not immediate. For example, pre-existing proteins must first be 'used up' before an effect is observed.

As well as binding to receptors, the sex hormones bind to transport proteins in the blood to facilitate their movement through the circulation. The sex hormone-binding globulin carries mostly oestradiol, corticosteroid-binding globulin carries mostly progesterone and albumin can carry both hormones.

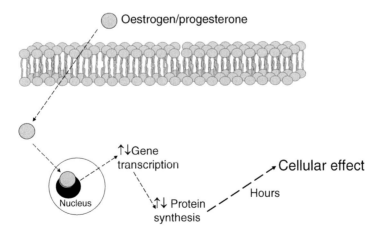

FIGURE 32.3 Cellular mechanism of action of oestrogen and progesterone.

FORMULATIONS OF OESTROGENS AND PROGESTERONES

Natural (oestradiol and oestriol) and synthetic (mestranol, ethinylestradiol [EE]) oestrogens are available in many different preparations for a wide range of indications. Natural and synthetic oestrogens are absorbed well from the gastrointestinal tract. Natural oestrogens are rapidly metabolised in the liver by the CYP450 system, synthetic oestrogens less so. This means that synthetic oestrogens are more potent and more likely to affect liver function. Oestrogens undergo a variable amount of enterohepatic cycling.

There are two main types of progestogen: the naturally occurring hormone (progesterone) and its derivatives (e.g., medroxyprogesterone acetate and levonorgestrel), and the testosterone derivatives (e.g., norethisterone, ethinodiol and norgestrel). Naturally occurring progesterone is virtually inactive due to first-pass metabolism; medroxyprogesterone is an injectable formulation. The testosterone derivatives can be administered orally. Some have androgenic activity and are metabolised to oestrogenic products. Newer products such as desogestrel and gestodene are now being used in contraception. Progestogens are also metabolised by the CYP450 system and are excreted in urine after conjugation, but do not undergo enterohepatic recycling.

STOP AND THINK

What does the ability to use transdermal administration tell us about the chemical composition of oestrogen?

HORMONAL CONTRACEPTION

There are currently seven types of hormonal contraception available in the UK; there is no cost to the individual for a prescription for contraception.

The subdermal implant, levonorgestrel intrauterine device and progestogen-only injection are long-acting reversible contraceptives. The combined hormonal contraceptives (CHCs), which include combined oral contraception (COC), transdermal patch and the ring, and progestogen-only pills (POPs) are short-acting methods. The subdermal implant and levonorgestrel intrauterine device should only be prescribed by a competent clinician who has attained a qualification in the fitting procedures. For this reason, these methods will not be discussed further in this chapter.

All contraceptives available in the UK are safe for most individuals that they will be prescribed for. As when prescribing any medication, this needs to be a shared decision-making process where the prescriber considers all elements that will affect the individual's health alongside their preferences. There will be lifestyle factors, personal and family health conditions, and other medications where the benefits of an individual contraceptive method may be outweighed by the risks. Prescribers should be guided by the Faculty of Sexual and Reproductive Health (FSRH) UK Medical Eligibility Criteria for Contraceptive Use (UKMEC) (FSRH 2016) and the FSRH individual method guidelines. A discussion with a clinical specialist or referral to a specialist sexual and reproductive health service may be needed when guidance is unavailable or outside the scope of practice of the prescriber.

PRACTICE APPLICATION

Contraception may be used by any individual who is having vaginal sex. It is necessary to consider the needs of transgender and non-binary patients. Testosterone treatment does not provide effective contraception and its use is an absolute contraindication to pregnancy. Use of CHCs is not recommended in trans women as this may counteract the effects of testosterone. All other methods of contraception are currently considered safe to prescribe.

COMBINED HORMONAL CONTRACEPTION AND THE PROGESTOGEN-ONLY PILL

CHCs and POPs are the most commonly used methods of contraception in the UK. CHCs contain oestrogen and progesterone, the POP contains only progesterone. These are short-acting, user-dependent contraceptives, with a first-year perfect (following the directions for use) and typical (used incorrectly or inconsistently) use failure rates of 0.3% and 9%, respectively. The failure rate can be increased due to drug interactions, diarrhoea and vomiting with COC and POPs, or a weight over 90 kg with the transdermal patch. There is some concern that the effectiveness of COC and POPs may be reduced following bariatric surgery (Shawe et al. 2019).

COMBINED HORMONAL CONTRACEPTION

CHCs contain an oestrogen and a progestogen. Most CHCs prescribed in the UK contain EE (a synthetic oestrogen) and a synthetic progestogen. There are a small number of newer COCs that contain oestradiol.

CHCs offer benefits and risks to those who use this method of contraception.

Individuals who use CHCs have a significantly reduced risk of ovarian and endometrial cancers, which persists for many years following discontinuation of these methods. There is also a reduced risk of colorectal cancer (FSRH 2019).

Other benefits include a reduction in heavy menstrual bleeding, management of premenstrual syndrome, and the management of endometriosis and symptoms of polycystic ovary syndrome.

There are health risks associated with the use of CHCs. These are rare and can be reduced by:

- history taking identifying those whose risk of use outweighs the benefits

- counselling those who can use this method so that they can make an informed choice to accept the small risks and be aware of signs and symptoms that require medical attention.

The increased risks are venous thromboembolism (VTE), arterial thromboembolic disease (ATE), and breast and cervical cancers. The rate of VTE is different dependent on the combination of oestrogen and progestogen included in the CHC. The risk of developing a VTE in CHC users is five to 12 per 10 000 women in a year (European Medicines Agency 2014). In current users of CHCs there is a slight increased risk of myocardial infarction and ischaemic stroke. There is also a small increase in the risk of breast cancer, which declines within 10 years of stopping, and a small increased risk of cervical cancer if CHCs are used for more than 5 years.

STOP AND THINK

Is your patient taking any other medication, prescribed or otherwise, that may affect the efficacy of oral contraception? Is oral contraception the best choice for this patient? Would another route of administration or a different method be more suitable?

How would you discuss the risks of CHC use to your patients? What steps should you take as a prescriber to minimise these risks?

There are different ways that your patient can use CHCs. Consider the options and how you would support them in making this decision.

To understand the mechanism of action of CHCs, we must return to the hormonal control of the ovarian and uterine cycles (Figure 32.4). Oestrogen and progesterone provide negative feedback to the pituitary to modulate the secretion of LH and FSH. By administering extra oestrogen and

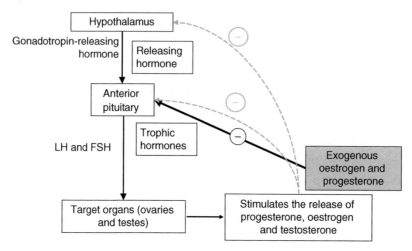

FIGURE 32.4 Mechanism of action of the oral contraceptives. By providing an extra exogenous source of oestrogens and or progestogen, the negative feedback to the pituitary is enhanced. FSH, follicle-stimulating hormone; LH, luteinising hormone.

progesterone, there is increased negative feedback to the pituitary gland. Oestrogen specifically inhibits FSH secretion; suppressing development of the primary follicle. Progestogens inhibit secretion of LH, which prevents the LH surge mid-cycle, therefore inhibiting ovulation. This inhibition of FSH and LH is the primary mechanism of CHCs. It is important to remember that these effects are generated by the molecular activity of oestrogens and progestogens at their nuclear receptors (Figure 32.4).

CHCs also cause changes to the reproductive tract. The progestogen makes the cervical mucus more hostile to sperm penetration and the endometrial lining becomes more resistant to implantation. However, there is little good-quality evidence regarding the biochemical/cellular changes that prevent implantation.

PROGESTOGEN-ONLY PILLS

There are four different POP combinations currently available to prescribe in the UK. Pills containing desogestrel (DSG) and drospirenone work predominantly by inhibiting ovulation. Pills containing levonorgestrel (LNG) and norethisterone work predominantly by thickening cervical mucus, thinning the endometrium and affecting tubal motility. The DSG pill is the most widely prescribed POP in the UK and became a pharmacy medicine in 2021.

Guidance in relation to risk when using POPs has been updated following the findings by Fitzpatrick et al. (2023) that current or recent use of progestogen-only contraception may be associated with a slight increase in breast cancer risk.

PRACTICE APPLICATION

COC is not recommended after the age of 50 or for individuals with health or lifestyle factors that contraindicate its use. The POP is a good alternative for most of these individuals until the age of 55, when contraception is no longer required.

PROGESTOGEN-ONLY INJECTION

There are currently three progestogen-only injections available to prescribe in the UK. Depo-Provera and Sayana Press contain medroxyprogesterone acetate, and Net-En contains norethisterone enanthate. Net-En is not routinely prescribed for contraception in the UK.

Depo-Provera contains 150 mg of medroxyprogesterone acetate (MPA) in 1 ml and is administered as a deep intramuscular injection. Sayana Press contains 104 mg of MPA in 0.65 ml and is administered subcutaneously. These are long-acting reversible contraceptives with first-year perfect and typical use failure rates of 0.2% and 6%, respectively. Both have a primary action of inhibiting ovulation, but also make cervical mucus unfavourable to penetration and thin the endometrium.

The benefits of MPA can include reduction in menstrual bleeding and pain, with almost 50% of individuals becoming amenorrhoeic by the end of the first year of use. There may be a reduction in pain in individuals suffering from endometriosis and those with sickle crisis (FSRH 2014).

The risks of MPA use have predominantly been related to a reduction in bone mineral density. For this reason, it is not recommended as a first-line contraceptive for individuals under the age of 18 years but can be used if other methods are inappropriate. There is some evidence to suggest that use of MPA for more than 5 years can slightly increase the risk of cervical cancer and, as with the POP, there may be a slight increased risk of breast cancer (Fitzpatrick et al. 2023).

STOP AND THINK

How would you discuss potential bleeding problems and other side effects with your patients?

What are the timings for repeat injections of MPA? If your patient is using Depo-Provera and unable to attend for appointments, what options could you consider?

DRUG INTERACTIONS

There are several significant drug–drug interactions that can reduce the efficacy of the hormonal contraceptives. Many of the effects of the drug–drug interactions involve EE, the oestrogen in many CHCs. The interactions can be divided by the stage of pharmacokinetics that is affected. As the potential outcome of contraceptive failure is an unwanted pregnancy, all potential drug interactions must be taken seriously. As well as drug interactions where the hormonal contraceptive is the 'victim', EE can also alter the pharmacokinetics of co-administered drugs, that is, act as a 'perpetrator'.

ABSORPTION

Oral contraceptives are absorbed across the wall of the small intestine so if vomiting occurs within 3 hours of taking the COC or POP or the individual suffers with severe diarrhoea, the efficacy of the drug may be reduced due to incomplete absorption. Missed pill guidance should be followed according to NHS guidelines (NHS 2021).

METABOLISM

EE and progestogens undergo extensive first-pass metabolism.

The enzyme CYP3A4 is the most abundant subtype of cytochrome P450 found in adult hepatocytes and is responsible for phase I metabolism of EE in the liver and the small intestine. EE also undergoes extensive phase II metabolism comprising conjugation via sulphation and glucuronidation.

STOP AND THINK

Which route of administration allows EE and progestogens to be absorbed directly into the bloodstream, thus bypassing first-pass metabolism?

ENZYME INHIBITION AND INDUCTION

The CYP450 enzymes may be induced or inhibited by certain drugs. Inhibition of CYP450, for example by fluconazole or grapefruit juice, produces a reduction in the metabolism of hormonal contraceptives. While toxicity is thought to be rare, one must be conscious of the potential side effects of high doses of EE, such as venous thromboembolism.

Induction of CYP450 by co-administered drugs is a much more serious consideration in contraceptive pharmacology. A range of drugs (Table 32.3) are known to induce (or speed up) the activity of CYP450 and therefore increase the metabolism of EE and progestogens. The potential consequence of co-administration of the CHC or POP with a CYP450 inducer is contraceptive failure.

The progestogen-only injectable contraceptive is, however, unaffected by enzyme-inducing drugs. FSRH provides guidance on the management of women taking enzyme-inducing drugs.

STOP AND THINK

Is your patient taking any other medication, prescribed or otherwise, that may affect the efficacy of oral contraception? Is oral contraception the best choice for this patient? Would another route of administration be more suitable?

OESTROGEN'S EFFECTS ON CO-ADMINISTERED DRUGS

Hormonal contraceptives may also affect the metabolism of certain co-administered drugs (Table 32.4). Depending on the nature of these drugs, there may be significant clinical effects.

COC induces glucuronosyltransferase activity (an enzyme which promotes glucuronidation during phase II metabolism), which may increase the excretion of drugs that are metabolised by

Table 32.3 Drugs which induce the metabolism of ethinylestradiol

Anti-epileptic drugs	Carbamazepine, phenytoin, phenobarbital, primidone
Antifungal drugs	Griseofulvin
Antiretroviral drugs	Ritonavir, amprenavir
Enzyme-inducing antibiotics	Rifampicin, rifabutin
Immunosuppressants	Tacrolimus
Gastrointestinal drugs	Lansoprazole (very weak effect)
Herbal supplements	St John's wort (not much good-quality evidence)

Table 32.4 Effect of combined oral contraception on co-administered drugs

Decreased clinical effect	Increased clinical effect
Tricyclic antidepressants	Ciclosporin
Lamotrigine	Theophylline
	Ropinirole

this pathway. The co-prescription of lamotrigine (an antiepileptic drug) with CHCs is particularly problematic as CHCs can substantially reduce the plasma levels of lamotrigine (40–60%) if the patient is not already on an enzyme-inducing antiepileptic drug.

CHCs may also inhibit CYP3A4, thus increasing the plasma concentration of other drugs that utilise this method of metabolism. An example of a drug whose concentration is increased with co-administration of CHCs is ciclosporin.

PRACTICE APPLICATION

Contraception may be compromised pharmacologically if:

- vomiting occurs <3 hours post oral dose
- liver enzyme-inducing drugs are taken concurrently.

EMERGENCY CONTRACEPTION

Emergency contraception (EC) can be used to reduce the risk of pregnancy after unprotected sexual intercourse (UPSI), where no contraception has been used or where a method of contraception has been misused. This section provides a brief insight and full guidance can be found in the FSRH Guideline on Emergency Contraception (FSRH 2017).

There are three methods of EC available in the UK: the copper intrauterine device (Cu-IUD), ulipristal acetate EC (UPA-EC) and levonorgestrel EC (LNG-EC). The Cu-IUD is the most effective method, with a failure rate of 0.093% (Goldstuck and Cheung 2019). This can only be fitted by a competent clinician.

UPA-EC and LNG-EC work by delaying ovulation for up to 5 days. UPA-EC is a selective progesterone receptor modulator that can be taken up to 120 hours after UPSI. It is effective during the LH surge until it reaches its peak. LNG-EC is a high dose of synthetic progestogen that can be taken up to 96 hours after UPSI. It is only effective if taken prior to the LH surge. Neither method has an effect after ovulation, but it is still recommended that they are offered to the individual due to the possibility of a delay in ovulation in any cycle. UPA-EC is more effective than LNG-EC, pregnancy rates after use being 1–2% and 0.6–2.6%, respectively (FSRH 2017). There are many variables besides the use of EC that will affect the risk of pregnancy, including the time of sexual intercourse, the fertility of either partner, the effectiveness of the contraception used and the age of the woman. The main risk of EC is failure as it is less effective than regular methods of contraception. Vomiting within 3 hours requires a further dose of the original EC taken if still within 120 (UPA-EC) or 96 (LNG-EC) hours.

Hormonal EC is safe and can be used by most individuals, but there are some limitations. Risk of failure is increased in relation to weight and body mass index, and the use of liver enzyme-inducing drugs taken at the time or in the preceding 28 days. When considering UPA-EC, there are drug interactions with other hormones, oral glucocorticoids being taken for severe asthma and caution recommended with drugs that increase gastric pH.

STOP AND THINK

Consider the complexities of a consultation for emergency contraception (EC).

You refer your patient to a specialist service for an EC IUD fit. If not contraindicated, would you prescribe hormonal EC prior to the patient leaving your consultation?

What medicines can inhibit the effects of oral EC?

What medications does ulipristal acetate EC interact with?

How many times can the individual take oral EC within a cycle?

Is there a risk to the foetus if oral EC fails?

Is oral EC safe for breast-feeding women?

NON-CONTRACEPTIVE USES OF OESTROGEN AND PROGESTERONE

Oestrogens can be used to treat primary ovarian failure to stimulate secondary sexual characteristics and menstruation. Progesterone alone is used in the treatment of endometriosis and as a second- or third-line treatment of breast cancer, or endometrial or renal carcinoma.

HORMONE REPLACEMENT THERAPY

The use of oestrogen and progesterone within hormone replacement therapy (HRT) to treat the symptoms of perimenopause and menopause has increased significantly in recent years; between 2020–2021 and 2021–2022 there was a 35% rise in prescribed items (NHS Business Services Authority 2022). HRT is used to supplement declining oestrogen and progesterone levels experienced in women during the peri-menopause and menopause, providing relief for short-term symptoms such as hot flushes, vaginal dryness and sweating as well as longer-term protection against cardiovascular disease, dementia and osteoporosis (Vigneswaran and Hamoda 2022).

   The use of HRT is not without risk, but newer formulations such as body identical hormones, micronized progesterone and transdermal oestrogen are associated with lower risks of cancer, cardiovascular disease and thromboembolism (Vigneswaran and Hamoda 2022).

SUMMARY

- The female reproductive system is regulated primarily by the hormones oestrogen and progesterone.

- Oestrogen and progesterone are secreted from the ovaries following stimulation by follicle-stimulating hormone (FSH) and luteinising hormone (LH). Negative feedback by oestrogen and progesterone provides fine tuning of FSH and LH secretion.

- Contraceptive drugs mimic oestrogen and progesterone to provide exogenous negative feedback to the pituitary gland, thereby reducing release of LH and FSH; this is the primary mechanism of action.

- Oestrogen and progesterone also have direct contraceptive effects on the reproductive system, which are classified as secondary mechanisms of action.

- Contraception can be prescribed safely for most individuals who require it by referring to Faculty of Sexual and Reproductive Health guidelines, the UK Medical Eligibility Criteria for Contraceptive Use or a specialist provider.

- Drug interactions with contraception can reduce the effectiveness of hormonal contraception, leading to an unplanned pregnancy.

- Hormonal contraception can alter the effectiveness of other drugs, leading to potentially serious health implications.

- Emergency contraception should be offered to all individuals who have had unprotected vaginal sex or where their contraception method has been compromised.

- Carefully prescribed hormone replacement therapy can reduce the short- and long-term symptoms of the declining sex hormones during perimenopause and menopause.

ACTIVITY

1. Luteinising hormone is secreted from which endocrine gland?

   (a) Hypothalamus

   (b) Pituitary

   (c) Ovary

2. Negative feedback of oestrogen to the pituitary reduces secretion of FSH. True/False

3. Progesterone acts primarily via membrane-bound receptors. True/False

4. The POP is suitable for women with breast cancer. True/False

5. Liver enzyme-inducing drugs may increase the efficacy of CHCs and hormonal emergency contraception. True/False

REFERENCES

European Medicines Agency (2014) Benefits of combined hormonal contraceptives (CHCs) continue to outweigh risks. https://www.ema.europa.eu/en/documents/referral/benefits-combined-hormonal-contraceptives-chcs-continue-outweigh-risks_en.pdf.

Fitzpatrick, D., Pirie, K., Reeves, G., Green, J. and Beral, V. (2023) Combined and progestogen-only hormonal contraceptives and breast cancer risk: A UK nested case-control study and meta-analysis. *PLoS Med* 20(3):e1004188.

FSRH (2014) FSRH Clinical Guideline: Progestogen-only Pills. Faculty of Sexual and Reproductive Healthcare. https://www.fsrh.org/standards-and-guidance/documents/cec-guideline-pop/.

FSRH (2016) UK Medical Eligibility Criteria for Contraceptive Use (UKMEC). Faculty of Sexual and Reproductive Healthcare. https://www.fsrh.org/standards-and-guidance/uk-medical-eligibility-criteria-for-contraceptive-use-ukmec/.

FSRH (2017) FSRH Clinical Guideline: Emergency Contraception. Faculty of Sexual and Reproductive Healthcare. https://www.fsrh.org/standards-and-guidance/documents/ceu-clinical-guidance-emergency-contraception-march-2017/.

FSRH (2019) FSRH Clinical Guideline: Combined Hormonal Contraception. Faculty of Sexual and Reproductive Healthcare. (January 2019, Amended October 2023) https://www.fsrh.org/standards-and-guidance/documents/combined-hormonal-contraception/

Goldstuck, N.D. and Cheung, T.S. (2019) The efficacy of intrauterine devices for emergency contraception and beyond: a systematic review update. *Int J Women's Health* 11:471–479.

NHS (2021) Your contraception guide. https://www.nhs.uk/conditions/contraception/.

NHS Business Services Authority (2022) Hormone Replacement Therapy – England. https://www.nhsbsa.nhs.uk/statistical-collections/hormone-replacement-therapy-england.

Ritter, J.M., Flower, R., Henderson, G., et al. (2023) *Rang and Dale's Pharmacology*, 10th edn. Elsevier, Amsterdam.

Shawe, J., Ceulemans, D., Akhter, Z., et al. (2019) Pregnancy after bariatric surgery: Consensus recommendations for periconception, antenatal and postnatal care. *Obesity Rev* 20:1507–1522.

Vigneswaran, K. and Hamoda, H. (2022) Hormone replacement therapy – Current recommendations. *Best Pract Res Clin Obstet Gynaecol* 81:8–21.

FURTHER READING

British National Formulary (online). Joint Formulary Committee. London: BMJ and Pharmaceutical Press. http://www.medicinescomplete.com.

FSRH (2022) Drug Interactions. Faculty of Sexual and Reproductive Healthcare. https://www.fsrh.org/standards-and-guidance/fsrh-guidelines-and-statements/drug-interactions/.

USEFUL WEBSITES

Hormone Replacement Therapy – England – April 2015 to June 2022. NHSBSA Statistics and Data Science. https://www.nhsbsa.nhs.uk/statistical-collections/hormone-replacement-therapy-england/hormone-replacement-therapy-england-april-2015-june-2022.

CLINICAL GUIDANCE

Endocrine Society (2021) Diagnosis and Treatment of Polycystic Ovary Syndrome: An Endocrine Society Clinical Practice Guideline. https://academic.oup.com/jcem/article/98/12/4565/2833703.

FSRH (2014) FSRH Clinical Guideline Progestogen-only Injectable. Faculty of Sexual and Reproductive Healthcare. https://www.fsrh.org/standards-and-guidance/documents/cec-ceu-guidance-injectables-dec-2014/.

FSRH (2016) UK Medical Eligibility Criteria for Contraceptive Use (UKMEC). Faculty of Sexual and Reproductive Healthcare. https://www.fsrh.org/standards-and-guidance/uk-medical-eligibility-criteria-for-contraceptive-use-ukmec/.

FSRH (2017) FSRH Clinical Guideline: Emergency Contraception. Faculty of Sexual and Reproductive Healthcare. https://www.fsrh.org/standards-and-guidance/documents/ceu-clinical-guidance-emergency-contraception-march-2017/.

FSRH (2020) FSRH Clinical Guideline: Combined Hormonal Contraception. Faculty of Sexual and Reproductive Healthcare. https://www.fsrh.org/standards-and-guidance/documents/combined-hormonal-contraception/.

FSRH (2022) FSRH Clinical Guideline: Progestogen-only Pills. Faculty of Sexual and Reproductive Healthcare. https://www.fsrh.org/standards-and-guidance/documents/cec-guideline-pop/.

FSRH (2022) Drug Interactions. Faculty of Sexual and Reproductive Healthcare. https://www.fsrh.org/standards-and-guidance/fsrh-guidelines-and-statements/drug-interactions/.

National Institute for Health and Care Excellence (2017) Endometriosis: diagnosis and management. NICE guideline [NG73]. https://www.nice.org.uk/guidance/ng73.

National Institute for Health and Care Excellence (2019) Menopause: diagnosis and management. NICE guideline [NG23]. https://www.nice.org.uk/guidance/ng23.

National Institute for Health and Care Excellence (2021) Heavy menstrual bleeding: assessment and management. NICE guideline [NG88]. https://www.nice.org.uk/guidance/ng88.

NHS (2021) Your contraception guide. https://www.nhs.uk/conditions/contraception/.

Royal College of Obstetrics and Gynaecology (2016) Management of Premenstrual Syndrome. Green-top Guideline No. 48. https://obgyn.onlinelibrary.wiley.com/doi/full/10.1111/1471-0528.14260.

Cancer Pharmacotherapy

Michael Randall

LEARNING OUTCOMES

By the end of this chapter the reader should be able to:

- describe the principles of cytotoxic anticancer chemotherapy

- describe the modes of action of:

  o antimetabolite anticancer drugs

  o false substrates

  o alkylating agents

  o antibiotics used in anticancer chemotherapy

  o platinum compounds

  o topoisomerase inhibitors

  o mitotic inhibitors

  o hormone-based therapy

- describe the key side effects associated with cytotoxic agents and how they might be mitigated against

- describe the principles of targeted anticancer therapy

- describe the relevance of human epidermal growth factor receptor-2 as a target in anticancer treatment

- describe the role of tyrosine kinase inhibitors in anticancer treatment

- describe the role of (poly(adenosine diphosphate-ribose)polymerase) inhibitors in anticancer treatment

- describe the role of proteasome inhibitors in anticancer treatment

- describe the role of antivascular endothelial growth factor-based drugs in anticancer treatment.

CANCERS

Cancers encompass a range of diseases affecting many bodily systems and involving the uncontrolled proliferation of abnormal cells. It is estimated that in the UK, one in two people will develop cancer in their lifetime. Cancers differ considerably in prognosis and Cancer Research UK provides an excellent resource outlining the prevalence and survival rates of many cancers. For example, breast cancer is relatively common, with a lifetime occurrence in women of around one in seven. The 5-year survival of patients with breast cancer ranges from 100% in early disease to 25% in advanced disease. By contrast, the survival rates for lung cancer and pancreatic cancer are less positive, with 5-year survival rates for lung cancer of 55% in early disease and 5% in advanced disease, and pancreatic cancer 3-year survival rates are 25% in localised disease and 1% in distant disease (data from Cancer Research UK).

Although cancers are often thought of as diseases of ageing, certain lifestyle habits are associated with cancers. It was established in the 1950s that there was a direct link between smoking and lung cancer, and smoking has now been associated with oral, oesophageal, bladder, stomach

The New Prescriber: An Integrated Approach to Medical and Non-medical Prescribing, Second Edition.
Edited by Joanne Lymn, Alison Mostyn, Roger Knaggs, Michael Randall, and Dianne Bowskill.
© 2024 John Wiley & Sons Ltd. Published 2024 by John Wiley & Sons Ltd.

and colon cancers, and certain types of leukaemia. Diet, obesity and alcohol are also associated risk factors for a range of cancers. Lifestyle measures such as smoking cessation, screening (e.g., mammography in breast cancer, faecal occult blood screening in colorectal cancer, prostate-specific antigen in prostate cancer) and awareness of alerting symptoms in patients play a vital role in prevention and early detection. In the case of cervical cancer, which is associated with the human papillomavirus, vaccination around puberty is proving successful in prevention.

Cancers involve the uncontrolled multiplication of cells, with replication of altered or damaged DNA. In health, the cell cycle is tightly regulated. Following mitosis, cells are in G_0 and only re-enter to G_1 in the presence of growth signals. In G_1, there is a restriction point to check for damage to the DNA. The cell then enters the S phase, where DNA is replicated, and then the G_2 phase, where the integrity of the replicated DNA is checked. In the pathogenesis of cancer, there may be the loss of essential genes (including loss of tumour suppressors), the inactivation of cell cycle regulators and prevention of apoptosis leading to the uncontrolled proliferation of cells. This may lead to a primary tumour at the initial site, but cancerous cells can invade locally, spreading to the local lymph nodes and then to distant sites via metastasis. It is this latter event that is often associated with the terminal disease.

CANCER PHARMACOTHERAPY

Cancer chemotherapy has been used for the past six decades. The conventional cytotoxic treatments are relatively non-selective but over the past 20 years, with increased understanding of cancer biology, there has been the introduction of more selective 'targeted' therapies.

Pharmacotherapy for cancers may be curative (e.g., in the treatment of testicular cancer following surgery), is sometimes used to shrink tumours prior to surgery (neoadjuvant chemotherapy) or may be used in addition to surgery, for example after the removal of a solid tumour, courses of chemotherapy may be used to prevent recurrence or suppress the growth of any metastases. Chemotherapy may also be used in palliative care to reduce tumour size or growth and to prolong life. There are a number of chemotherapy agents and these are often used in specific combinations, generally involving three agents. The purpose of using combinations is to attack different pharmacological targets and so limit both toxicity and the development of resistance.

CYTOTOXIC ANTICANCER CHEMOTHERAPY

Chemotherapy is the use of cytotoxic drugs to kill rapidly growing cells and the target is generally associated with DNA structure, function or replication (Figure 33.1 and Table 33.1). This is quite a poor targeting strategy and affects rapidly dividing healthy cells, leading to widespread side effects, notably on bone marrow. Drugs used in anticancer chemotherapy generally target:

- the synthesis of nucleotides: the purine (adenine and guanine) and pyrimidine (cytosine and thymine) base pairs which form the genetic code

- the structure and function of DNA: the double helix and its role in expressing the genetic code and cell replication

- mitosis: the division of somatic cells.

ANTIMETABOLITES

FOLATE ANTAGONISTS (E.G. METHOTREXATE)

Folate antagonists are folic acid analogues that cause inhibition of dihydrofolate reductase to decrease thymidylate synthesis and interfere with DNA synthesis. They also reduce pyrimidine synthesis and hence limit DNA synthesis and cell division. By interfering with folate metabolism, these agents may cause megaloblastic anaemia and patients are often given a rescue course of folates (such as folinic acid)

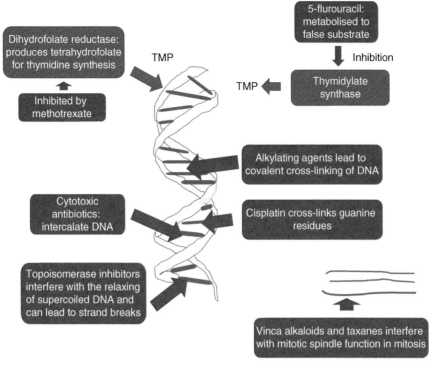

FIGURE 33.1   Key pharmacological targets in cytotoxic chemotherapy, showing inhibition of nucleotide synthesis, false metabolites, direct chemical damage of the DNA, inhibition of DNA replication and inhibition of mitosis. TMP, thymidine monophosphate.

Table 33.1   Summary of the key pharmacological targets for cytotoxic anticancer chemotherapy and the respective pharmacological agents

Drug target	Pharmacological therapies
Nucleotide synthesis	Folate antagonists
	Pyrimidine analogues
	Purine analogues
DNA structure and function	Alkylating agents
	Platinum compounds
	Anthracycline antibiotics
	Topoisomerase inhibitors
Inhibition of mitosis	Microtubule inhibitors

to limit this side effect. Methotrexate is sometimes given intrathecally to improve access to the central nervous system and attack cancerous cells that may have spread to 'sanctuary' sites.

PYRIMIDINE ANALOGUES (E.G., 5-FLUOROURACIL, CAPECITABINE, GEMCITABINE)

5-fluorouracil inhibits thymidylate synthase. It is administered parenterally to treat many solid tumours and is also used topically in some dermatological neoplasms. Capecitabine is given orally and metabolized to 5-flurouracil.

PURINE ANALOGUES (E.G., MERCAPTOPURINE AND THIOGUANINE)

Purine analogues are activated by hypoxanthine phosphoribosyltransferase to form toxic metabolites. They interfere with purine synthesis and become incorporated into DNA (and RNA) as false metabolites that lead to damage of the DNA, such as breaks in the double strand. Mercaptopurine is inactivated via thiopurine S-methyltransferase and pharmacogenetic differences mean that some patients are more susceptible to its effects and toxicity.

ALKYLATING AGENTS (E.G., CYCLOPHOSPHAMIDE, BUSULPHAN)

These agents cause chemical cross-linking of DNA, leading to defective DNA replication. They are widely used in combination therapy in a number of haematological malignancies and solid tumours.

PLATINUM COMPOUNDS (E.G., CISPLATIN)

These compounds cause cross-linking guanine DNA and residues, thus inhibiting DNA synthesis. Platinum compounds are associated with a high level of emesis.

ANTHRACYCLINE ANTIBIOTICS (E.G., DOXORUBICIN, EPIRUBICIN AND DAUNORUBICIN)

These substances interfere with nucleotide synthesis by intercalating between DNA strands, inhibiting topoisomerase and generating free radicals. They are widely used in a variety of haematological malignancies and solid tumours. Doxorubicin is associated with cardiac toxicity.

TOPOISOMERASE INHIBITORS (E.G., ETOPOSIDE)

Inhibition of topoisomerase II prevents ligation of DNA, leading to breaks in the DNA strand.

MICROTUBULE INHIBITORS

These agents interfere with mitosis. Vinca alkaloids (vincristine and vinblastine) inhibit the formation of the mitotic spindle, whereas taxanes (paclitaxel and docetaxel) lead to stabilisation of spindle fibres. Vinca alkaloids are powerful neurotoxins and have been associated with fatalities when they have been inadvertently given by the intrathecal route.

STOP AND THINK

Anticancer drugs are toxic drugs and using the correct route of administration is essential in drug safety and prevention of medication errors. The World Health Organization has produced an excellent video entitled 'Vincristine Error' (https://www.who.int/teams/integrated-health-services/patient-safety/guidance).

SIDE EFFECTS OF CYTOTOXIC ANTICANCER DRUGS

Cytotoxic drugs do not differentiate between healthy and cancerous cells, and this lack of selectivity of gives rise to a wide range of side effects, including myelosuppression leading to pancytopenia, which is associated with anaemia, increased susceptibility to infections due to neutropenia and increased bleeding due to thrombocytopenia.

MYELOSUPPRESSION

Myelosuppression is a common occurrence with many cytotoxic agents and is a reason to carry out chemotherapy in cycles to allow the bone marrow to recover between cycles. Colony-stimulating factors may be used under some circumstances to increase the white cell count and reduce the time between cycles. Prophylactic antimicrobial agents may also be required.

STOP AND THINK

Why is neutropenic sepsis such an important consideration? What might raise suspicion of neutropenic sepsis and how should it be managed?

As a result of the toxic nature of cytotoxic agents, they may exhibit a range of other side effects which, depending on the agent, may include those shown in Table 33.2.

Given the toxicity of cytotoxic anticancer drugs, they are often used in combination to reduce the doses required and also the possibility of resistance. Many regimens involve three or four agents that target different stages in the cell cycle, for example DNA synthesis (e.g., an anti-metabolite), DNA structure and replication (e.g., an alkylating agent) and cell division (e.g., a microtubule inhibitor). Regimens are often given in cycles (e.g., every 21 days) so that the body and especially the bone marrow can recover between doses. A core principle in this approach is that an initial treatment might lead to a substantial reduction in cancer cell number but be associated with side effects due to other, healthy rapidly dividing cells (e.g., bone marrow) being killed off. The body is then allowed to recover and the next phase leads to another substantial reduction in the number of cancer cells. The ideal goal is total destruction of the cancer cell load or at least a remission.

Table 33.2 Key side effects associated with a range of cytotoxic agents (side effects vary between agents and patients)

Other key side effects	Comments and mitigations
Alopecia	Prevention can involve cold caps to limit scalp blood flow during chemotherapy to reduce exposure
Nausea and vomiting	Particularly problematic with platinum compounds May be limited by the use of antiemetic drugs (Chapter 16)
Mouth ulcers	Close attention should be paid to dental hygiene, e.g., use of antiseptic mouth washes and relief using ice
Renal damage	A particular problem with cisplatin; patients should be well hydrated before treatment
Bladder damage	Often local irritation (cystitis) due to the toxic effects of the drugs and their metabolites
Neuropathy	Can be treated with the antidepressant duloxetine
Memory	Some agents may impair memory, which is referred to as 'chemo brain'
Infertility	Sperm or eggs may be harvested
Lung damage	Be vigilant for changes in respiratory symptoms and function
Cardiotoxicity	This is a particular problem with anthracycline antibiotics; cardiac function should be monitored and there is lifetime maximum dose
Carcinogenic effects	Many agents are mutagenic and can lead to the development of cancers later in life

Table 33.3 Examples of chemotherapy combination regimens

Regimen	Constituents
CHOP (e.g., for non-Hodgkin's lymphoma)	• Cyclophosphamide
	• Doxorubicin
	• Vincristine
	• Prednisolone
ABVD (e.g., for Hodgkin's lymphoma)	• Doxorubicin
	• Bleomycin
	• Vinblastine
	• Dacarbazine
EC (e.g., for small-cell lung cancer)	• Etoposide
	• Cisplatin
FEC (e.g., for breast cancer)	• Flurouracil
	• Epirubicin
	• Cyclophosphamide

REGIMENS

Some commonly used regimens include those shown in Table 33.3.

TARGETED CANCER THERAPY

With a greater understanding of the biology of cancer, newer targeted therapies have been introduced and often target cell signalling. In general, these newer agents target 'weaknesses' in the tumour cells, such as overexpression of receptors and signalling mechanisms. This increased selectivity means that targeted therapy is less likely to be associated with widespread side effects. Targeted anticancer drugs are divided into monoclonal antibodies (e.g., trastuzumab for breast cancer) and small molecules (e.g., imatinib for chronic myeloid leukaemia). Monoclonal antibodies inhibit the cell surface receptor and facilitate an immune response. Small molecules are designed to inhibit various enzymic activities associated with cell signalling.

HORMONAL-BASED THERAPIES

Breast cancers are common tumours and in patients who overexpress the oestrogen receptor (ER+) breast cancer the growth of the cancerous cells is driven by oestrogen. Tamoxifen is a selective oestrogen-receptor modulator that has been used to prevent breast cancer for many years. It is a receptor modulator and has an additional benefit in preventing bone loss. Tamoxifen is associated with endometrial changes and unexplained vaginal bleeding should be investigated.

An additional or alternative approach is the use of aromatase inhibitors (such as anastrozole). In post-menopausal women there is peripheral conversion of androgens to oestrogen via aromatase and inhibition of this enzyme is effective at inhibiting oestrogen-stimulated tumour growth.

HUMAN EPIDERMAL GROWTH FACTOR RECEPTOR 2

Human epidermal growth factor receptor 2 (HER2) is naturally present at low levels but can be overexpressed in some cancers (e.g., breast cancer, ~25%), especially in older patients. The overexpression is due to the oncogene ERBB2, and affects both gene transcription and the cell cycle.

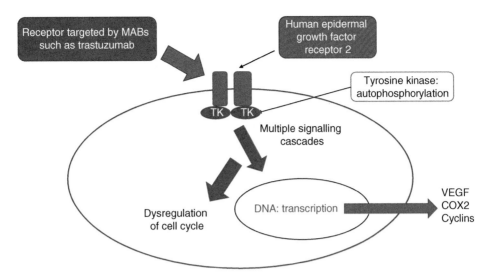

FIGURE 33.2   The human epidermal growth factor receptor 2 is overexpressed in some breast cancers and is the target for trastuzumab. COX2, cyclo-oxgenase-2; HER2, Human epidermal growth factor receptor 2; MABs, monoclonal antibodies; TK, tyrosinse kinase; VEGF, vascular endothelial growth factor.

Trastuzumab is a monoclonal antibody that selectively targets HER2, interfering with signal transduction, slowing it down, and also induces immune cell-mediated cytotoxicity (Figure 33.2). It is used early breast cancer and in metastatic breast cancer with HER2-positive tumours. Trastuzumab is associated with cardiotoxicity, leading to heart failure.

EGF RECEPTOR KINASE

Epidermal growth factor (EGF) receptors have tyrosine kinase activity associated with epithelial cell growth and differentiation (Figure 33.3a). Inhibition of the EGF kinase by small molecules such as erlotinib is a newer approach in the treatment of lung and pancreatic cancers (Figure 33.3b). The receptor is also the target for monoclonal antibodies, such as cetuximab, which inhibit cell signalling and growth.

EGRF inhibitors such as erlotinib are associated with keratitis and can rarely cause corneal proliferation so prescribers should be vigilant for changes in vision.

TYROSINE KINASE INHIBITORS

Imatinib is a tyrosine kinase inhibitor that has revolutionised the management of chronic myeloid leukaemia. In this condition there is a translocation between chromosomes 9 and 22, known as the Philadelphia chromosome, which results in fusion of two proteins to form BCR-ABL, a constitutively active tyrosine kinase that leads to uncontrolled cell proliferation.

Imatinib has been associated with reactivation of hepatitis B and so viral status should be determined before treatment.

POLY (ADENOSINE DIPHOSPHATE-RIBOSE) POLYMERASE PARP) INHIBITORS (OLAPARIB)

Olaparib has recently been introduced for ovarian cancers with the breast cancer (BRCA) gene mutations that are resistant to platinum-based therapy. Poly(adenosine diphosphate-ribose)-polymerase (PARP) is a DNA repair enzyme. BRCA genes are important in DNA repair at

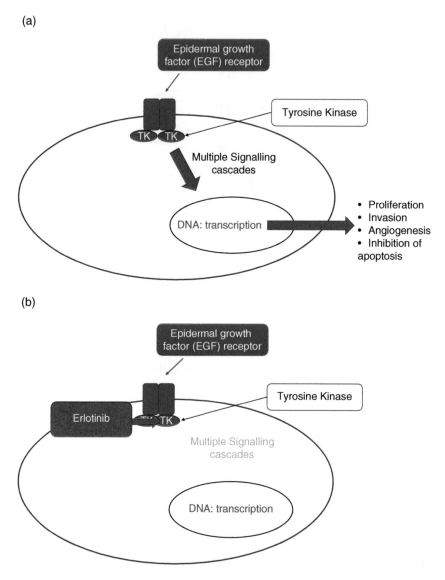

FIGURE 33.3 (a) The epidermal growth factor (EGF) receptor is expressed in some cancers. (b) Its tyrosine kinase activity is the target for small molecules, such as erlotinib. TK, tyrosinse kinase.

double-strand breaks and PARP repairs single-strand breaks. In patients with BRCA gene mutations, inhibition of PARP leads to the inability of cancer cells to repair double-strand breaks, leading to cell death.

PROGRAMMED DEATH-1 RECEPTOR INHIBITORS

Pembrolizumab is a monoclonal antibody that blocks the programmed death-1 receptor on T-lymphocytes and promotes an immune response to attack cancer cells. It is used either alone or in combination with cytotoxic agents in the management of non-small-cell lung, colorectal, oesophageal and renal cancers, and Hodgkin's lymphoma.

PROTEOSOME INHIBITORS

Proteosomes are cellular structures that degrade proteins. Some proteins, such pro-apoptotic factors, kill cancer cells and so inhibition of proteasomes alters the regulation of intracellular proteins. Bortezomib is a proteosome inhibitor used in multiple myeloma.

ANTI-ANGIOGENIC APPROACHES

Vascular endothelial growth factor (VEGF) is secreted to promote angiogenesis, the growth of blood vessels that supports the development of metastasis. Bevacizumab is a monoclonal antibody that targets this receptor and is used in advanced colonic and breast cancer.

Sunitinib is a small molecule that inhibits VEGF-associated receptor tyrosine kinase and is used in advanced renal carcinoma.

GUIDANCE

The pharmacotherapy of cancers is very much driven by guidance, often with evidence-based local protocols that have been developed to integrate pharmacotherapy with radiotherapy and surgery as appropriate. Supporting local protocols, the National Institute for Health and Care Excellence should be consulted for both specific cancers and a vast array of technological appraisals.

PRACTICE POINTS

- Chemotherapy is a specialised area of therapeutics.
- Cytotoxic chemotherapeutic agents have narrow therapeutic windows, so doses may be determined by body weight or body surface area and in relation to adverse events. Specialist literature and local protocols should be consulted.
- In terms of drug safety, the route of administration is critical. For example, practitioners are registered to administer drugs via the intrathecal route and protocols are in place to avoid inadvertent administration of neurotoxic drugs ('never ever events').
- Cytotoxics are associated with many side effects, the profile and extent of which varies between agents and patients.
- Myelosuppression is a key adverse event of many cytotoxic chemotherapeutic drugs and practitioners should be vigilant for the development of neutropenia.
- Recovery of neutropenia may be promoted by the use of colony-stimulating factors.

SUMMARY

- Cytotoxic anticancer chemotherapy targets the uncontrolled proliferation of cancer cells by preventing the synthesis of nucleotides, damaging DNA structure and function, and inhibiting microtubules in mitosis.
- Cytotoxic anticancer drugs are often given in combination to limit toxicity and target different sites of DNA.
- Cytotoxic anticancer drugs are poorly selective and have many side effects, especially on rapidly dividing healthy cells, such as bone marrow.

- Many cytotoxic anticancer regimens are given in cycles to allow the body, especially the bone marrow, to recover.

- Targeted anticancer therapy has emerged, with both monoclonoal antibodies and small molecules being used to target molecular weaknesses in cancer cells.

ACTIVITY

Methotrexate is a metabolic inhibitor used to inhibit the production of purines and pyrimidines.

1. Methotrexate inhibits which ONE of the following enzymes?

   (a) Caspase

   (b) Dihydrofolate reductase

   (c) Topoisomerase II

   (d) Thymidylate synthase

   (e) Tyrosine kinase

2. Anthracycline antibiotics (such as doxorubicin) are used in anticancer therapy. Anthracycline antibiotics act by which ONE of the following mechanisms?

   (a) Inhibition of dihydrofolate reductase

   (b) Inhibition of DNA synthase

   (c) Inhibition of the 80S ribosomal subunit

   (d) DNA intercalation

   (e) Stabilisation of mitotic spindle fibres

3. Cytotoxic anticancer chemotherapy is carried out in cycles, often of 21 days. Which ONE of the following is the best explanation for this?

   (a) Enables the bone marrow to recover

   (b) Enables folate levels to return to normal

   (c) To enable regrowth of hair

   (d) To limit cardiotoxicity

   (e) To limit renal toxicity

4. Human epidermal growth factor receptor 2 (HER2) is associated with which ONE of the following enzyme activities?

   (a) Adenylyl cyclase

   (b) Guanylyl cyclase

   (c) Phospholipase A_2

   (d) Topoisomerase II

   (e) Tyrosine kinase

5. Vascular endothelial growth factor (VEGF) is targeted by the mononclonal antibody bevacizumab. VEGF is associated with regulating which ONE of the following?

(a) Angiogenesis

(b) Apoptosis

(c) Proteasomal degradation

(d) The cell cycle

(e) Uncontrolled proliferation of epithelial tumours

USEFUL WEBSITES

British National Formulary (online) London: BMJ Group and Pharmaceutical Press. https://bnf.nice.org.uk/.

www.cancerresearchuk.org is an excellent resource for cancers and their treatment.

FURTHER READING

Brunton, L. and Knollmann, B. (2022). *Goodman and Gilman's The Pharmacological Basis of Therapeutics*, 14th edn. New York: McGraw Hill,.

Ritter, J.M., Flower, R., Henderson, G. et al. (2023) *Rang and Dale's Pharmacology*, 10th edn. Elsevier, Amsterdam.

CHAPTER 34

Musculoskeletal Disease

Sana Awan and David Andrew Walsh

LEARNING OUTCOMES

By the end of this chapter the reader should be able to:

- define the breadth of musculoskeletal disorders and the role of drugs in their management

- describe the pathophysiology of osteoarthritis, inflammatory arthritis, spinal pain and crystal arthritis

- explain which pharmacological agents can improve symptoms or reduce tissue damage in musculoskeletal disorders

- understand the use of glucocorticoids (systemic and locally administered) in practice

- understand the pharmacology, benefits and risks of conventional, biologic and targeted synthetic disease-modifying antirheumatic drugs in inflammatory arthritis

- select optimal pharmacological approaches to reduce symptoms in people with musculoskeletal disease

- describe strategies that minimise risk of side effects from the use of pharmacological agents for musculoskeletal disorders.

RHEUMATIC AND MUSCULOSKELETAL DISORDERS

Rheumatic and musculoskeletal disorders (RMDs) are amongst the most common reasons for primary care consultations in the UK, and are major burdens to the individual, carers, health and social care providers, and employers. Pain, physical disability, fatigue and psychological distress are amongst their predominant symptoms. RMDs encompass many different diseases (Table 34.1) and can affect all age groups.

Discrete diagnoses, such as osteoarthritis, rheumatoid arthritis or spinal pain, may be considered prototypic examples of structural, inflammatory and biopsychosocial RMDs. However, both pathological mechanisms and symptoms overlap between these conditions. Osteoarthritis and spinal pain are by far the most common RMDs, each affecting the majority of us at some time of our lives. Rheumatoid arthritis is the most prevalent chronic inflammatory RMD, affecting about 1% of adults in the UK. Rarer connective tissue diseases such as systemic lupus erythematosus (prevalence 0.1%) have specific immunological mechanisms and greater potential to damage tissues beyond the musculoskeletal system, including kidneys and lungs.

Musculoskeletal disorders may be acute, for example following trauma or associated with crystal deposition in the joint, or chronic, lasting many years. Chronic RMDs pose a risk of `flare', with acute increases in symptoms. Conditions such as osteoarthritis or inflammatory arthritis are currently without cure, and lifelong management aims to control symptoms and maintain function.

The New Prescriber: An Integrated Approach to Medical and Non-medical Prescribing, Second Edition.
Edited by Joanne Lymn, Alison Mostyn, Roger Knaggs, Michael Randall, and Dianne Bowskill.
© 2024 John Wiley & Sons Ltd. Published 2024 by John Wiley & Sons Ltd.

Table 34.1 The breadth of rheumatic and musculoskeletal disorders (conditions addressed in this chapter are shown in bold)

	Subclassifications	
	Anatomical distribution	**Aetiology/pathogenesis**
Osteoarthritis	**Knee, hip, centralised nodal osteoarthritis**	**Primary, secondary, e.g. to inflammatory arthritis**
Spinal pain	**Low back, neck, radiculopathy**	**Spondylosis, intervertebral disc disease, osteoarthritis**
Inflammatory arthritis	**Monoarthritis, oligoarthritis, polyarthritis**	**Rheumatoid arthritis, psoriatic arthritis, enteropathic arthritis, reactive arthritis, ankylosing spondylitis**
Crystal arthropathies	**Monoarthritis, polyarticular, tophaceous gout**	**Gout, pseudogout**
Connective tissue diseases		*Inflammatory:* e.g. systemic lupus erythematosus, scleroderma, mixed connective tissue
		Non-inflammatory: e.g. hypermobility syndromes
Vasculitic syndromes	Large vessel arteritis (e.g., giant cell arteritis)	Antineutrophil cytoplasmic antibody-associated vasculitis
	Medium vessel vasculitis (e.g., polyarteritis nodosum)	
	Small vessel vasculitis (e.g., microscopic polyangiitis)	
Inflammatory muscle disease		
Bone diseases		Osteoporosis, Paget's disease

Pharmacological treatment can not only relieve symptoms, but also reduce the progressive joint damage from inflammation, and therefore help to maintain long-term function. Medicines, however, comprise only one component of the toolbox used to manage RMDs. Exercise- and psychological-based therapies, orthoses (e.g., knee braces, shoe inserts), mobility and other aids, social interventions including support from carers and significant others, injections and surgery each can play important roles at appropriate stages of RMD management. Pharmacological and non-pharmacological interventions should be coordinated. Medicines often require the involvement of a professional prescriber, and concordant education and training can empower the patient and enable self-management.

This chapter presents an overview of the pharmacological management of prevalent RMDs, and then provides more detailed descriptions of the pharmacological management of inflammatory arthritis.

OVERVIEW OF PREVALENT RMDs

OSTEOARTHRITIS

Osteoarthritis causes joint pain, stiffness and loss of function. Clinical features include crepitus (`grating' on joint movement), local tenderness, bony swelling, and restricted and painful movement. Increased synovial fluid within the joint (effusion) and inflammation (synovitis) can

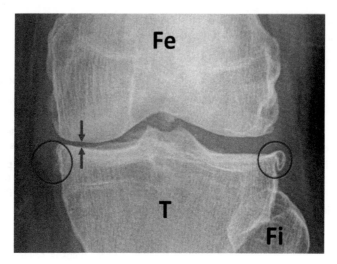

FIGURE 34.1 Radiographic appearance of knee osteoarthritis. Posteroanterior weightbearing radiograph of a left knee. Arrows indicate reduced joint space at the medial tibiofemoral compartment, consistent with articular cartilage loss and meniscal extrusion. Circles indicate marginal new bone formation (osteophytes). Fe, femur; T, tibia; Fi, fibula.

cause soft tissue swelling. Radiographs (Figure 34.1) may reveal joint space narrowing and osteophytes. At arthroscopy, articular cartilage may appear swollen and fibrillated, with fissures or defects. Magnetic resonance imaging can reveal subchondral bone marrow lesions (areas of high signal on T2-weighted images) and synovitis. Osteoarthritis can be both distressing and disabling, although even advanced radiographic osteoarthritis may sometimes cause few symptoms.

Osteoarthritis may involve any synovial joint, but most commonly causes problems with weightbearing joints in the lower limbs. The earliest symptoms of osteoarthritis might be intermittent pain, for example when weightbearing. Pain that persists at rest and disturbs sleep may result from sensitisation of nerves within the joint (peripheral sensitisation). Sensitisation within the central nervous system can increase pain severity, psychological aspects including anxiety and low mood, fatigue, sleep disturbance and cognitive dysfunction, and extend pain to additional sites beyond the osteoarthritic joint.

Exercise remains the cornerstone of osteoarthritis management, reducing pain and improving function, and often is more effective than pharmacological agents (National Institute for Health and Care Excellence, 2022). Osteoarthritis is an aberrant repair response, and activity can facilitate repair. Pharmacological management can help maintain activity and facilitate exercise by relieving activity-induced pain. Most episodes of knee pain will settle with conservative management, although surgery (e.g., knee arthroplasty) can be helpful in some cases.

INFLAMMATORY ARTHRITIS

In inflammatory arthritis joint inflammation is driven by lymphocytes. Rheumatoid arthritis and seronegative arthropathies are the most prevalent inflammatory arthritides. Pain is the predominant symptom, but stiffness, fatigue and loss of function also occur. Synovitis can lead to joint damage, causing radiographic erosion and joint space narrowing, and may eventually lead to secondary osteoarthritis.

Rheumatoid arthritis is a symmetrical polyarthritis particularly affecting small joints of the hands, wrists, elbows, shoulders, knees and feet. It may also affect the cervical spine, eyes (Sjogren's syndrome causing dry eyes and mouth), lungs (interstitial lung disease) and blood vessels (vasculitis). Systemic rheumatoid disease may cause fever, malaise and weight loss, and blood dyscrasias (Felty's syndrome). Rheumatoid arthritis may sometimes be associated with autoantibodies (rheumatoid factor, anticitrullinated peptide antibodies) and subcutaneous rheumatoid nodules.

Seronegative arthritides include *psoriatic arthritis, enteropathic arthritis* (in ulcerative colitis or Crohn's disease), *reactive arthritis* (following gastrointestinal or reproductive tract infection) and *ankylosing spondylitis*. Ocular inflammation (uveitis) and inflammatory spinal disease (spondylitis) may be present. Seronegative arthritides differ from rheumatoid arthritis, with discrete genetic associations, comorbidities, joint distribution (typically asymmetrical, involving predominantly large joints) and pathology (absent autoantibodies, inflammation localised to tendon and ligament insertions at joint margins). Inflammation may affect sacroiliac joints, lumbar and thoracic and cervical spine, with or without involvement of peripheral joints.

Some pharmaceuticals might relieve disease in multiple organs, but others might be specific for joints or for extra-articular disease. Tumour necrosis factor (TNF) is implicated in both rheumatoid and seronegative spondylarthropathies, but other mediators may be specific for one disease. B-cell targeted rituximab may selectively reduce rheumatoid arthritis inflammation, whereas interleukin (IL)-17 inhibitors can suppress spinal and joint inflammation in psoriatic and enteropathic arthritis, but without demonstrated benefit for rheumatoid arthritis.

SPINAL PAIN

Low back or cervical (neck) pain are highly prevalent. Most acute spinal pain cannot be linked to objective evidence of structural change. Muscle spasm is extremely painful and disabling, but typically settles within days. `Red flag' features should trigger medical review (Box 34.1). Spinal pain severity is a weak indicator of underlying pathology or prognosis.

Nerve root irritation causes neuropathic pain radiating or shooting into the leg (sciatica) or arm (brachalgia). Acute nerve root irritation might be due to intervertebral disc prolapse, although radiculopathy pain is more often driven by inflammatory mediators than by physical nerve root compression. Pain can improve as inflammation subsides. Back pain often occurs without radiculopathy, and radiculopathy may occur in the absence of any spinal pain.

Chronic spinal pain may follow previous episodes of acute pain or might develop insidiously without an acute episode. Associations between symptoms and imaging findings are often at best weak. Radiographic spondylosis (disc space narrowing, facet joint osteoarthritis) and magnetic resonance imaging abnormalities of intervertebral discs or vertebral endplates have been associated with spinal pain, but may be present in the absence of pain.

Initial treatment of acute spinal pain is with analgesia (see Chapter 26) and exercise. For most, acute back pain and radiculopathy will resolve with conservative management. Management of chronic spinal pain may also involve analgesia and exercise, although the benefits of analgesic medications are less well established for chronic than acute spinal pain. Non-pharmacological approaches may include physiotherapy, cognitive behavioural therapy, and interventional or surgical procedures in selected cases.

GOUT AND PSEUDOGOUT

Crystals within synovial tissue or fluid can trigger acute inflammation, characterised by a red, hot, swollen joint, severe pain, mild pyrexia, and raised acute phase and neutrophilia on blood tests. This resembles acute infection, which should be urgently excluded by joint aspiration, microscopy and synovial fluid and blood culture. Infection and crystals can coexist.

Crystals may comprise monosodium urate (gout) or calcium pyrophosphate dihydrate (CPPDH, pseudogout). Urate deposits may be subcutaneous (tophi), and may cause joint erosions

BOX 34.1	RED FLAG SYMPTOMS AND SIGNS THAT INDICATE A NEED FOR MEDICAL REVIEW IN PEOPLE WITH SPINAL PAIN

The relative rarity of reversible or progressive underlying pathologies poses a diagnostic challenge. The clinician must repeatedly review diagnosis, particularly if clinical features change or do not settle as expected. Acute compression of nerves within the cauda equina, resulting in saddle anaesthesia, bladder or bowel dysfuntion, requires immediate surgical intervention to avoid permanent deficits.

Significant neurological compromise

Saddle anaesthesia around the anus, perineum or genitals

Recent onset of bladder dysfunction or faecal incontinence

Widespread or progressive weakness

Gait disturbance (back pain)

Altered cognitive status, ataxia, visual loss (neck pain)

Spinal fracture

Major trauma (e.g., fall from height, road traffic accident) or surgery

Minor trauma (if osteoporosis or advanced ankylosing spondylitis)

Infection or cancer

Constitutional symptoms (fever, unexplained weight loss)

Thoracic pain

Previous or current cancer

Recent bacterial infection

Intravenous drug use

Immune suppression

---

and secondary osteoarthritis. Very high serum urate levels may be a consequence or cause of renal impairment. Low serum urate levels do not preclude crystal deposition within the joint. CPPDH deposition might be detected as chondrocalcinosis (radio-opaque deposits on plain radiographs) and might be a consequence or cause of osteoarthritis.

The severe pain of acute crystal arthritis should be treated with non-steroidal anti-inflammatory drugs (NSAIDs) or colchicine (Neilson et al. 2022). A course of colchicine should be of limited dose and duration (see *British National Formulary* for details) to minimise risks of diarrhoea or neuropathy. Glucocorticoids (oral, systemic or intra-articular) also reduce inflammation and pain. IL-1 inhibitors may also abort an acute attack of gout. Glucocorticoids or IL-1 inhibitors should not be used unless septic arthritis has been definitively excluded.

Urate-lowering therapy is indicated for people with recurrent attacks of gout, impaired renal function, and those requiring diuretic therapy, or with chronic gouty arthritis or subcutaneous tophi (Neilson et al. 2022). Titrate urate-lowering therapy to achieve serum urate levels in the lower half of the normal range to prevent acute attacks. Allopurinol is first line, and usually well tolerated, but may cause rashes or liver dysfunction. Allopurinol is renally excreted and dosage is adjusted in severe renal impairment. Febuxostat may be considered if allopurinol is contraindicated or not tolerated. Febuxostat has been associated with angina, myocardial infarction and stroke. Initiation of urate-lowering therapy may precipitate or prolong acute attacks of gout. NSAIDs or low-dose colchicine may therefore be given alongside urate-lowering therapies until serum urate levels have been stable for 3 weeks.

FIBROMYALGIA AND NOCIPLASTIC PAIN

Chronic pain can only rarely be entirely explained by objective evidence of peripheral tissue pathology. Nociceptive signals are modulated by both peripheral and central nervous systems (Figure 26.4). Sensitisation augments, whereas endogenous analgesic pathways supress nociceptive signals. Peripheral neuronal sensitisation may result from acute inflammatory mediators such as prostaglandins and bradykinin. Central pain facilitation results from enhanced spinal transmission. Descending control by brain and brainstem activity can suppress spinal nociceptive transmission, for example during exercise, but may be deficient in some people with chronic pain. Increased functional connectivity between brain regions responsible for sensory and emotional components of pain, sleep regulation and cognitive function may, in part, explain the broader characteristics and often widespread nature of chronic pain. Peripheral sensitisation might also contribute to widespread pain in polyarticular disease or in the presence of systemic inflammation.

This plasticity of nociceptive neuronal transmission contributes to discordance between pain and objective evidence of tissue damage, leading to the recent mechanistic classification of 'nociplastic pain' as distinct from, but often coexisting with, nociceptive and neuropathic pain (Kosek et al. 2021). Nociplastic pain may occur without obvious tissue pathology, as in fibromyalgia, or alongside other RMDs such as rheumatoid arthritis, osteoarthritis and spinal pain. The presence of nociplastic pain predicts poor response to peripherally targeted treatments such as NSAIDs, joint injection and arthroplasty. Other treatments such as antidepressants aim to restore deficient endogenous descending inhibitory control. Identifying nociplastic features of pain in RMDs is a key component of optimising treatment.

PHARMACOLOGICAL MANAGEMENT OF INFLAMMATORY ARTHRITIS

Pharmacological management of inflammatory arthritis can broadly be categorised as acute or maintenance. Both aim to reduce symptoms and joint damage. Acute treatment may focus on immediate symptom control, whereas maintenance treatment aims to prevent future acute symptom flares, tissue damage, and long-term pain and disability.

Management of inflammatory arthritis therefore comprises sequential treatments that (1) quickly relieve acute symptoms, particularly pain, and (2) suppress ongoing disease, thereby reducing joint damage and long-term symptoms and disability. Once disease is supressed, acute symptomatic treatments should be withdrawn to minimise the risk of side effects. However, people with chronic inflammatory arthritis remain susceptible to acute flares, and relief for acute symptoms may need to be reintroduced periodically.

SYMPTOM CONTROL IN INFLAMMATORY ARTHRITIS

Rapid symptom relief is often the highest priority for people with inflammatory arthritis. Pain and stiffness can respond exquisitely to glucocorticoids or NSAIDs (Allen et al. 2018). Maximum symptomatic benefit from glucocorticoids or NSAIDs might be expected within 2 weeks. Simple analgesics such as paracetamol and opioids may also provide some short-term pain relief and can be co-administered with anti-inflammatory drugs if necessary. More detailed information on NSAIDs and their possible side effects can be found in Chapter 26. Rheumatoid arthritis pain can also be mechanical or, more rarely, neuropathic, therefore inadequate symptom relief from anti-inflammatory treatments should lead to review of possible pain mechanisms and consideration of other treatment options. Fatigue in rheumatoid arthritis is usually linked to pain, and fatigue and sleep management strategies may be more effective at improving fatigue than anti-inflammatory drugs.

Short-term bridging glucocorticoids can manage flares by rapidly decreasing inflammation. Intra-articular, intra-muscular or intravenous glucocorticoids may provide symptomatic benefit for around 6 weeks, often sufficient for an inflammatory flare to naturally remit, or for a disease-modifying agent to suppress underlying inflammation and symptoms. In established rheumatoid arthritis, glucocorticoids should only continue long term if the risks and complications of glucocorticoids have been fully discussed with the patient and all other treatment options have been considered. There is little evidence of any disease-modifying benefit from glucocorticoids in established rheumatoid arthritis, and symptomatic benefit wanes after 3 months treatment (McWilliams et al. 2021). As soon as inflammatory disease is controlled, glucocorticoids should be tapered to discontinuation. People who have received glucocorticoids for several weeks may have impaired endogenous production, and abrupt discontinuation may lead to malaise, hypotension and hyponatraemia.

STOP AND THINK

A patient with rheumatoid arthritis presents to you and mentions he has suddenly stopped his long-term oral prednisolone of 10 mg daily because he ran out of tablets. What advice would you give?

Minimising drug exposure minimises the risk of side effects, and symptomatic treatments should be used at the lowest effective dose over the shortest necessary time. People are not all the same in how they balance the benefits and risks of treatment. A key role of the prescriber is to explain what might be expected, and patients should be empowered to make informed decisions about whether to initiate or continue treatment. Review (by both patient and prescriber) of response after treatment initiation is essential.

INFLAMMATORY ARTHRITIS DISEASE SUPPRESSION AND REMISSION

Intensive target-driven immunosuppressive treatment of inflammatory arthritis is aimed at disease remission(Allen et al. 2018). Disease suppression and remission might be achieved by selecting from a range of disease-modifying antirheumatic drugs (DMARDs) (Table 34.2). In early disease, the first DMARD is usually a conventional synthetic (cs)DMARD, initiated as monotherapy alongside symptomatic treatments. In the UK, methotrexate is usually recommended as first-line DMARD treatment(Allen et al. 2018). Patients with an inadequate response to csDMARDs, due to inefficacy or side effects, should be screened for contraindications to biologic (b)DMARD or targeted synthetic (ts)DMARD therapy. Prioritisation of the various available DMARDs within treatment pathways depends on cost as well as likely clinical outcomes. bDMARDs are large, complicated molecules that pose manufacturing challenges. Biosimilars that share specificity (e.g., for TNF), despite molecular differences from originator molecules, may be available at lower cost and therefore may be considered for first-line bDMARD therapy.

DMARDs may be used alone (monotherapy). Combination therapy aims to use two or more DMARDs, each acting on different pathogenic mechanisms. Some combinations have evidence of superiority compared to either agent alone (e.g., methotrexate plus TNF inhibitors(Bechman et al. 2020). Other combinations have evidence of safety, permitting licensed co-prescription, but not of greater efficacy than the more potent drug administered alone. Some combinations do not currently have evidence for either efficacy or safety and should be avoided. Some bDMARDs (e.g., rituximab) might be approved only for use in combination with methotrexate. Tocilizumab

Table 34.2 Disease-modifying antirheumatic drugs used for inflammatory arthritis

DMARD	Indications	Selected adverse events
Conventional synthetic DMARDs		
Methotrexate	Rheumatoid arthritis Seronegative inflammatory arthritis	Neutropenia, thrombocytopenia, hepatitis, liver cirrhosis, pneumonitis
Sulphasalazine	Rheumatoid arthritis Seronegative inflammatory arthritis	Severe rashes, neutropenia, thrombocytopenia, hepatitis
Leflunomide	Rheumatoid arthritis	Hypertension, neutropenia, thrombocytopenia, hepatitis
Hydroxychloroquine	Rheumatoid arthritis	Maculopathy
Ciclosporin A	Rheumatoid arthritis	Renal impairment
Azathioprine	Rheumatoid arthritis	Hepatitis, neutropenia, lymphopenia, thrombocytopenia
Biologic DMARDs		
Tumour necrosis factor alpha inhibitors		
Monoclonal antibodies: Infliximab[a-e] Adalimumab[a-e] Certolizumab[a-c,e] Golimumab[a,c-e]	[a]Rheumatoid arthritis [b]Juvenile idiopathic arthritis [c]Psoriatic arthritis [d]Ankylosing spondylitis [e]Enteropathic arthritis	Infection
IgG-TNFR2 fusion protein: Etanercept	Rheumatoid arthritis Polyarticular juvenile idiopathic arthritis Psoriatic arthritis Ankylosing spondylitis	Infection
T-cell co stimulator		
Abatacept	Rheumatoid arthritis Psoriatic arthritis Juvenile idiopathic arthritis	Infection
Interleukin-6 inhibitors		
Sarilumab[a] Tocilizumab[a,b]	[a]Rheumatoid arthritis [b]Juvenile idiopathic arthritis	Infection, hepatitis, neutropenia, thrombocytopenia, dyslipidaemia
Interleukin-12/23 inhibitor		
Ustekinumab	Psoriatic arthritis	Infection
CD20 inhibitor B-cell modulator		
Rituximab	Rheumatoid arthritis	Infection, hypogammaglobulinaemia
Interleukin-17a inhibitor		
Secukinumab	Psoriatic arthritis Ankylosing spondylitis	Infection
Targeted synthetic DMARDs		
Janus kinase inhibitors		
Baricitinib[a] Toficitinib[a] Upadicitinib[a-c] Filgotinib[a]	[a]Rheumatoid arthritis [b]Psoriatic arthritis [c]Ankylosing spondylitis	Infection, neutropenia, thrombocytopenia, hepatitis, dyslipidaemia, thrombosis
Phosphodiesterase type-4 inhibitor		
Apremilast	Psoriatic arthritis	Diarrhoea, nausea, vomiting Depression, loss of weight Infection

DMARD, disease-modifying antirheumatic drug.

may be equally efficacious whether administered alone or in combination with methotrexate. Combination therapy might be expected to at least summate the risks of each individual drug, and combinations of multiple bDMARDs or tsDMARDs are not currently recommended due to likely synergistic risk of infection. When initiating bDMARDs or tsDMARDs in people who can tolerate but have inadequate response to methotrexate, methotrexate may be continued initially, then withdrawal considered once an adequate response is achieved.

SCREENING AND COUNSELLING PRIOR TO DMARD INITIATION

Individual DMARDs have specific risks of side effects (Table 34.2), and close attention to possible contraindications underpins recommendations and patient choice. Pre-treatment screening evaluates individual risk factors through both history/examination (Box 34.2) and investigations (Table 34.3). Individual risk factors should be discussed with the patient to permit an informed shared decision on the right treatment for them. Advice on screening and monitoring may vary: always review local guidelines. Tests routinely monitored following DMARD initiation also should be taken at baseline. Conditions that may increase risks from specific DMARDs should be investigated and, where appropriate, treated.

When counselling patients, all bDMARD and tsDMARDs should be assumed to increase risks from infection (Sepriano et al. 2023). Patients should be advised to seek assessment early if

---

BOX 34.2	CLINICAL ASSESSMENT INFORMING DMARD CHOICE

Inflammatory disease activity: Consider symptoms (pain, stiffness), joint swelling and tenderness, blood tests for acute phase reactants (e.g., C-reactive protein or erythrocyte sedimentation rate). Composite measures of disease activity are recommended (e.g., DAS28 for rheumatoid arthritis).

Previous DMARD exposure: Including response, adverse events

Comorbidities:

- Alcohol use (current and lifetime: risk of cirrhosis with methotrexate)

- Hypertension (may be destabilised by leflunomide)

- Lung disease (increased risk of respiratory adverse events if respiratory reserve is low)

- Congestive cardiac failure (TNF inhibitors cautioned if severe)

- Thrombosis (JAKi contraindicated if past or high risk of thromboembolic disease)

- Demyelinating disease (contraindicates TNF inhibitors)

- Uveitis (contraindicates some TNF inhibitors)

Infection: Latent, active or risk of infection (e.g., diabetes mellitus, skin ulcers, drug or alcohol abuse, immunosuppression).

Malignancy: Current or risk factors, including past history.

Vaccination status: Recommend complete recommended vaccination programmes before commencing bDMARD or tsDMARD, i.e., influenza (annual), pneumococcus (5-yearly), shingles (age ≥50 years) and COVID-19.

Fertility: Recommend effective contraception in women of childbearing age who use methotrexate, leflunominde, bDMARDs or tsDMARDs. Antibodies (bDMARDs) are actively transported across the placenta and into milk

---

bDMARD, biologic disease-modifying antirheumatic drug; DAS28,; DMARD, disease-modifying antirheumatic drug; JAKi,; TNF, tumour necrosis factor; tsDMARD, targeted synthetic disease-modifying antirheumatic drug.

Table **34.3** Pre-treatment screening tests aiming to minimise adverse events when commencing or continuing DMARDs

Screening	Targeted adverse event	DMARD
Risk assessment		
Lipids	Cardiovascular risk	IL-6 inhibitors, JAKi
Mycobacterial T-cell reactivity (e.g., Quantiferon Gold)	Tuberculosis	bDMARDs and tsDMARDs
Viral and serology screen for hepatitis B, C and human immunodeficiency virus	Infection	bDMARDs and tsDMARDs
Varicella serology	Shingles	bDMARDs and tsDMARDs
Chest radiograph	Interstitial lung disease, latent infection (bronchiectasis, tuberculosis)	Methotrexate, leflunomide, bDMARDs and tsDMARDs
Monitoring tests		
Blood pressure	Hypertension	Leflunomide
Full blood profile	Cytopenia	All
Serum folate	Cytopenia	Methotrexate
Creatinine	All	Methotrexate
Creatinine	Nephrotoxicity	Ciclosporin A
Liver function (transaminase)	Hepatotoxicity	All
Antinuclear antibody	Drug-induced lupus	bDMARDs
Acute phase (e.g., erythrocyte sedimentation rate or C-reactive protein)	Inefficacy	All
Immunoglobulins[a]	Infection	Rituximab

[a] Infection risk on rituximab increased if IgG <6 g/L. Check pre and post each infusion.
bDMARD, biologic disease-modifying antirheumatic drug; DAS28,; DMARD, disease-modifying antirheumatic drug; IL, interleukin; JAKi,; tsDMARD, targeted synthetic disease-modifying antirheumatic drug.

infection is suspected. Treatment is contraindicated during significant active infection, and caution should be exercised in those with high risk of infection. Occult infection may be revealed after bDMARD or tsDMARD introduction. Examples include bronchiectasis, diverticular disease, dental or joint prosthesis bacterial infections, or viral hepatitis. Infection risk may be high in people with diabetes mellitus or leg ulcers. Risks from COVID-19 might also be increased, for example with rituximab. bDMARDs may also suppress immune response to vaccination, reducing vaccine efficacy, and live vaccines are contraindicated in people on bDMARDs or tsDMARDs.

Despite previous concerns, the risk of primary or recurrent malignancy might not be increased by bDMARD therapy, although rheumatoid arthritis itself has been associated with risk of lymphoproliferative disorders (Sepriano et al. 2023).

MONITORING FOR DMARD BENEFITS AND RISKS

DMARDs have a variable time to benefit after commencing treatment, but all should be considered 'slow acting'. Early symptomatic benefit may precede objective evidence of synovitis suppression, although part of this early response might be attributable to placebo effects. Maximum benefit may be not experienced until 3 months. Where patients have an apparently good response, but are taking glucocorticoids, a further 3 months of steroid tapering and withdrawal may be required before the adequacy of disease control can be definitively assessed.

After commencing DMARDs, recommended monitoring tests and frequency depend on the DMARD that is used (Ledingham et al. 2017). Monitoring might be fortnightly initially after commencing or increasing dose of a csDMARD, then less frequent (e.g., monthly or 3-monthly) in patients on stable treatment without overt side effects. Disease activity should also be monitored and might include the 28 joint Disease Activity Score (DAS28) with bloods tests for acute phase reactants (erythrocyte sedimentation rate [ESR] or C-reactive protein [CRP]). Periodic hand and foot radiographs (e.g., annually in early disease, increasing intervals to every 3 years in established disease) may reveal unexpected progression of erosive damage and indicate potential benefits from DMARD escalation. Repeated ultrasound scans may reveal residual inflammation despite low DAS28, although the value of imaging alone for determining DMARD escalation is currently unproven.

If the response to DMARDs is inadequate, review whether residual symptoms might be attributable to post-inflammatory pain rather than active synovitis (Ishida et al. 2018). An absence of swollen joints and normal CRP or ESR might indicate that residual symptoms are not attributable to inflammation, although ultrasound imaging may be necessary to exclude clinically relevant residual synovitis.

PRACTICE APPLICATION

It is not possible to accurately predict which DMARD will produce an optimal response in any individual with inflammatory arthritis. DMARD optimization can require time, even years. Regimens that are most likely to provide benefit should be used alongside symptomatic treatments. Patients, significant others and employers should expect eventually a lifestyle similar to the normal population. It is important to avoid unnecessary acceptance of disability. Inflammatory arthritis, although not currently curable, can be controlled in remission with long-term treatment and specialist support.

DMARDs might need to be withheld due to intercurrent illness, emergent adverse events or contraindications, or to facilitate concurrent treatment. A risk assessment should be taken to balance the likely adverse consequences of continuing the DMARD, against the risk of disease reactivation following DMARD withdrawal.

PRACTICE APPLICATION

In an attempt to minimise the risk of surgical infection, bDMARDs are typically withheld before surgery for a variable washout period depending on their half-life. They can be restarted postoperatively once the wound is healed and stitches/sutures are removed.

A patient presenting on bDMARDs or tsDMARDs with an active infection should temporarily have those medicines withheld until the antibiotic course has been completed and they have recovered from infection. After clinically serious infections, bDMARDs and tsDMARDs might be contraindicated for 12 months.

Patients taking a janus kinase inhibitor (JAKi) who present with a confirmed thromboembolic event should permanently discontinue the JAKi.

Patients on tocilizumab or JAKi presenting with diverticulitis should consider the medication as a cause. DMARDs may sometimes be cautiously continued or changed to an alternative.

Once optimal disease control has been achieved, dose tapering or withdrawal of DMARDs should be considered to minimise the risk of side effects, while maintaining adequate disease control (Kuijper et al. 2015). Patients should be reviewed at least annually, and changes to treatment considered if side effects or additional risk factors emerge, if inflammatory disease recurrently or persistently flares, or if serial radiographs demonstrate progressive structural damage. For patients who have sustained remission without glucocorticoids, cDMARD dosing should be cautiously reduced in a step-down regimen. Complete remission for 3 years may predict natural remission sustained after complete withdrawal of DMARD monotherapy. Prompt return to the previous or an alternative DMARD is required if remission is not maintained after tapering or withdrawal. Symptomatic treatments (e.g., glucocorticoids) may be necessary to bridge between drug initiation and regaining disease control.

DMARDS COMMONLY PRESCRIBED FOR INFLAMMATORY ARTHRITIS

Further information on commonly prescribed DMARDs in current clinical practice is presented in the following sections.

Methotrexate

The considered treatment standard is administration orally or subcutaneously up to 25 mg once weekly. Do not conclude ineffective unless used for 12 weeks at a dose of at least 20 mg weekly. Folic acid (5 mg) is co-prescribed to minimise the risk of side effects. Folic acid regimens vary from once per week to daily, but it should not be taken on same day as methotrexate.

Mechanism of action Folic acid antagonist, competitively inhibiting dihydrofolate reductase. This reduces cell proliferation and increases T-cell apoptosis and endogenous adenosine release, whilst altering the expression of cellular adhesion molecules. It also might influence cytokine production and humoral responses.

Pharmacokinetics Therapeutic dose ranges from 10 to 25 mg once weekly, with a variable time to therapeutic effect of 8–12 weeks. Serum concentration peaks within 1–2 hours and is absorbed rapidly, with a high bioavailability ranging from 80% to 100% with all routes. However, bioavailability decreases at oral doses above 25 mg due to saturation of absorption.

PRACTICE APPLICATION

Methotrexate is mainly excreted renally with an elimination half-life of 3–10 hours. Impaired renal function can lead to rapid methotrexate accumulation. Review methotrexate dosing if unstable renal function. Dosage should be reduced if the eGFR is below 60 ml/min/1.73m^2 and consider discontinuation if the eGFR is below 30.

Monitoring Guidelines for monitoring vary, but may be fortnightly full blood count and liver function tests during the first 6 weeks of treatment or after dosage escalation, then monthly, then reducing to 3-monthly for those on stable treatment with normal test results.

Hydroxychloroquine

Mechanism of action Traditionally used as an antimalarial, hydroxycholoroquine may interfere with antigen presentation, release of cytokines and activation of the immune response by increasing the pH within macrophage phagolysosomes.

Pharmacokinetics The oral therapeutic dose is usually 200 mg twice daily, with a maximum dose based on ideal bodyweight (maximum 6.5 mg/kg/day). It is rapidly absorbed, with a mean peak concentration after 2 hours and a half-life of 3–4 hours.

Monitoring Side effects are uncommon with hydroxychloroquine and blood monitoring is not required. Monitoring might include fundoscopy after treatment for a year and periodically thereafter. More frequent ophthalmological monitoring might be recommended in people using concomitant tamoxifen therapy, impaired renal function eGFR (<60 mL/min/1.73 m^2) or high-dose hydroxychloroquine >5 mg/kg/day).

Leflunomide

Mechanism of action Suppression of cell proliferation by inhibiting dihydro orotate dehydrogenase and reducing pyrimidine synthesis. Relative selectivity for lymphocytes.

Pharmacokinetics Therapeutic oral maintenance doses may be 10 or 20 mg daily. Leflunomide is well absorbed, with a peak plasma concentration after 6–12 hours. However, the active metabolite has a long half-life of 2 weeks. Steady-state plasma levels may not be reached before 20 weeks of regular dosing. Leflunomide undergoes enterohepatic recycling and may persist in plasma for 6 months after treatment discontinuation. Elimination can be accelerated to 10 days by administration of cholestyramine or activated charcoal, which prevent reabsorption in the gut.

Monitoring Monitoring regimens may include full blood count, liver function tests and blood pressure, initially fortnightly and reduced to monthly then 3-monthly on stable treatment.

Sulfasalazine

Mechanism of action Unclear, but may inhibit transcription factors, which are increased in inflammation. Sulphasalazine is cleaved in the colon by bacterial enzymes to release 5-aminosalicylic acid and sulfapyridine, but is not believed to act through cyclooxygenase inhibition nor as an antibacterial agent.

Pharmacokinetics The therapeutic oral dose ranges from 1.5 to 3 g daily, in divided twice-daily doses. Peak serum levels occur after 3–5 hours and a half-life of 5–10 hours.

Monitoring Monitoring regimens may include full blood count and liver function tests, initially fortnightly, and reduced to 3-monthly for the first year of treatment.

BIOLOGIC AND TARGETED SYNTHETIC DMARDS

'Biologics' are highly complex biological products of living cells or organisms, with precise molecular actions, but which lack precise characterisation of their molecular structures. The first biologics used for inflammatory arthritis specifically bound TNF, thereby preventing it from activating its receptor. TNF-specific antibodies (e.g., adalimumab) or soluble TNF receptor fusion proteins (etanercept) bind TNF with high affinity. Biologics have been engineered to optimise bioavailability and pharmacokinetics for intravenous or subcutaneous delivery. Side effects might be predicted from the specific action of bDMARDs (e.g., infection due to immunosuppression) or are general to antibody-based drugs (e.g., hypersensitivity reactions). Biosimilar molecules are not exact copies of the original biologic, but are anticipated to behave similarly in vivo.

bDMARDs have relatively long pharmacological half-lives, enabling administration at intervals between 1 and 4 weeks without loss of pharmacological benefit. Rituximab has a prolonged biological effect, depleting B cells and reducing antibody production for 6–12 months after intravenous administration. Dosing intervals for bDMARDs are therefore long and effects are not easily reversed by treatment discontinuation.

tsDMARDs became available in the European Union for inflammatory arthritis in 2017. Inhibitors of the Janus kinase pathways (JAKi) modulate T-cell function (Cohen and Reddy 2023). Baricitinib inhibits with similar potency both JAK1 and JAK2 subtypes, with 10-fold lower affinity for tyrosine kinase 2. Tofacitinib significantly inhibits both JAK and JAK3 kinases. Different specificities might be expected to associate with different therapeutic efficacies in different diseases, and with unique side effect profiles. However, empirical evidence of this awaits adequately powered head-to-head trials. The phosphodiesterase type 4 inhibitor apremilast has recently received a license for treating psoriatic arthritis.

SUMMARY

- Pharmacological treatment of rheumatic and musculoskeletal disorders aims to reduce current and future pain and disability.

- Treatment choice requires balancing likely benefits against risks. The prescriber should provide information to facilitate treatment choice, matching treatment to the patient's diagnosis, symptoms and evidence of inflammatory disease activity, within the context of individual- and treatment-specific risk factors.

- Patients should be empowered to monitor benefits, risks and adverse events before and during treatment.

- Crystal arthritis requires rapid and effective management of acute inflammation, and gout attacks can be prevented by adequately titrated urate-lowering therapy.

- The pain of inflammatory arthritis may respond better to immunomodulatory treatments than to simple analgesics such as opioids.

- Glucocorticoids may relieve symptoms but usually do not prevent joint damage, and with continued treatment benefits wane and adverse events emerge.

- Immunosuppressive disease-modifying antirheumatic drugs may reduce both symptoms and tissue damage.

- Pharmacological treatment should only be provided within the context of holistic care, and non-pharmacological interventions such as physiotherapy may improve symptoms more effectively than medications alone.

- Rheumatic and musculoskeletal disorders often cannot be cured, but the prescriber can enable patients to live normal and high-quality lives.

ACTIVITY

1. Match the most appropriate long-term medication to each of the following cases. Each medication may be used for one case only, for multiple cases or not at all.
   Colchicine
   Methotrexate
   Adalimumab

Sulphasalazine
Allopurinol
Naproxen
Sekukinumab
Prednisolone
Hydroxychloroquine
Rituximab

Case 1: An otherwise healthy 40-year-old man who 4 weeks ago suffered an acute attack of gout for the third time this year.

Case 2: A 35-year-old woman who is keen to start a family 'before it is too late', but has recently developed rheumatoid arthritis and has radiographic evidence of erosive joint damage.

Case 3: A 50-year-old otherwise healthy man who continues to have severely active rheumatoid arthritis despite previous treatment with methotrexate and sulphasalazine.

Case 4: A 55-year-old lady with severe psoriatic spondyloarthritis affecting knees, spine and skin that has not adequately responded to a combination of methotrexate and adalimumab.

Case 5: A 60-year-old man who regularly drinks 5 units of alcohol per day, has severely active rheumatoid arthritis and has not responded adequately to sulphasalazine or hydroxychloroquine.

Case 6: A 95-year-old lady with a past history of severe bronchiectasis, tuberculosis and pulmonary embolus, chronic renal impairment and active rheumatoid arthritis despite previous treatment with methotrexate, sulphasalazine and hydroxychloroquine.

2. Match each of the following routine monitoring tests with each DMARD. Each test may be matched to one, more than one or no DMARDs in the list.

   (a) Full blood count

   (b) Ophthalmological examination

   (c) Blood pressure

   (d) Liver function tests (transaminases)

   (e) Blood lipid profile

   (f) Urinalysis

   (g) Creatinine/glomerular filtration rate

   (h) Serum immunoglobulins

   Methotrexate
   Sulphasalazine
   Hydroxychloroquine
   Rituximab
   Baricitinib
   Leflunomide

REFERENCES

Allen, A., Carville, S. and McKenna, F. (2018) Diagnosis and management of rheumatoid arthritis in adults: summary of updated NICE guidance. *BMJ* 362:k3015.

Bechman, K., Oke, A., Yates, M., et al. (2020) Is background methotrexate advantageous in extending TNF inhibitor drug survival in elderly patients with rheumatoid arthritis? An analysis of the British Society for Rheumatology Biologics Register. *Rheumatology* 59(9):2563–2571.

Cohen, S. and Reddy, V. (2023) Janus kinase inhibitors: efficacy and safety. *Curr Opin Rheumatol* 35(6):429–434.

National Institute for Health and Care Excellence (2022) Osteoarthritis in over 16s: diagnosis and management NICE guideline NG226.

Ishida, M., Kuroiwa, Y., Yoshida, E., et al. (2018) Residual symptoms and disease burden among patients with rheumatoid arthritis in remission or low disease activity: a systematic literature review. *Mod Rheumatol* 28(5):789–799.

Kosek, E., Clauw, D., Nijs, J., et al. (2021) Chronic nociplastic pain affecting the musculoskeletal system: clinical criteria and grading system. *Pain* 162(11):2629–2634.

Kuijper, T.M., Lamers-Karnebeek, F.B., Jacobs, J.W., Hazes, J.M. and Luime, J.J. (2015) Flare rate in patients with rheumatoid arthritis in low disease activity or remission when tapering or stopping synthetic or biologic DMARD: a systematic review. *J Rheumatol* 42(11):2012–2022.

Ledingham, J., Gullick, N., Irving, K., et al. (2017) BSR and BHPR guideline for the prescription and monitoring of non-biologic disease-modifying anti-rheumatic drugs. *Rheumatology* 56(6):865–868.

McWilliams, D.F., Thankaraj, D., Jones-Diette, J., et al. (2021) The efficacy of systemic glucocorticosteroids for pain in rheumatoid arthritis: a systematic literature review and meta-analysis. *Rheumatology* 61(1):76–89.

Neilson, J., Bonnon, A., Dickson, A. and Roddy, E. (2022) Gout: diagnosis and management-summary of NICE guidance. *BMJ* 378:o1754.

Sepriano, A., Kerschbaumer, A., Bergstra, S.A., et al. (2023) Safety of synthetic and biological DMARDs: a systematic literature review informing the 2022 update of the EULAR recommendations for the management of rheumatoid arthritis. *Ann Rheum Dis* 82(1):107–118.

USEFUL WEBSITES

National Institute for Health and Care Excellence (2016) Adalimumab, etanercept, infliximab, certolizumab pegol, golimumab, tocilizumab and abatacept for rheumatoid arthritis not previously treated with DMARDs or after conventional DMARDs only have failed. Technology appraisal guidance TA375. https://www.nice.org.uk/guidance/ta375.

National Institute for Health and Care Excellence (2021) Adalimumab, etanercept, infliximab and abatacept for treating moderate rheumatoid arthritis after conventional DMARDs have failed. Technology appraisal guidance TA715. https://www.nice.org.uk/guidance/ta715.

National Institute for Health and Care Excellence (2022) *Osteoarthritis: care and management. Clinical guideline CG177.* https://www.nice.org.uk/guidance/cg177.

National Institute for Health and Care Excellence (2020) *Rheumatoid arthritis in adults: management. NICE guideline NG100.* https://www.nice.org.uk/guidance/ng100.

National Institute for Health and Care Excellence (2012) *Tocilizumab for the treatment of Rheumatoid arthritis.* Technology appraisal guidance *TA247.* https://www.nice.org.uk/guidance/ta247.

National Institute for Health and Care Excellence (2022) Gout: diagnosis and management. NICE guideline NG219. https://www.nice.org.uk/guidance/ng219.

British Society for Rheumatology. A professional organisation that has supported guidelines and service development in rheumatology. https://www.rheumatology.org.uk/.

American College of Rheumatology. A professional organisation with a strong track record in supporting patients and developing evidence-based guidelines. https://www.rheumatology.org/.

European Alliance of Associations for Rheumatology. A professional organisation with a strong track record in supporting patients and developing evidence-based guidelines. https://www.eular.org/index.cfm.

Versus Arthritis. A charity that provides resources for patients and funds research into rheumatic and musculoskeletal disorders. https://www.versusarthritis.org.

National Rheumatoid Arthritis Society. A charity that supports patients with rheumatoid arthritis. https://www.nras.org.uk/.

BMJ Best Practice. Provides regularly updated information on the diagnosis and management of most of the rheumatic and musculoskeletal diseases discussed in this chapter. https://bestpractice.bmj.com/.

Pharmacology Glossary

Absorption: The passage of a drug from its site of administration to the plasma. Important for all drugs except those given intravenously (not strictly required for inhalation of bronchodilators.

Acetylcholine: Neurotransmitter in both the autonomic nervous system and the central nervous system.

Acetylcholinesterase: Enzyme present in the synaptic cleft that inactivates acetycholine by breaking it down into acetate and choline.

Acid-glycoprotein: An example of a plasma protein; binds basic drugs (particularly propranolol, tricyclics and lidocaine).

Adenosine diphosphate (ADP): Pro-aggregatory chemical released by activated platelets.

Adrenaline: Endocrine hormone produced by the adrenal medulla following stimulation by the sympathetic nervous system.

Adrenergic receptors (adrenoceptors): Receptors of the sympathetic nervous system. Stimulated by endogenous adrenaline and noradrenaline. Can be divided into α- and β-receptors, which have differential affinity for adrenaline and noradrenaline.

Adverse drug reaction (ADR): A noxious or unintended reaction to a drug that is administered in standard doses by the proper route for the purpose of prophylaxis, diagnosis or treatment (World Health Organization definition).

Affinity: Likelihood of drug binding to a receptor.

Afterload: The force against which the heart has to pump (peripheral vascular resistance).

Agonist: Binds to a receptor and elicits a response (has affinity and efficacy). Full agonists induce a maximal tissue response.

Albumin: An example of a plasma protein; binds mainly acidic drugs. Most important plasmabinding protein, binds warfarin, aspirin, phenytoin, furosemide and so on.

Aldosterone: Hormone produced by the action of angiotensin II on the adrenal cortex. Promotes the retention of sodium ions in the plasma.

Angiotensin II: Potent vasoconstrictor produced by the action of angiotensin-converting enzyme on angiotensin I.

Antagonist: Binds to a receptor but does not elicit a response (has affinity but no efficacy).

Autocrine hormone: Hormone that is released from and acts on the same cell.

Autonomic nervous system: The nervous system responsible for regulating involuntary body systems.

β-globulin: An example of a plasma protein; binds basic drugs.

Biliary excretion: Major route of excretion of large ionised molecules (often glucuronide or sulphate conjugates).

Bioavailability: Indicates the proportion of administered drug that passes into the systemic circulation and can therefore have a therapeutic effect, taking into account absorption and first-pass metabolism. Important for orally administered drugs.

Blood pressure (BP): BP = cardiac output × peripheral vascular resistance.

Bradykinin: Inflammatory mediator.

The New Prescriber: An Integrated Approach to Medical and Non-medical Prescribing, Second Edition.
Edited by Joanne Lymn, Alison Mostyn, Roger Knaggs, Michael Randall, and Dianne Bowskill.
© 2024 John Wiley & Sons Ltd. Published 2024 by John Wiley & Sons Ltd.

Cardiac output (CO): Cardiac output = heart rate × stroke volume.

Carrier protein: One of the four groups of protein drug targets.

Central nervous system (CNS): The brain and the spinal cord.

Chemical antagonism: Binding of 'antagonist' and drug in solution to produce an inactive complex.

Cholesterol: Lipid produced by the liver which is a key component of cell membranes and forms the basis of a number of hormones.

Clearance: Rate of drug elimination divided by plasma concentration. Concerned with the rate at which an active drug is removed from the body. Involves metabolism and excretion.

Cockcroft–Gault equation: This equation allows for rapid estimation of creatinine clearance. Incorporates patient's weight.

Competitive antagonism: Antagonist competes with agonist for receptor binding. Binding is only weak (hydrogen bonds, etc.). Agonist receptor occupancy is reduced in the presence of competitive antagonist, can be overcome by increasing agonist concentration. Inhibition is surmountable.

Creatinine clearance: $\dfrac{U \times V}{P} \times 100$ where U is the urine concentration of creatinine, V is the rate of urine flow and P is the plasma concentration of creatinine. An estimation of GFR.

Cyclooxygenase: Enzyme that is important in the production of prostaglandins from arachidonate. Activity is inhibited by NSAIDs.

Cytochrome P450: Large family of drug-metabolising enzymes found mainly in the liver.

Distribution: Refers to the localisation of drug throughout the body. Each drug has a specific pattern of localisation/distribution.

DNA: Long threadlike molecule made up of a large number of deoxyribonucleotides (themselves made up of a base [ATCG], a sugar and a phosphate). The bases carry the genetic information, found in the cell nucleus.

Dopamine: One of the principal neurotransmitters in the CNS.

Efficacy: The likelihood of drug binding to activate the receptor, resulting in an effect.

E_{max}: The maximal response to a drug.

Endocrine hormone: Hormone released into the bloodstream that acts on distant targets.

Endocrine system: Diverse range of organs, tissue and cells that release hormones to regulate most body systems.

Endogenous: Naturally occurring (within the body) product or mediator.

Enterohepatic recycling: Recycling of metabolised drugs in the bile. Transported from the liver to the gut, drugs are then hydrolysed in the gut, releasing parent drug, which is then reabsorbed into the hepatic portal system and transported back to the liver, where it is metabolised again.

Enzyme: A protein that speeds up chemical reactions within the body without being chemically altered itself. Enzymes are one of the four groups of protein drug targets.

Estimated GFR (e-GFR): Prediction of patient's GFR based on a formula that takes into account the patient's age, gender, ethnicity and creatinine levels.

Excretion: The removal of drug from the body.

Exocrine secretions: Secretions stimulated by the parasympathetic nervous system (with the exception of sweat, which is a sympathetic response).

Fibrin: An insoluble protein that cross-links platelets and stabilises the platelet plug. The end-product of the coagulation cascade.

First-pass metabolism: Metabolism that occurs in the liver and gut wall prior to a drug reaching the systemic circulation. Significant feature of orally administered drugs. Reduces bioavailability.

Forebrain: Largest part of the brain. Area where conscious thought and action are initiated.

Full agonist: Binds to a receptor and induces a maximal tissue response.

Gamma-amino butyric acid (GABA): The major inhibitory neurotransmitter in the CNS.

Gastrin: Endocrine hormone that stimulates gastric acid production.

Glial cells: Cell type found in the brain. Do not directly take part in electrical communication but can modulate and support neuronal function.

Glomerular filtration: Fundamental process of drug excretion. Diffusion of drug through glomerular capillaries into filtrate.

Glomerular filtration rate (GFR): A measure of the rate at which blood is filtered by the kidneys.

Glutamate: The major excitatory neurotransmitter in the CNS.

Glycogenolysis: Breakdown of glycogen to glucose for energy.

Glycolipids: Lipids contained in the plasma membrane of the cell.

Haemostasis: Arrest of blood loss from damaged blood vessels. Normal physiological response.

Half-life ($t_{1/2}$): The half-life of a drug is the time taken for the plasma concentration of the drug to fall by 50%.

Heart rate (HR): Measure of cardiac activity. CO = HR × stroke volume.

Hindbrain: Located at the top of the spinal cord. Consists of three structures (medulla oblongata, pons, cerebellum).

Histamine: Inflammatory mediator, released from mast cells.

Hydrophilic: Water loving. Drugs that are hydrophilic do not readily cross cell membranes (polar, ionised, lipophobic).

Hydrophobic: Water hating. Hydrophobic drugs readily cross cell membranes (unionised, non-polar, lipophilic).

Inducer: Drug/chemical that speeds up the activity of specific cytochrome P450 enzymes.

Inhibitor: Drug/chemical that inhibits the activity of specific cytochrome P450 enzymes.

Inotrope: Acts directly on the heart muscle.

Ion channels: Proteins which act as gated tunnels allowing passage of ions across cell membranes. Ion channels are one of the four groups of protein drug targets.

Ionised: Drug that is charged, lipophobic and hydrophilic. Will not readily cross cell membranes.

Irreversible antagonist: A drug that binds to the receptor using strong covalent bonds. Dissociates from the receptor only slowly or not at all.

Leukotrienes: Inflammatory mediators that cause bronchoconstriction.

Lipolysis: The breakdown of fats to produce fuel molecules.

Lipophilic: Lipid loving. Lipophilic drugs can readily cross cell membranes (unionised, nonpolar, hydrophobic).

Lipophobic: Lipid hating. Lipophobic drugs do not readily cross cell membranes (ionised, polar, hydrophilic).

Mediators: Chemicals/drugs that modulate biological processes, for example neurotransmitters, hormones, inflammatory mediators.

Metabolism: The enzymatic conversion of one chemical entity to another. Transformation of drugs within the body with the purpose of making them more hydrophilic.

Midbrain: Smallest processing region of the brain. Connects hindbrain to forebrain.

Monoamine oxidase: Enzyme that acts to break down monoamines once they have been taken back up into the presynaptic nerve cell.

Muscarinic receptors: Postsynaptic cholinergic receptors of the parasympathetic nervous system. Also found in the CNS.

Neonate: Newborn infant (particularly less than 1 month old).

Neuron: Nerve cell.

Neurotransmitter: Chemical that is released from nerve cells and transmits signal either to another nerve cell or to an effector organ.

Nicotinic acetylcholine receptors: Presynaptic cholinergic receptors of the autonomic nervous system. Also found in the CNS.

Non-competitive antagonist: An antagonist does not act at receptor level but instead interferes with the cellular response to an agonist.

Non-polar: Substances which dissolve freely in lipids, move readily across cell membranes (unionised, lipophilic, hydrophobic).

Noradrenaline: Neurotransmitter released from postganglionic neurons in the sympathetic system and in the CNS.

Paracrine hormone: Local hormone that is released from specialised cells and acts on neighbouring cells.

Parasympathetic nervous system: Branch of the autonomic nervous system, usually active during satiation and repose (rest and digest system).

Parenteral: Describes the route of administration of drugs given by injection (subcutaneous, intramuscular, intravenous).

Partial agonist: Binds to receptor and induces a submaximal tissue response. Less efficacious than full agonists.

Passive diffusion: Fundamental process of drug excretion. Reabsorption of plasma and drug as it passes through renal tubule.

Peripheral nervous system: Connects the CNS and body tissues. Made up of the autonomic nervous system and the somatic nervous system.

Peripheral vascular resistance (PVR): Degree of vasoconstriction/vasodilation of the peripheral arteries. BP = CO × PVR.

pH: Measure of the acidity or alkalinity of a solution.

Pharmacogenetics: Clinically important hereditary variation in response to drugs. May result, for example, in increased or decreased activity of cytochrome P450 enzyme activity.

Pharmacokinetics: How the body handles the drug (absorption, distribution, metabolism, excretion).

Pharmacokinetic antagonism: Situation where an antagonist acts to either reduce

absorption of the drug or increase its metabolism and/or excretion.

Phase I metabolism: Consists of three types of chemical reaction (oxidation, reduction, hydrolysis). Often involves the cytochrome P450 family of enzymes. Phase I metabolites may still be active.

Phase II metabolism: Involves the process of conjugation. Phase II metabolites are generally inactive.

Phospholipids: Lipids contained in the plasma membrane of cells.

Physiological antagonism: Situation where an antagonist has the opposite effect to the drug such that they cancel each other out. Occurs more frequently in polypharmacy.

pKa: The pH at which a drug exists in a 50:50 equilibrium between unionised and ionised forms.

Plasma proteins: Proteins found in the plasma that bind drugs. Drug–protein binding interaction is rapid, reversible and saturable. Does not represent a drug target. Non-selective. Has no physiological effect.

Plasmin: The end-product of the fibrinolytic cascade. Acts to break down fibrin.

Polar: Drug that is ionised, lipophobic, hydrophilic. Will not readily cross cell membranes.

Postganglionic neuron: The second neuron in the autonomic nervous system.

Potency: Affinity × efficacy.

Preganglionic neuron: The first neuron in the autonomic nervous system. Has its cell body in the CNS.

Preload: Volume load of the heart.

Pro-drug: Drug that is not active until it has been metabolised.

Prostaglandins: Lipid-derived mediators that have a wide variety of roles within the body.

Proton pump: K^+/H^+ ATP-ase, which actively pumps hydrogen ions into the lumen of the stomach.

Receptor: Naturally occurring body protein that acts as a recognition site for the body's normal mediators. Found either within the cell (nuclear receptors) or on the cell surface. Receptors are one of the four groups of protein drug targets.

Renin: Enzyme secreted from the juxtaglomerular cells of the kidney. Acts to convert angiotensinogen to angiotensin I.

Serotonin (5HT): One of the principal neurotransmitters of the CNS.

Smooth endoplasmic reticulum: Large membranous structure and, in hepatocytes, the location of the cytochrome P450 enzyme system.

Somatic nervous system: Relays messages from the central nervous system to the skin and skeletal muscles. Regulates voluntary responses.

Specificity: Describes the likelihood of a drug acting on a subsection of targets.

Stroke volume (SV): The volume of blood pumped from the heart. $CO = HR \times SV$.

Sympathetic nervous system: Branch of the autonomic nervous system, activity increased during times of stress (fight/flight/fright system).

Synapse: Gap between two nerve cells or between a nerve cell and an effector organ.

Therapeutic index: The ratio between the minimum effective dose and the maximum tolerated dose of a drug.

Thrombosis: The pathological formation of a blood clot in the absence of bleeding.

Thromboxane A_2 (TXA$_2$): Pro-aggregatory chemical secreted from platelets.

Tubular secretion: Fundamental process of drug excretion. Drug molecules are carried into tubular lumen by carrier systems.

Type A ADR: Adverse drug reaction that represents an augmented, or exaggerated, response to the pharmacological action of the drug. Predictable, usually dose related and known prior to marketing.

Type B ADR: Bizzare effects which can occur at any dose, not predictable, usually immunologically mediated.

Unconjugated: Free drug that is released following hydrolysis of conjugated drug by bacteria in the small intestine.

Unionised: Substances that dissolve freely in lipids, move readily across cell membranes (non-polar, lipophilic, hydrophobic).

Volume of distribution (Vd): Volume of plasma that would be required to contain the total body content of a drug at the same concentration as that present in the plasma.

The Patient Glossary

Act: Primary legislation that is considered as a Bill and debated by both UK Houses of Parliament.

Administrative law: Statutory law delegating power to public bodies and setting out their accountability for quality; the body itself may be fined or contractors may be fined with the money passing to the public body.

Artificial intelligence: computer systems able to perform tasks normally requiring human intelligence, such as visual perception, speech recognition and decision-making.

Black triangle: Symbol in the *British National Formulary* denoting newly licensed medicines that are monitored intensively by the Medicines and Healthcare products Regulatory Agency.

Civil law: Law expressing duties owed by citizens to one another, particularly duty of care.

Clinical management plan: A written patient-specific agreement between independent and supplementary prescribers, which details the condition(s) to be managed and the medicines that may be prescribed.

Clinical negligence: The branch of law dealing with the duty of care between health professionals and their users and alleged failures in care. If there was breach in that duty of care, compensation may be ordered.

Conscience clauses: Part of many codes of ethics in healthcare that respect the personal (including religious) beliefs of individuals and broadly exempt individuals from undertaking acts that conflict with their conscience.

Controlled drug: Any dangerous or otherwise harmful substance included in the Misuse of Drugs Act 1971 or subsequent Misuse of Drugs Regulations.

Cost impact analysis: An examination of both the costs and health outcomes of one or more interventions.

Criminal law: Statutory law with criminal sanctions, such as fines going to the Treasury and prison, generally enforced by the police service.

Deontology: Ethical theories that claim individuals have certain duties that must be followed at all times, irrespective of the outcome.

Determinants of health: The range of personal, social, economic and environmental factors that determine the health of individuals or communities.

Distributive justice: A concern, usually ethical, about how resources and money should be allocated amongst individuals and in society in the fairest way.

Duty of care: An obligation to provide care to a reasonable standard; the duty relates to both acts and omissions.

ECT: Electroconvulsive therapy. A treatment for depression which involves the passing of an electric current across the brain to induce an epileptic-type seizure.

Ethics: Ethics, or moral philosophy as it is often also called, involves questioning and justifying what individuals do, and particularly what actions are thought right or wrong, or what sort of person one should try to be.

Four principles of bioethics: Influential ethical theory which argues that four key principles – autonomy, beneficence, non-maleficence and justice – can be applied to decide the ethical problems that arise in healthcare.

The New Prescriber: An Integrated Approach to Medical and Non-medical Prescribing, Second Edition.
Edited by Joanne Lymn, Alison Mostyn, Roger Knaggs, Michael Randall, and Dianne Bowskill.
© 2024 John Wiley & Sons Ltd. Published 2024 by John Wiley & Sons Ltd.

Independent prescribing: Prescribing by a practitioner responsible and accountable for the assessments of patients with undiagnosed or diagnosed conditions and for decisions about the clinical management required, including prescribing.

Medicinal purpose: Marketed for the purpose of treating or preventing disease or related purposes.

Medicines compliance: A measure of patient behaviour: the extent to which patients take medicines according to the prescribed instructions.

Medicines concordance: A two-way consultation process: shared decision making about medicines between a healthcare professional and a patient, based on partnership, where the patient's expertise and beliefs are fully valued.

Negligence: Negligence is a tort involving a civil action for compensation arising from a breach of the duty of care which has caused damage.

Non-medical prescriber: A prescriber who is not a doctor.

Off-label, off-licence, outwith the licence: Using a licensed medicinal product in circumstances not covered by the licence.

Patient factors: Nonclinical factors that influence patient decision making, for example age, socioeconomic factors or previous experience.

Patient Group Direction: A written instruction for the supply and/or administration of a medicine(s) in an identified clinical situation, signed by a doctor or dentist and a pharmacist. It applies to groups of patients who may not be individually identified before presenting for treatment.

Patient-specific direction: The traditional written instruction, from a doctor, dentist, nurse or pharmacist independent prescriber, for medicines to be supplied or administered to a named patient.

Professional law: Statutory law with professional sanctions, such as being struck off a professional register.

Public health: 'The science and art of preventing disease, prolonging life and promoting health through organised efforts of society' (Acheson, 1988).

Regulations: Secondary or subordinate legislation that implements the details of an Act; usually laid before Parliament only.

Remote prescribing: Prescribing following a telephone or video assessment of a patient or other online communication. Remote prescribing can potentially expose a non-medical prescriber to additional risk.

Statute: Instruments of legislation passed by Parliament, i.e. Acts, Regulations and Orders.

Statutory law: Law that has been made by Parliament.

Statutory administrative law: Statutory law delegating power to public bodies and setting out their accountability for quality; the body itself may be fined or contractors may be fined, with the money passing to the public body.

Statutory criminal law: Statutory law with criminal sanctions, such as fines going to the Treasury and prison, generally enforced by the police service.

Statutory professional law: Statutory law with professional sanctions, such as being struck off a professional register.

Supplementary prescribing: A voluntary partnership between an independent prescriber (a doctor or dentist) and a supplementary prescriber to implement an agreed patient-specific clinical management plan with the patient's agreement.

Tort: A tort is a civil wrong.

Unlicensed: Using a product or substance that does not have a licence for a medicinal purpose.

Utilitarianism: Ethical theory that deems acts right only if they lead to the greatest overall happiness (or welfare in some versions) for the greatest number of individuals.

Vicarious liability: The liability held by employers for the actions of their employees, specifically in relation to costs for harm caused to patients.

Written directions: The form of instruction for prescribing medicines to hospital inpatients (bed chart, ward chart, etc.).

Yellow Card scheme: Medicines and Hleathcare products Regulatory Agency-administered scheme for reporting and monitoring the occurrence of adverse drug reactions.

Activity Answers

CHAPTER 1

1. What sort of preparation should you make in advance of a patient consultation?

   Study all the information available to you about the patient prior to the consultation. Pay particular attention to referral letters and available medical records for information, including the patient's past history, medications and allergies. Ensure that the environment is set up appropriately with adequate lighting and privacy.

2. List the seven elements of a traditional medical history.

   Presenting complaint, past medical and surgical history, family history, medications drug history and allergies. Personal and social history, systems review.

3. The purpose of the physical examination and near-patient tests is diagnosis. Is this statement true or false?

   False: the purpose of the physical examination and near-patient tests is to supplement your findings from the history and to support or refute your diagnostic hypothesis.

4. Identify two generic 'red flag' features.

   Any of the following: unexplained weight loss, night sweats, unexplained chronic pain, pain that keeps the patient awake at night.

5. There are a number of 'bottom liners' that are considered essential elements for safe prescribing. List as many bottom liners as you can.

   Ascertain the patient's name, date of birth, address, hospital or NHS number. Check weights where appropriate, particularly when prescribing for children. Check for allergies, check there are no interactions with other medicines the patient is taking. Ensure the patient has no other medical condition that might be exacerbated by the medication. Inform the patient of any mild or more serious side effects of the medication.

CHAPTER 2

Answer True or False to the following.

1. The Health and Care Professions Council, Nursing and Midwifery Council and General Pharmaceutical Council all act to protect the interests of the profession they represent.   True/***False***

2. You cannot be held accountable for omissions in your prescribing.   True/***False***

3. Maintaining your clinical knowledge and competence is only a professional requirement.   ***True***/False

The New Prescriber: An Integrated Approach to Medical and Non-medical Prescribing, Second Edition.
Edited by Joanne Lymn, Alison Mostyn, Roger Knaggs, Michael Randall, and Dianne Bowskill.
© 2024 John Wiley & Sons Ltd. Published 2024 by John Wiley & Sons Ltd.

4. The Bolam test means that as a prescriber, you have not breached
   your duty of care if other prescribers would have done the same thing.   True/**False**

5. An error in prescribing resulting in a patient's death may result in
   criminal proceedings against the prescriber.   **True**/False

6. Tort of negligence is covered by criminal law.   True/**False**

7. In ethical practice I can always act with no harm to the patient.   True/**False**

CHAPTER 3

1. Which one of the following is a non-medical prescriber not accountable to?

   (a) Society

   (b) Themselves

   (c) The patient

   (d) Their employer

2. What is now regarded as the main source of medicines law in the UK?

   (a) The Medicines Act 1968

   (b) The Consumer Protection Act 1987

   (c) The Prescription Only Medicines (Human Use) Order 1997

   (d) The Human Medicines Regulations 2012

3. The main source of law regulating a non-medical prescriber's authority to prescribe
   controlled drugs is:

   (a) The Misuse of Drugs Act 1971

   (b) The Misuse of Drugs Regulations 2001

   (c) The Misuse of Drugs (Amendment No 2) Regulations 2012

   (d) The Human Medicines Regulations 2012

4. Which of the following non-medical prescribers can issue a Patient Specific Direction in a
   community setting?

   (a) A community practitioner prescriber

   (b) A physiotherapist independent prescriber

   (c) A paramedic independent prescriber

   (d) A pharmacist independent prescriber

5. Consent is a defence against an allegation of trespass to the person:

   (a) True

   (b) False

6. The element(s) of a real consent are:

   (a) It is free, full and reasonably informed.

   (b) It is specific, the patient's choice and in writing.

   (c)   The patient tells the prescriber what treatment they want.

   (d)   Prescriber's professional judgement, patient's permission, consent form

7. A patient with capacity who refuses treatment can be treated if it is in their best interests.

   (a)   True

   (b)   False

8. The duty to warn of risks is based on:

   (a)   What a reasonable body of prescribers would mention to a patient with this condition.

   (b)   What a reasonable person in the patient's situation would want to know about risks.

   (c)   Whether the patient would be too afraid to have treatment if told about risks.

   (d)   Whether the patient askes specific questions about specific risks.

9. Which of the following forms part of a non-medical prescriber's duty of care?

   (a)   The standard of their handwriting.

   (b)   Giving advice about medicines and adverse reactions.

   (c)   Acting on allergy information.

   (d)   All of the above.

10. The condition for a lawful prescription requires a prescriber to handwrite their signature.

   (a)   True

   (b)   False

CHAPTER 4

Answer True or False to each of the following.

1. Prescribers must never act in an ethically justifiable way that is contrary to the law.   True/**False**

2. Duty based deontological justification involves considering the overall consequences of a proposed action.   True/**False**

3. 'Top down' ethical reasoning involves applying a particular ethical theory consistently to different problems.   **True**/False

4. If a prescriber conscientiously objects to prescribing a certain medicine, they may still have to appropriately refer the patient to an alternative prescriber.   **True**/False

5. If using the four principles of bioethics, only one principle can be considered at a time when making an ethical decision.   True/**False**

CHAPTER 5

1. Look carefully at the descriptions of independent and supplementary prescribing. Can you identify the differences between them?

   Under independent prescribing the prescriber is accountable for the diagnosis, the decision to prescribe and drug choice.

2. What benefits might you, patients, colleagues and the organisation gain from you becoming a prescriber?

   It is useful to consider what your new knowledge and skills will bring to your patients and the team within which you will prescribe.

3. What approach will you take to prescribing in your practice and who in your clinical team might need to be aware of your approach to prescribing?

   Making others aware if you are to restrict your prescribing is essential for safe prescribing in teams.

4. Under repeat prescribing who is accountable for the diagnosis of the condition(s) for which you prescribe medication therapy?

   Under repeat independent prescribing it is the prescriber who is accountable for the diagnosis for which the prescribing decision is made. Under repeat supplementary prescribing it is the doctor who holds accountability for the diagnosis.

5. Are any of the drugs you are likely to prescribe or are listed in your personal formulary on the government list as likely to impair capacity to drive safely?

   It is important that you are aware if you are to prescribe drugs that may impair safe driving. Knowing will enable you to counsel patients for whom you prescribe.

CHAPTER 6

1. What are the three domains of public health?

   Health improvement

   Healthcare public health: improving services

   Health protection

2. In which Canadian city was the World Health Organization's Charter for Health Promotion launched?

   Ottowa

3. What is the name of the latest public health strategy for England?

   All our Health (2021)

4. What are the three criteria for a health-promoting pharmacy?

   Healthy work environment, appropriate care for clients and staff, and a strong sense of community.

5. What is the public health initiative supporting lifestyle change called?

   Making Every Contact Count (MECC)

CHAPTER 7

1. Which of the following is not a drug target?

   (a) Receptor

   (b) Carrier protein

   (c) *Lipid*

   (d) Enzyme

2. Which of the following statements about partial agonists is true?

   (a) They can achieve a maximal response.

   (b) They have similar efficacy to a full agonist.

   (c) The dose–response curve of a partial agonist is shifted to the left of the dose–response curve of a full agonist.

   (d) *They have similar affinity to a full agonist.*

3. Which of the following drugs acts as an irreversible receptor antagonist?

   (a) Salbutamol

   (b) Bisoprolol

   (c) Atorvastatin

   (d) *Candesartan*

4. Which of the following forms of drug antagonism describes the action of protamine on heparin?

   (a) Receptor blockade

   (b) Non-competitive antagonism

   (c) *Chemical antagonism*

   (d) Pharmacokinetic antagonism

5. Which of the following drugs acts to irreversibly inhibit enzyme activity?

   (a) *Aspirin*

   (b) Ibuprofen

   (c) Atorvastatin

   (d) Ramipril

6. Which of the following statements is correct?

   (a) *Agonists mimic the body's normal physiological response.*

   (b) Agonists have affinity but no efficacy.

   (c) Irreversible antagonists use hydrogen binding.

   (d) Antagonists have similar efficacy to agonists.

CHAPTER 8

1. The passage of a drug molecule across a lipid membrane is influenced by the:

• lipid solubility of the drug	***True***/False
• route of administration	True/***False***
• degree of ionisation of the molecule	***True***/False
• pH of the surrounding medium	***True***/False
• presence of carrier molecules	***True***/False

2. With regard to drug absorption, which of the following statements are correct?

- Drug absorption is required for drugs given by all routes — True/**False**

- The rate and extent of absorption following oral administration are dependent on the pH of the gut — **True**/False

- Drug absorption always starts in the stomach — True/**False**

- Drug absorption is unaffected by the lipid solubility of a drug — True/**False**

- The rate of absorption of very polar drugs may depend on carrier molecules — **True**/False

3. With regard to plasma protein binding, which of the following statements are correct?

- Drugs bound to plasma proteins readily cross cell membranes — True/**False**

- Albumin, acid-glycoprotein and beta-globulin are all plasma proteins — **True**/False

- Plasma protein concentrations can be reduced in severe malnutrition — **True**/False

- Plasma proteins are important drug targets — True/**False**

- Plasma protein binding can restrict the pattern of drug distribution — **True**/False

4. With regard to volume of distribution, which of the following statements are correct?

- It represents the total volume of the body. — True/**False**

- It is generally larger for lipid-soluble compared to polar drugs. — **True**/False

- It is important for calculating a loading dose. — **True**/False

- It is not affected by the size of the drug or its plasma protein binding. — True/**False**

- It describes the ability of a drug to distribute throughout body tissues. — **True**/False

CHAPTER 9

1. Which of the following statements regarding drug metabolism are correct?

- It is increased in children compared to adults. — **True**/False

- It is decreased by rifampicin. — True/**False**

- It is decreased by grapefruit juice. — **True**/False

- It is decreased in elderly patients. — **True**/False

- It is more important for lipid-soluble drugs. — **True**/False

2. Which of the following statements regarding first-pass metabolism are correct?

- It affects bioavailability. — **True**/False

- It affects drugs given SC and IM. — True/**False**

- It never affects drugs administered IV. — **True**/False

- It occurs prior to the drug entering the systemic circulation. — **True**/False

- It can be reduced in elderly patients. — **True**/False

3. Which of the following statements regarding passive diffusion of drug in the renal tubule are correct?

- It depends on the pH of the urine.   ***True***/False
- It depends on the rate of glomerular filtration.   True/***False***
- It depends on the degree of plasma protein binding.   True/***False***
- It depends on the age of the patient.   True/***False***
- It depends on the lipid solubility of the drug.   ***True***/False

4. Which of the following statements regarding biliary excretion and enterohaptic recycling are correct?

- It affects drugs which undergo only phase I metabolism.   True/***False***
- It can be disrupted by broad-spectrum antibiotics.   ***True***/False
- It results in drug excretion in the faeces.   ***True***/False
- It is more important for unionised molecules.   True/***False***

5. Which of the following statements regarding half-life are correct?

- It determines the time to reach steady state.   ***True***/False
- It increases with increasing drug clearance.   True/***False***
- It is longer in drugs with a large volume of distribution.   ***True***/False
- It determines the dosing schedule of drugs.   ***True***/False
- It can be affected by increasing age.   ***True***/False

CHAPTER 10

1. Which of the following routes are routinely used to give systemic effects?

- Oral   ***True***/False
- Intravenous   ***True***/False
- Inhalation   True/***False***
- Ocular   True/***False***
- Transdermal   ***True***/False

2. Which of the following routes are routinely used for parenteral administration?

- Oral   True/***False***
- Subcutaneous   ***True***/False
- Intramuscular   ***True***/False
- Rectal   True/***False***
- Sublingual   True/***False***

3. Drug absorption from the oral route can be decreased by which of the following?

- Diarrhoea   ***True***/False
- Use of metoclopramide   True/***False***

- Gastric stasis **True**/False
- Antacids **True**/False
- Taking with food **True**/False

4. Which of the following routes of drug administration avoid first-pass metabolism?

- Inhaled **True**/False
- Oral True/**False**
- Sublingual **True**/False
- Transdermal **True**/False
- Intramuscular **True**/False

5. Which of the following statements concerning intramuscular drug administration are correct?

- Results in 100% bioavailability True/**False**
- Is affected by blood flow **True**/False
- Is unaffected by shock True/**False**
- Is used to produce systemic effects **True**/False
- Is dependent on the pH of the injected solution **True**/False

CHAPTER 11

1. Which of the following statements regarding drug dosing in neonatal patients are correct?

- The skin is more permeable to agents. **True**/False
- Body systems are mature. True/**False**
- Plasma albumin concentration is reduced. **True**/False
- Gentamicin dose intervals are increased. **True**/False
- Therapeutic drug monitoring is not performed. True/**False**

2. Which of the following statements regarding drug dosing in children are correct?

- The skin is more permeable to agents. **True**/False
- Young children have a higher amount of body water than adults. **True**/False
- Doses of albumin-bound drugs may need altering. **True**/False
- The adult BNF can be used for children's doses. True/**False**
- Children's doses are usually quoted in mg/kg. **True**/False

3. Which of the following statements regarding drug dosing in the elderly are correct?

- Generally lower doses are used. True/**False**
- Generally shorter dosage intervals are used. True/**False**

- Renal function improves with age.   True/**False**
- Lower loading doses of warfarin are used.   **True**/False
- Short-acting benzodiazepines are preferred.   **True**/False

4. Which of the following statements regarding drug dosing in renal impairment are correct?

- No dose amendments are required.   True/**False**
- Renal function cannot be easily categorised.   True/**False**
- NSAIDs are drugs of choice.   True/**False**
- Drug dose is not affected by dialysis.   True/**False**
- Generally longer dosage intervals are used.   **True**/False

5. Which of the following statements regarding drug dosing in liver impairment are correct?

- NSAIDs are drugs of choice.   True/**False**
- Degree of liver impairment can be calculated.   True/**False**
- Long-acting drugs are preferred.   True/**False**
- Drugs which cause drowsiness are preferred.   True/**False**
- Enzyme activity can be affected by drugs.   **True**/False

CHAPTER 12

1. Polypharmacy can be both appropriate and problematic.   **True**/False

2. Reduced kidney function can decrease the half-life of medication, thereby increasing the likelihood of adverse effects.   True/**False**

3. STOMP is a national project helping to stop the overmedication of people with a learning disability, autism or a dual diagnosis.   **True**/False

4. Patient discharge is an example of a healthcare interface where the propensity for polypharmacy and/or medication errors increases.   **True**/False

5. Caucasian patients are more likely to have kidney failure compared to Black African or Black Caribbean patients.   True/**False**

6. Drugs implicated in polypharmacy are almost exclusively prescription-only medicines.   True/**False**

7. Proton pump inhibitors (e.g., omeprazole) can cause drug interactions due to being mild enzyme inducers.   **True**/False

8. The process of medicines optimisation comprises four key principles.   **True**/False

9. Medicines reconciliation is a process which ensures that prescribed medication synchronises with pre-admission/discharge practice.   **True**/False

10. The STOPP/START criteria are an example of a medicine's optimisation tool.   **True**/False

CHAPTER 13

1. Which of the following statements regarding type A adverse drug reactions are correct?

   They are predictable. ***True*/False**

   They have low incidence. **True/*False***

   They have low mortality. ***True*/False**

   They can be managed by dose reduction. ***True*/False**

   They have low morbidity. **True/*False***

2. Which of the following statements regarding the pharmacokinetic mechanisms of adverse drug reactions are correct?

   Dose reduction may be necessary in renal impairment. ***True*/False**

   Increases in drug plasma concentrations result in type A ADRs. ***True*/False**

   The cytochrome P450 enzyme system is important in ADRs. ***True*/False**

   Pharmacokinetic ADRs result mainly in type B ADRs. **True/*False***

   There is genetic variation in the way isoniazid is metabolised. ***True*/False**

3. Which of the following statements about how ADRs should be managed are correct?

   The patient will know exactly which drug is causing their ADR. **True/*False***

   The causative drug must always be stopped. **True/*False***

   The causative drug must always be slowly withdrawn. **True/*False***

   You must only report definite ADRs to the MHRA. **True/*False***

   Anyone can report an ADR to the MHRA. ***True*/False**

4. Which of the following statements about drug interaction mechanisms are correct?

   Synergy is where the effects of two drugs cancel each other out. **True/*False***

   The formation of chelates in the GI tract aids drug absorption. **True/*False***

   Methotrexate and aspirin have an important interaction. ***True*/False**

   Cytochrome P450 interactions affect the metabolism of various drugs. ***True*/False**

   Patients taking oral contraceptives must use extra contraceptive methods when they are taking rifampicin. ***True*/False**

5. Which of the following statements about the management of drug interactions are correct?

   Patients taking MAOIs must not excessively eat foods containing tyramine. ***True*/False**

   When starting new drugs, prescribers must disregard any other drugs the patient is taking. **True/*False***

   The BNF is a useful reference source for identifying drug interactions. ***True*/False**

   Patients taking simvastatin should drink lots of grapefruit juice. **True/*False***

   There are no drug interactions with warfarin. **True/*False***

CHAPTER 14

Are the following statements true of false:

1. The two main neurotransmitters that operate in the autonomic nervous system are acetylcholine and adrenaline. True/**False**

2. The sympathetic and parasympathetic nervous systems have opposing effects on gastrointestinal smooth muscle motility. **True**/False

3. The sympathetic and parasympathetic nervous systems both act to stimulate sweat production. True/**False**

4. Neurotransmitters in the autonomic nervous system are released into the synapse by exocytosis. **True**/False

5. Acetylcholine is inactivated by enzymes within the synaptic cleft. **True**/False

6. Side effects of muscarinic agonists include constipation and urinary retention. True/**False**

7. Drugs that act as agonists at adrenoceptors activate the 'fight/flight/fright' response. **True**/False

8. Drugs acting at nicotinic receptors affect both the sympathetic and parasympathetic nervous systems. **True**/False

9. Drugs that act as antagonists at β-adrenoceptors induce bronchodilation. True/**False**

10. The action of noradrenaline is curtailed by reuptake into the nerve terminal. **True**/False

11. Sympathetic nervous system stimulation to the bladder relaxes the detrusor muscle and constricts the sphincter. **True**/False

12. The parasympathetic nervous system stimulates glycogenolysis in the liver. True/**False**

13. There is direct sympathetic innervation of the lungs. True/**False**

14. Drugs which bind to β-1-receptors modulate heart rate. **True**/False

15. Muscarinic receptors are located on the postganglionic neuron of the parasympathetic nervous system. True/**False**

CHAPTER 15

1. Tropicamide, a muscarinic antagonist, is used as eye drops to facilitate the examination of the fundus of the eye. Why do you think tropicamide is useful in these circumstances?

   Tropicamide binds to muscarinic receptors in the eye, preventing the binding of acetylcholine to these receptors. This blocks the constriction of the pupil usually stimulated by acetylcholine. This effectively dilates the pupil, allowing eye examination to be performed.

2. Why is bradycardia listed as a caution for the use of anticholinesterase drugs?

   Anticholinesterase drugs prevent the breakdown of acetylcholine in the cleft, which increases acetylcholine levels. The acetylcholine reduces heart rate by stimulating the activation of muscarinic receptors in the heart, which may therefore result in heart block.

3. Salbutamol mimics the action of which of the following chemicals?

   (a) Noradrenaline

   (b) *Acetylcholine*

   (c) Adrenaline

4. One of the most common side effects of salbutamol use is fine tremor. Can you explain why this might be the case?

   If overused, salbutamol can be absorbed into the systemic circulation and act on other β_2-adrenoceptors in the body, including those located on the skeletal muscle. Stimulation of these receptors results in fine tremor.

5. Why would the use of β-adrenoceptor antagonists lessen the effect of salbutamol in the lungs?

   β-adrenoceptor antagonists compete with salbutamol for binding to the β_2-adrenoceptors in the lungs, thus reducing the ability of salbutamol to promote bronchodilation. This action is much reduced for β_1-selective agents but still occurs at higher doses.

6. Why would ephedrine be useful for the treatment of nasal congestion?

   Ephedrine constricts the blood vessels in the nasal mucosa, resulting in reduced oedema.

CHAPTER 16

1. A patient is prescribed a proton pump inhibitor. Which ONE of the following is a relevant counselling point?

   (a) A dry cough is a common side effect.

   (b) Avoid alcohol as the medicine interacts with alcohol.

   (c) Do not take with aspirin-containing products.

   (d) Swallow the capsule whole.

   (e) You should expect rapid relief within a few minutes.

   D: Proton pump inhibitor capsules should be swallowed whole because they are enterically coated with a pH-sensitive polymer to prevent degradation by gastric acid but to facilitate dissolution in the duodenum, where the drug is absorbed.

2. In choosing triple therapy, which ONE of the following would influence the choice of antibacterials?

   (a) Concurrent asthma

   (b) Penicillin allergy

   (c) The co-prescribed proton pump inhibitor

   (d) The microbiome

   (e) The presence of MRSA in the gastric mucosa

   B: Penicillin precludes using amoxicillin as part of triple therapy.

3. For which ONE of the following classes of drugs would you counsel a patient that constipation is a common side effect?

   (a) Metformin

   (b) Opioids

(c) Paracetamol

(d) Prostaglandin analogues

(e) Proton pump inhibitors

B: Opioids cause presynaptic inhibition of parasympathetic nerves, reducing motility, which leads to constipation.

CHAPTER 17

1. Which ONE of the following classes of drugs is associated with causing hyperkalaemia?

    (a) AT1 receptor antagonists (e.g., losartan)

    (b) Calcium channel inhibitors (e.g., amlodipine)

    (c) Loop diuretics (e.g., furosemide)

    (d) Potassium channel activators (e.g., nicorandil)

    (e) Thiazide-like diuretics (e.g., indapamide)

    A: AT1 receptor antagonists (and ACE inhibitors) are both associated with hyperkalaemia due to reductions in aldosterone.

2. Which ONE of the following is a common side effect of ACE inhibitors (e.g., ramipril)?

    (a) Ankle swelling

    (b) Constipation

    (c) Cough

    (d) Hyperglycaemia

    (e) Negative inotropy

    C: Cough is a common side effect due to potentiation of bradykinin.

3. Which ONE of the following classes of drug is now being used in the management of chronic heart failure?

    (a) Endocannabinoids (e.g., anandamide)

    (b) Peroxisome proliferator–activated receptor γ agonists (e.g., pioglitazone)

    (c) Potassium channel activators (e.g., nicorandil)

    (d) Rate-limiting calcium channel inhibitors (e.g., verapamil)

    (e) Sodium-glucose co-transporter 2 inhibitors (e.g., dapagliflozin)

    E: Sodium-glucose co-transporter 2 inhibitors are beneficial in chronic heart failure.

4. Which ONE of the following is a key counselling point for statin therapy?

    (a) Ankle swelling is a key side effect.

    (b) Dizziness on standing is a common side effect.

    (c) Headaches are a common side effect.

    (d) Report unexplained muscle pain.

    (e) Statins should be taken first thing in the morning.

    D: Unexplained muscle pain may indicate myopathy, which can rarely lead to rhabdomyolysis.

CHAPTER 18

1. Atrial fibrillation is a key risk factor for which one of the following?

   (a) Deep vein thrombosis

   (b) Fibrinolysis

   (c) Ischaemic stroke

   (d) Haemorrhage

   (e) Hypertension

   C: Cardioembolic stroke is associated with atrial fibrillation.

2. Which one of the following is an integral part of the coagulation cascade?

   (a) Adhesion of platelets.

   (b) Factor X activates fibrinogen.

   (c) Thrombin activates fibrinogen.

   (d) Thrombin is converted to fibrinogen.

   (e) Thrombin is the final product.

   C: Thrombin converts fibrinogen to form fibrin.

3. Which one of the following is a clear advantage of direct oral anticoagulants (DOACs) compared to warfarin?

   (a) DOACs have fewer drug interactions.

   (b) DOACs are selective for the vitamin K epoxide reductase complex.

   (c) DOACs are cheaper.

   (d) DOACs are more easily reversed.

   (e) DOACs are not associated with causing bleeding.

   A: DOACs have fewer drug interactions but interactions should always be checked for.

4. Which one of the following is an important issue in the use of warfarin?

   (a) It acts almost immediately.

   (b) It is given by injection.

   (c) It is unaffected by inhibitors of cytochrome P450.

   (d) It opposes the actions of vitamin K.

   (e) It requires monitoring via the activated partial thromboplastin time.

   D: It is a vitamin K antagonist at the vitamin K epoxide reductase complex.

5. Which one of the following promotes platelet aggregation?

   (a) Adenosine triphosphate

   (b) Endothelial cyclooxygenase

   (c) Nitric oxide

(d) Prostacyclin

(e) Thromboxane

E: Thromboxane is released by platelets to promote aggregation.

6. Which one of the following is thought to contribute towards the antiplatelet activity of low dose aspirin?

(a) Aspirin inhibits the expression of glycoprotein IIb-IIIa

(b) Aspirin is a thromboxane receptor antagonist

(c) Aspirin is selective for endothelial cyclooxygenase

(d) Endothelial cells are resistant to aspirin

(e) Platelets lack a nucleus

E: The non-nucleated platelets cannot regenerate cyclooxygenase once it is inhibited, whereas endothelial cells have a nucleus and so can regenerate cyclooxygenase.

7. Which one of the following is the principal use of the thrombolytic drug alteplase?

(a) Atrial fibrillation

(b) Haemorrhagic stroke

(c) Hypertension

(d) Ischaemic stroke

(e) Secondary prevention of myocardial infarction

D: It is the primary treatment of ischaemic stroke and contraindicated in haemorrhagic stroke.

CHAPTER 19

1. In addition to its regulatory and excretory roles, the kidney is also a synthetic and metabolic organ. **True**/False

2. Kidney disease is more common amongst Caucasian populations. True/**False**

3. The molecular weight and electronic charge of a molecule partly determine if it is filtered by the kidney. **True**/False

4. Creatinine is a substance produced by the body that is both filtered and actively secreted by the kidneys. **True**/False

5. The Cockcroft–Gault equation gives an estimation of creatinine clearance normalised for body surface area. True/**False**

6. Renal impairment can affect all four ADME pharmacokinetic parameters. **True**/False

7. The MDRD equation is the recommended method of estimating renal function for use in modifying drug doses in patients at extremes of weight. True/**False**

8. Dosing of opiates should be adjusted in renal impairment due to their narrow therapeutic index and method of elimination from the body. **True**/False

9. Potassium-sparing diuretics are the diuretic of choice in patients with renal impairment. True/**False**

10. A reduction in kidney function due to ramipril could be described as an idiosyncratic reaction. **True**/False

CHAPTER 20

1. Which ONE of the following is part of the second messenger system associated with activation of β_2-adrenoceptors?

   (a) ***Activation of adenylyl cyclase***

   (b) Decrease in cAMP

   (c) Increase in calcium

   (d) Increase in cGMP

   (e) Opening of calcium channels

2. Which ONE of the following is a feature of inhaled corticosteroids?

   (a) ***An initial response is delayed by a few days.***

   (b) Standard doses are associated with significant suppression of the hypothalamus- pituitary- adrenal axis.

   (c) They act via G-protein-coupled receptors.

   (d) They are contraindicated in hypertension.

   (e) They are used to relieve asthmatic attacks.

3. Which ONE of the following drugs should be avoided in asthma?

   (a) ACE inhibitors (e.g., ramipril)

   (b) β_2-adrenoceptor agonists (e.g., salbutamol)

   (c) ***β_1-adrenoceptor antagonists (e.g., bisoprolol)***

   (d) Muscarinic receptor antagonists (e.g., tiotropium)

   (e) Phosphodiesterase inhibitors (e.g., theophylline)

CHAPTER 21

1. The brain is divided into three major areas (hindbrain, midbrain and forebrain). ***True***/False

2. The tectum is only involved with auditory processing. True/***False***

3. The limbic system is important in emotion and decision making. ***True***/False

4. Glial cells take no direct part in electrical communication in the CNS. ***True***/False

5. An EPSP is a local hyperpolarisation of the membrane of the receiving neuron. True/***False***

6. A small-diameter axon has the fastest transmission of action potentials. True/***False***

7. Noradrenaline and dopamine have different synthesis pathways. True/***False***

8. Serotonin is more prevalent in the CNS than in any other part of the body. True/***False***

9. Dopamine and serotonin are broken down by the same monoamine oxidase enzyme. True/***False***

10. Glutamate is the major excitatory neurotransmitter in the CNS. ***True***/False

CHAPTER 22

1. Parkinson's disease is associated with a loss of dopaminergic neurons in the substantia nigra. *True*/False

2. Parkinson's disease is associated with decreased acetylcholine activity. True/*False*

3. Monoamine oxidase-B inhibitors inhibit the metabolism of all monoamines. True/*False*

4. Dopamine agonists act to replenish the body's supply of dopamine. True/*False*

5. Levodopa has fewer side effects if administered with a decarboxylase inhibitor. *True*/False

6. Levodopa can exhibit cardiovascular side effects due to the nature of its synthesis path. *True*/False

7. Age does not play a contributory role in the development of Alzheimer's disease. True/*False*

8. Acetylcholinesterase inhibitors have only limited side effects as their effects are restricted to the central nervous system. True/*False*

9. Memantine is a NMDA receptor antagonist. *True*/False

10. All drugs used to treat Alzheimer's disease increase acetylcholine levels. True/*False*

CHAPTER 23

1. Stressful life events are a trigger for major depression. *True*/False

2. The monoamine theory suggests that depression is associated with an increase in serotonin levels. True/*False*

3. SSRIs preferentially inhibit the reuptake of serotonin into the presynaptic neuron. *True*/False

4. Tricyclic antidepressants exhibit antimuscarinic side effects. *True*/False

5. Tricyclic antidepressants have a wide therapeutic index and are safe to use across a wide range of doses. True/*False*

6. Venlafaxine is a widely used selective serotonin reuptake inhibitor. True/*False*

7. Serotonin and noradrenaline reuptake inhibitors and tricyclic antidepressant both inhibit noradrenaline and serotonin reuptake. True/*False*

8. Serotonin and noradrenaline reuptake inhibitors are sympathomimetic. *True*/False

9. Moclobemide exhibits the same dietary restrictions as phenelzine. True/*False*

10. St John's wort affects cytochrome P450 enzymes. *True*/False

11. Anxiety is associated with increased glutamate. *True*/False

12. Fast-acting benzodiazepines have high lipid solubility. *True*/False

13. Buspirone is a full agonist. True/*False*

14. β-blockers are useful in treating the underlying cause of anxiety. True/*False*

CHAPTER 24

1. The more closely related a person is to someone with schizophrenia, the more likely they are to show psychoses associated with schizophrenia. *True*/False

2. Risk factors for schizophrenia include environmental factors such as urbanicity. *True*/False

3. Antipsychotic drug efficacy is correlated to D_2 blocking activity. *True*/False

4. The complete blockade of D_2 receptors completely alleviates all schizophrenic symptoms. True/*False*

5. First-generation antipsychotic drugs are most effective in managing positive symptoms of schizophrenia. *True*/False

6. First-generation antipsychotics do not antagonise muscarinic, histaminergic or adrenergic receptors. True/*False*

7. First generation antipsychotics do not potentiate the action of opioids. True/*False*

8. Second-generation antipsychotics have fewer extrapyramidal side effects. *True*/False

9. Weight gain can be a major side effect of atypical antipsychotics. *True*/False

10. All second-generation antipsychotics act as full antagonists at D_2 receptors. True/*False*

CHAPTER 25

1. Which one of the following drugs is a powerful enzyme inducer, associated with a number of key drug interactions?

   (a) Carbamazepine

   (b) Clobazam

   (c) Lamotrigine

   (d) Levetiracetam

   (e) Sodium valproate

   A: Carbamazepine.

2. What pharmacokinetic effect is the combined oral contraceptive likely to have on lamotrigine?

   (a) Decrease in elimination

   (b) Decrease in plasma clearance

   (c) Decrease in volume of distribution

   (d) Increase in plasma half-life

   (e) Increase in plasma clearance

   E: The combined oral contraceptive accelerates the metabolism of lamotrigine and increases it plasma clearance.

3. Which one of the following is the site of action of carbamazepine?

   (a) AMPA (glutamate) receptor

   (b) Calcium channels

   (c) GABA

   (d) Sodium channels

   D: Inhibition of sodium channels.

4. In recommending anti-epileptic therapy, which one of the following should be monitored during treatment?

   (a) EEG

   (b) Lipid profile

   (c) Liver function tests

   (d) Plasma levels of α-fetoprotein

   (e) Potassium levels

   C: Liver functions tests.

5. Which one of the following is an appropriate treatment for the termination of status epilepticus?

   (a) A benzodiazepine (such a midazolam)

   (b) A Z-drug (such as intravenous zoplicone)

   (c) An antipsychotic (such as intramuscular haloperidol)

   (d) An opioid (such as intravenous diamorphine)

   (e) Ketamine

   A: Benzodiazepines (phenytoin is often used).

6. In discussing withdrawal of antiepileptic treatment, which ONE of the following is a key consideration?

   (a) During withdrawal, driving should be continued

   (b) Withdrawal is not possible as therapy is lifelong

   (c) Withdrawal is often accompanied by hallucinations

   (d) Withdrawal might be considered after a couple of years of seizure-free control

   (e) Withdrawal should be carried out under the cover of a benzodiazepine

   D: Gradual withdrawal might be considered with the neurologist.

CHAPTER 26

For each of the statements 1–10 choose the most appropriate option from A to L. Each option may be used once, more than once or not at all.

Options

(a) Morphine

(b) Dihydrocodeine

(c) Ibuprofen

(d) Amitriptyline

(e) Gabapentin

(f) Paracetamol

(g) Glyceryl trinitrate

(h) Aspirin

(i) Buprenorphine

(j) Tramadol

(k) Diamorphine

(l) Oxycodone

1. A drug that should not be given to children under the age of 16 due to the risk of Reye's syndrome.

2. A drug that treats the pain associated with angina pectoris.

3. A drug that would be appropriate to reduce fever in a 10-year-old boy who also has asthma.

4. A drug that would be appropriate to prevent further ischaemic events in a 65-year-old woman who has recently suffered a myocardial infarction.

5. An opioid drug used in the immediate treatment of a myocardial infarction.

6. A drug that would be appropriate to treat a 36-year-old man suffering from tennis elbow.

7. An opioid that is formulated for transdermal administration.

8. An opioid drug that is contraindicated in epilepsy.

9. An antiepileptic drug used in the management of neuropathic pain.

10. An opioid used almost exclusively in palliative care because of high water solubility that allows smaller volumes to be infused by the subcutaneous route.

1. *Aspirin (H)*

2. *Glyceryl trinitrate (G)*

3. *Paracetamol (F)*

4. *Aspirin (H)*

5. *Morphine (A)*

6. *Ibuprofen (C)*

7. *Buprenorphine (I)*

8. *Tramadol (J)*

9. *Gabapentin (E)*

10. *Diamorphine (K)*

CHAPTER 27

1. The cannabis or the cannabinoid system has which one of the following features?

   (a) Anandamide is the endogenous ligand.

   (b) Cannabinoids are all highly addictive.

   (c) Cannabinoids do not have therapeutic uses.

   (d) Cannabis is used injected intravenously.

   (e) Δ9-tetrahydrocannabinol is a cannabinoid receptor antagonist.

   A: Anandamide is the natural ligand.

2. Which ONE of the following opposes the actions of opioids?

   (a) Codeine

   (b) Loperamide

   (c) Naloxone

   (d) Nandrolone

   (e) Nicotine

   C: Naloxone is an opioid receptor antagonist used to manage opioid overdoses.

3. Which ONE of the following describes the pharmacology of ketamine?

   (a) It is a selective μ-opioid receptor agonist.

   (b) It is a serotonin selective reuptake inhibitor.

   (c) It is a sympathomimetic.

   (d) It is a GABA modulator.

   (e) It is an NMDA receptor antagonist.

   E: It blocks NMDA receptors.

4. Which ONE of the following is helpful in mitigating the adverse effects of alcohol withdrawal?

   (a) Benzodiazepines

   (b) Carbamazepine

   (c) Disulfiram

   (d) Neuromuscular blockers

   (e) Opioids

   A: Benzodiazepines are used in the short term to reduce withdrawal reactions.

CHAPTER 28

1. Which of the following statements regarding bacteria and antibiotics are correct?

   (a) Ciprofloxacin is the first-line antibiotic to treat uncomplicated urinary tract infection.   True/***False***

   (b) Augmentin® can be used in patients allergic to a penicillin.   True/***False***

   (c) Trimethoprim and sulphonamides act on the same metabolic pathway and have synergy when used in combination.   ***True***/False

   (d) *Staphylococcus aureus* is a Gram-positive organism.   ***True***/False

   (e) Gentamicin's efficacy is linked to the amount of time its concentration is above the bacteria's MIC   True/***False***

2. Which two of the following antibiotics would be effective against respiratory atypicals?

   (a) Co-amoxiclav

   (b) Cefuroxime

   (c) *Clarithromycin*

   (d) *Doxycycline*

   (e) Vancomycin

3. Which three of the following antibiotics act by inhibiting peptidoglycan synthesis?

   (a) *Co-amoxiclav*

   (b) *Cefuroxime*

   (c) Clarithromycin

   (d) Doxycycline

   (e) *Vancomycin*

4. Which two of the following organisms commonly cause skin and soft tissue infections (e.g. cellulitis)?

   (a) *Staphylococcus aureus*

   (b) *Haemophilus influenzae*

   (c) *Moraxella catarrhalis*

   (d) *Streptococcus pyogenes* (group A β-haemolytic Strep.)

   (e) *Bacteroides* spp.

5. Which of the following bacteria can be treated by metronidazole?

   (a) *Staphylococcus aureus*

   (b) *Haemophilus influenzae*

   (c) Moraxella *catarrhalis*

   (d) Streptococcus *pyogenes* (group A β-haemolytic Strep.)

   (e) *Bacteroides spp.*

CHAPTER 29

1. Using a broader-spectrum antibiotic reduces the risk of resistance as it can treat more infections.   True/**False**

2. *Clostridioides difficile* infection can be induced by the use of any antibiotic.   **True**/False

3. The risk of contracting *Clostridioides difficile* infection increases with age.   **True**/False

4. The risk of relapse following *Clostridioides difficile* infection is low (<5%).   True/**False**

5. An extended-spectrum β-lactamase producer (ESBL) is:

   (a)   an antibiotic that kills most types of bacteria (e.g., meropenem)

   (b)   a Gram-negative bacteria with resistance against all current cephalosporins and penicillins

   (c)   a strain of *Clostridioides difficile* that produces more toxin, causing more severe disease

   (d)   a form of MRSA that is particularly difficult to eradicate

6. Which of these antibiotics are considered higher risk for inducing *Clostridioides difficile* infection?

   (a)   Ciprofloxacin

   (b)   Doxycycline

   (c)   Piperacillin/tazobactam

   (d)   Gentamicin IV

7. Which of these is NOT a resistance mechanism employed by bacteria to evade antibiotic attack?

   (a)   Hyperproduction of the target

   (b)   Efflux pumps

   (c)   Ribosomal inhibition

   (d)   Changing the cell permeability

CHAPTER 30

1. Invasive fungal infections only affect patients who have recently received chemotherapy.   True/**False**

2. The dermatophytes are a group of fungi that cause fungal lung infections.   True/**False**

3. Voriconazole is a broad-spectrum antifungal with good activity against *Candida* and *Aspergillus*.   **True**/False

4. Aciclovir has poor bioavailability, so the intravenous route should be used for treating life-threatening viral infections such as herpes simplex encephalitis.   **True**/False

5. Oseltamivir should be started as soon as possible after flu symptom onset but certainly within the first 48 hours.   **True**/False

6. Lipid-associated formulations of amphotericin B are more effective for treating fungal infections.   True/**False**

7. Fluconazole is the drug of choice for treating fungal nail infections.   True/***False***

8. Molnupiravir is first-line treatment for mild COVID-19 infection in high-risk patients.   ***True***/False

CHAPTER 31

1. Pancreatic β-cells produce which hormone?

    (a) Cortisol

    (b) Glucagon

    (c) *Insulin*

    (d) Tri-iodothyronine

2. Insulin promotes the storage of glucose in body tissues.   ***True***/False

3. Insulin is a protein.   ***True***/False

4. Which group of oral antidiabetic drugs increases plasma insulin?

    (a) Biguanides

    (b) *Sulphonylureas*

    (c) Thiazolidinediones

    (d) SGLT-2 inhibitors

    (e) DPP-4 inhibitors

5. Skeletal muscle uptake of glucose occurs through which channel?

    (a) Calcium channel

    (b) *GLUT4*

    (c) Sodium pump

6. SGLT-2 inhibitors reduce glucosuria.   True/***False***

7. Tri-iodothyronine (T3) is more active than thyroxine (T4)   ***True***/False

8. Carbamizole takes a few weeks to exert a clinical effect. Why?

    (a) Patients forget to take it.

    (b) *Preformed thyroid hormones are unaffected.*

    (c) The drug is taken very slowly from the gut to the thyroid gland.

CHAPTER 32

1. Luteinising hormone is secreted from which endocrine gland?

    (a) Hypothalamus

    (h) *Pituitary*

    (c) Ovary

2. Negative feedback of oestrogen to the pituitary reduces secretion of FSH.   ***True***/False

3. Progesterone acts primarily via membrane-bound receptors.   True/**False**

4. The POP is suitable for women with breast cancer.   True/**False**

5. Liver enzyme-inducing drugs may increase the efficacy of CHCs and hormonal emergency contraception.   True/**False**

CHAPTER 33

Methotrexate is a metabolic inhibitor used to inhibit the production of purines and pyrimidines.

1. Methotrexate inhibits which ONE of the following enzymes?

   (a) Caspase

   (b) Dihydrofolate reductase

   (c) Topoisomerase II

   (d) Thymidylate synthase

   (e) Tyrosine kinase

   B: Methotrexate is folate antagonist and inhibits dihydrofolate reductase, reducing the synthesis of both purines and pyrimidines.

2. Anthracycline antibiotics (such as doxorubicin) are used in anticancer therapy. Anthracycline antibiotics act by which ONE of the following mechanisms?

   (a) Inhibition of dihydrofolate reductase

   (b) Inhibition of DNA synthase

   (c) Inhibition of the 80S ribosomal subunit

   (d) DNA intercalation

   (e) Stabilisation of mitotic spindle fibres

   D: By slotting between DNA strands.

3. Cytotoxic anticancer chemotherapy is carried out in cycles, often of 21 days. Which ONE of the following is the best explanation for this?

   (a) Enables the bone marrow to recover

   (b) Enables folate levels to return to normal

   (c) To enable regrowth of hair

   (d) To limit cardiotoxicity

   (e) To limit renal toxicity

   A: Myelosuppression is a common side effect due to inhibition of rapidly dividing bone marrow cells. The bone marrow is often given 21 days to recover between treatments.

4. Human epidermal growth factor receptor 2 (HER2) is associated with which ONE of the following enzyme activities?

   (a) Adenylyl cyclase

   (b) Guanylyl cyclase

   (c) Phospholipase A$_2$

    (d)   Topoisomerase II

    (e)   Tyrosine kinase

E: HER has intrinsic tyrosine kinase activity, which is the target for drugs such as erlotinib

5. Vascular endothelial growth factor (VEGF) is targeted by the mononclonal antibody bevacizumab. VEGF is associated with regulating which ONE of the following?

    (a)   Angiogenesis

    (b)   Apoptosis

    (c)   Proteasomal degradation

    (d)   The cell cycle

    (e)   Uncontrolled proliferation of epithelial tumours

A: Tumour growth is supported by blood vessel growth (angiogenesis) and this is a target for bevacizumab.

CHAPTER 34

1. Match the most appropriate long-term medication to each of the following cases. Each medication may be used for one case only, for multiple cases or not at all.

Colchicine

Methotrexate

Adalimumab

Sulphasalazine

Allopurinol

Naproxen

Sekukinumab

Prednisolone

Hydroxychloroquine

Rituximab

Case 1: An otherwise healthy 40-year-old man who 4 weeks ago suffered an acute attack of gout for the third time this year.

Case 2: A 35-year-old woman who is keen to start a family 'before it is too late', but has recently developed rheumatoid arthritis and has radiographic evidence of erosive joint damage.

Case 3: A 50-year-old otherwise healthy man who continues to have severely active rheumatoid arthritis despite previous treatment with methotrexate and sulphasalazine.

Case 4: A 55-year-old lady with severe psoriatic spondyloarthritis affecting knees, spine and skin who has not adequately responded to a combination of methotrexate and adalimumab.

Case 5: A 60-year-old man who regularly drinks 5 units of alcohol per day, has severely active rheumatoid arthritis and has not responded adequately to sulphasalazine or hydroxychloroquine.

Case 6: A 95-year-old lady with a past history of severe bronchiectasis, tuberculosis and pulmonary embolus, chronic renal impairment and active rheumatoid arthritis despite previous treatment with methotrexate, sulphasalazine and hydroxychloroquine.

Suggested answers with explanations

Case 1: Allopurinol is the first-line urate-lowering therapy that aims to reduce risk of future gout attacks.

Case 2: Sulphasalazine possibly has the lowest risk for this lady and her future baby, and for some individuals can be a highly effective disease-modifying antirheumatic drug (DMARD). Some patients may choose to withhold DMARD initiation until after delivery. Hydroxychloroquine is less likely to be effective than hydroxychloroquine. Methotrexate is contraindicated. Prednisolone may be used as rescue medication, but risks adrenal suppression in the baby. Naproxen will not retard further joint damage.

Case 3: Adalimumab is usually the first-line biologic DMARD in someone who has failed to adequately benefit from at least two conventional synthetic DMARDs.

Case 4: Sekukinumab may be effective for peripheral and axial joint disease and cutaneous psoriasis.

Case 5: Adalimumab may be indicated, although chronic liver disease may be a risk factor for infection. Methotrexate should not be used due to risk of cirrhosis. The patient should be strongly advised to stop drinking alcohol, but treatment of his arthritis should not be withheld.

Case 6: Prednisolone might be the best option for this lady with multimorbidity. Long-term adverse events might be less of a concern than rapid relief of symptoms. Remaining DMARDs would each have high risk of adverse events in this patient.

2. Match each of the following routine monitoring tests with each DMARD. Each test may be matched to one, more than one or no DMARDs in the list.

   (a) Full blood count

   (b) Ophthalmological examination

   (c) Blood pressure

   (d) Liver function tests (transaminases)

   (e) Blood lipid profile

   (f) Urinalysis

   (g) Creatinine/glomerular filtration rate

   (h) Serum immunoglobulins

   Methotrexate

   Sulphasalazine

   Hydroxychloroquine

   Rituximab

   Baricitinib

   Leflunomide

Suggested answers

Methotrexate: *A, D, G*

Sulphasalazine: *A, D*

Hydroxychloroquine: *B*

Rituximab: *H*

Baricitinib: *A, D, E*

Leflunomide: *A, C, D*

Index

Printed and bound by CPI Group (UK) Ltd, Croydon, CR0 4YY

22/11/2024

14597714-0001